D0622265

Children's Speech and Literacy Difficulties

A Psycholinguistic Framework

Joy Stackhouse

Reader in Developmental Speech and Language Disorders

and

Bill Wells

Reader in Clinical Linguistics

Department of Human Communication Science
University College London

Consulting Editor: Professor Margaret Snowling
University of York

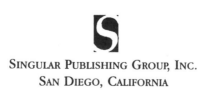

Singular Publishing Group, Inc.
San Diego, California

First published 1997 by
Whurr Publishers Ltd
19B Compton Terrace,
London N1 2UN,
England

Published and distributed in the
United States and Canada by
Singular Publishing Group, Inc.
401 West A Street, Suite 325
San Diego, CA 92101, USA

British Library Cataloguing in Publication Data
A catalogue record for this book is available from the British Library.

ISBN 1 86156 030 3

Singular Number 1-56593-795-3

Printed in Great Britain by
Antony Rowe Ltd, Chippenham, Wiltshire

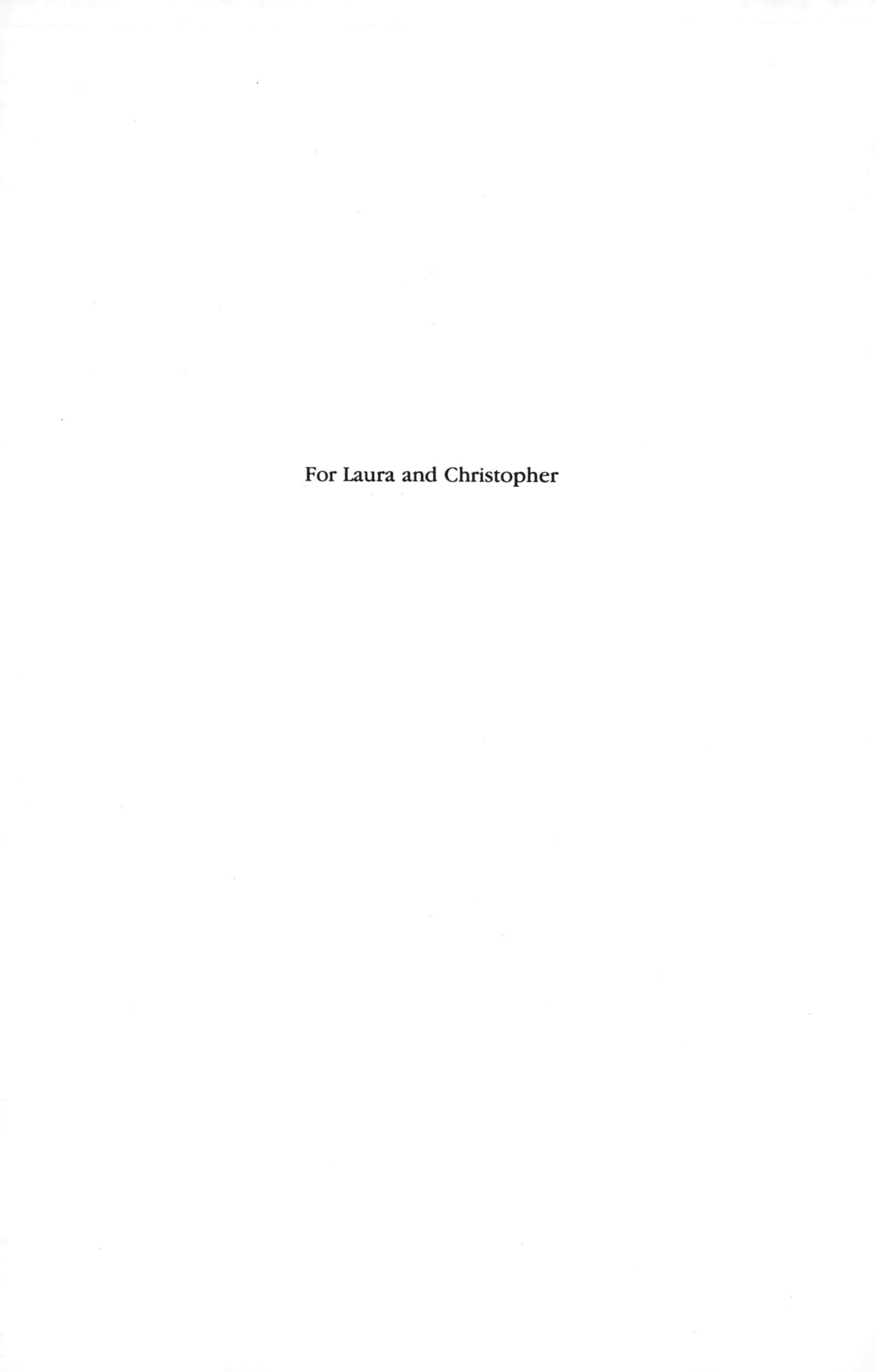

For Laura and Christopher

Contents

Preface

The framework for practice and research presented in this book has developed and continues to develop as a result of new research data and feedback from practitioners. It is being published now not because we believe it to be complete but because we feel that enough work has been carried out for it to be of use. This has been confirmed by the increasing interest shown by colleagues working in education and health. The framework is not confined to any single clinical population but can be used with any child. It can be used for the study of normal development as well as for investigating children with difficulties.

The work that has influenced our approach is not new: we draw on years of psycholinguistic and cognitive neuropsychological work by the research community. It was while working at Birmingham Polytechnic in the late 1980s that an opportunity arose for us to combine our own particular interests in speech and language therapy, developmental cognitive psychology and clinical linguistics. We carried out joint clinical consultancy assessments of children with persisting speech, language and literacy problems. As a result we set up a systematic hypothesis testing assessment procedure on which principled remediation programmes could be based. These programmes were then carried out by the child's local speech and language therapist and progress was monitored.

The framework was first presented publicly in 1989 at the Congress of the International Association of Logopaedics and Phoniatrics in Prague, and since then has been the subject of a number of papers and talks given in the UK and abroad. In addition, training courses to introduce the framework have been run in the Department of Human Communication Science, University College London (formerly the National Hospital's College of Speech Sciences) and around the UK. Although the target audience for our courses was originally speech and language therapists, there has been growing interest in our approach from teachers and psychologists – particularly those who are working with speech and language therapists. A pleasing result of this is that the assessment framework has fostered collaborative work across professions and our courses are now multidisciplinary.

We have based this book on these introductory training courses, in which principles of psycholinguistic assessment are introduced through a series of workshops aimed at heightening awareness of theoretical and practical issues. In writing it we have tried to emphasize the application of theory to practice and vice versa. We have kept in touch with users of the framework and have incorporated their feedback into this text. We would value ongoing feedback from users of the framework and readers of the text so that we can ensure that the content of subsequent texts meets the needs of the 'consumers', i.e. the practitioners and, most importantly, the children.

Joy Stackhouse and Bill Wells
June 1997

Acknowledgements

We are indebted to the therapists in the Birmingham Phonology Group for their stimulating questions and discussions which spurred us on in the initial stages of this work. We are grateful for financial support from the Association for All Speech Impaired Children (AFASIC), who along with Action for Dysphasic Adults (ADA) funded the clinic where this work initially took place, and to Jackie Stengelhofen, whose brainchild the clinic was. Further financial support has come from the Joint Research Advisory Committee of the National Hospital for Neurology and Neurosurgery and the Institute of Neurology, London (1993/4) to investigate the speech processing skills of normally-developing children; and the North Thames Regional Health Authority (1995–1999) to profile the speech processing skills of children with speech problems and to follow up their literacy development.

We are grateful to the team of tutors and researchers at the Department of Human Communication Science, University College London, who continue to develop the content and presentation of the framework: Alison Constable, Hilary Dent, Liz Nathan, Rachel Rees and especially Maggie Vance. Their feedback on various drafts of this text has been invaluable. We would also like to thank the therapists, teachers, psychologists and students who have given feedback on the framework and in particular, the clinicians who have piloted materials: Juliet Corrin, Nuffield Hearing and Speech Centre, London; Jill Popple, Rowan School, Sheffield; Jane Speake, Arbury Language Unit, Cambridge; Bridget Tempest, Dawn House School, Nottinghamshire; Wendy Wellington, Rowan School, Sheffield; and Pam Williams, Nuffield Hearing and Speech Centre, London; those who helped to collect data used in this text: Dr Nata Goulandris, Ian Bell and Jenny Horn; and also the many students who have carried out projects within the framework.

We would like to thank Professor Maggie Snowling in the Department of Psychology and Professor John Local in the Department of Language and Linguistic Science, both at the University of York, for their continuing support and collaboration. Finally, many thanks to Barbara Wilson for her invaluable help behind the scenes.

Information for the Reader

The broad aims of the book are:

(a) to present a systematic hypothesis testing approach to the investigation of speech processing skills in children with speech and literacy difficulties;
(b) to elaborate the theoretical foundations of the approach;
(c) to facilitate the development of analytical skills and theoretical knowledge in practitioners who need to administer and evaluate assessment materials;
(d) to provide a handbook for practice and research.

The book is intended for practitioners and researchers working with children who are having difficulties with the development of speech and/or literacy skills. We hope that it will be of particular interest to speech and language pathologists and therapists and we have assumed the level of background knowledge (for example in phonetics) that students and qualified therapists can be expected to have. At the same time, we have attempted to make the book accessible to other interested readers, such as teachers and psychologists working with children who have speech and literacy difficulties.

The chapters are cumulative and aim to show how theory can be applied to practice. Chapter 1 presents an introduction to the psycholinguistic approach, which is compared with other approaches to the assessment of children with speech and literacy difficulties; it also includes a discussion of the development of literacy and the relationship between speech processing deficits and literacy difficulties. In Chapters 2–5, the assessment framework is built up on the basis of an analysis of the psycholinguistic nature of speech and auditory processing assessments (Chapter 2) and assessments of phonological awareness (Chapter 3). The complete framework is presented in Chapter 4 and is illustrated in Chapter 5 through two contrasting case studies: a preschool child with apparent speech difficulties and an 11-year-old boy with specific learning difficulties (dyslexia).

In the second half of the book, the theoretical foundations for the assessment framework are elaborated. In Chapter 6, our assumptions about information processing are made more explicit in terms of a processing model. In Chapters 7 and 8, a developmental perspective on speech and literacy disorders is presented, firstly by exploring how the various components of the speech processing system develop in infancy, and then by discussing different types of speech impairment in childhood as instances of arrested development at earlier developmental phases. A detailed longitudinal case study is presented in Chapter 9, in which one child's speech processing deficits are investigated using the assessment framework and profile from Chapters 2–5, and are also related to the model and phases of development described in Chapters 6–8. In Chapter 10, the same child's later progress is described, with particular reference to the impact of speech processing deficits on her reading and spelling. Chapter 11 has a methodological focus, exploring some of the practicalities involved in designing tests of speech processing in children. Finally, directions for the future development of this approach are outlined in Chapter 12.

The book does not itself constitute an assessment package. Instead, examples are drawn from a range of assessment materials in order to illustrate the psycholinguistic approach. Each chapter includes paper and pencil activities, and a suggested key to each activity follows the chapter. These answers are not intended to be definitive in any sense, but are offered as a stimulus for reflection and discussion.

Conventions

TIE	spoken real word target / stimulus, as in real word repetition test, rhyme production test, spelling to dictation of real words; also used for picture target / stimulus, as in naming test, or silent rhyme detection.
/straɪ/	spoken nonword target, as in nonword repetition or discrimination test; spelling nonwords to dictation; also used for real word target when phonological information is required.
‹tie›	written target, as in a test of single word reading (real or nonword).
[taɪ]	spoken response, where phonetic information is required.
"tie"	spoken real word response, where phonetic information is not required.
‹tie›	written response, as in a test of spelling to dictation, or free writing.
→	'is realized as', e.g. /straɪ/ → [taɪ]; ‹tie› → "tie" ; TIE → ‹die›.

Chapter 1
Why Psycholinguistic Assessment?

Children with speech and language difficulties often have literacy problems. These include problems with reading comprehension, reading aloud, spelling and expressive writing. The reverse is also true. Children with literacy problems often have speech and language difficulties. These present as delayed speech and language development, persisting problems with articulation, word-finding and grammar (Snowling, 1987; Stackhouse, 1990). Although recent work has clarified how visual deficits may also affect reading performance, there is an overwhelming consensus that verbal skills are the most influential in literacy development (Catts, Hu, Larrivee, et al., 1994). The work of Vellutino (1979) in particular shifted the emphasis from visual to verbal processing deficits in children as an explanation of specific reading difficulties (dyslexia). Vellutino, Harding, Phillips, et al., (1975) demonstrated that children with dyslexia could visually match and select abstract shapes as well as normally-developing children in grades 4–6. The children with dyslexia, however, did less well at associating abstract shapes with a verbal response and had difficulty transferring their verbal codes to new tasks. This became known as the *verbal deficit hypothesis* of dyslexia.

A number of studies have demonstrated that speech, language and literacy problems co-occur, and that they are more common in males. In particular, there has been much interest in the tendency for these problems to run in families. Children with a family history of speech, language and/or literacy problems are more likely to have problems with their reading and spelling development; Crary (1984) reported that a high percentage of fathers of children with specific speech disorder, or paternal family members, have a history of delayed speech development, articulatory difficulties, stuttering or dyslexia. Studies of identical and fraternal twins have shown that some aspects of speech processing difficulties in particular are highly heritable (Olson, Wise, Conners, et al., 1989).

A number of studies have also attempted to identify predictors of literacy outcome in children with speech and language difficulties. These studies have had interesting but sometimes conflicting results. Some report that syntax performance is a particularly good predictor of literacy outcome (e.g. Bishop and Adams, 1990; Magnusson and Naucler, 1990), while others have emphasized aspects of speech production as being the strongest predictor (e.g. Webster and Plante, 1992; Bird, Bishop and Freeman, 1995). Indeed it is possible that normal speech production may compensate for other weaknesses. For example, Stothard, Snowling and Hulme (1996) have reported the case of LF, a 7-year-old girl who had proficient reading and spelling development despite specific deficits in auditory processing and phonological awareness. Catts (1993), emphasizing the importance of defining very precisely what was meant by literacy outcome, divided reading measures into (a) reading comprehension and (b) word recognition. His longitudinal study showed that receptive and expressive language skills were better predictors of reading comprehension, while speech processing skills were better predictors of word recognition.

Another explanation for conflicting result in studies that attempt to predict literacy outcome from spoken language skills, is that these spoken language skills are developing in young children and will change over time (Menyuk, Chesnick, Liebergott, et al., 1991). Scarborough (1990) carried out a longitudinal study of 20 children aged 30 months selected from families with a history of dyslexia. The children who went on to have literacy problems did indeed have early spoken language problems but the nature of these problems changed during the preschool years. At 2;6 the language deficit was most obvious in syntax and pronunciation. Lexical problems became more obvious at 3 years of age through deficits in receptive vocabulary and naming abilities. By 5 years of age, problems with sound awareness and letter-sound knowledge were apparent.

The co-occurrence of speech, language and literacy difficulties is not a mere coincidence. Before learning to read and spell, children have already established a speech processing system to deal with their spoken language (Pring and Snowling, 1986). This system is also the foundation for their written language development. Thus, any fault in the speech processing system will have repercussions for a child's literacy development. To some extent reading may progress if the child has intact visual processing skills and adequate verbal comprehension to compensate. Spelling development, however, is more dependent on speech processing skills and so persisting spelling difficulties may be more obvious than reading problems in children with speech and literacy difficulties. Figure 1.1 illustrates the relationship between speech and literacy development; both are rooted in the speech processing system.

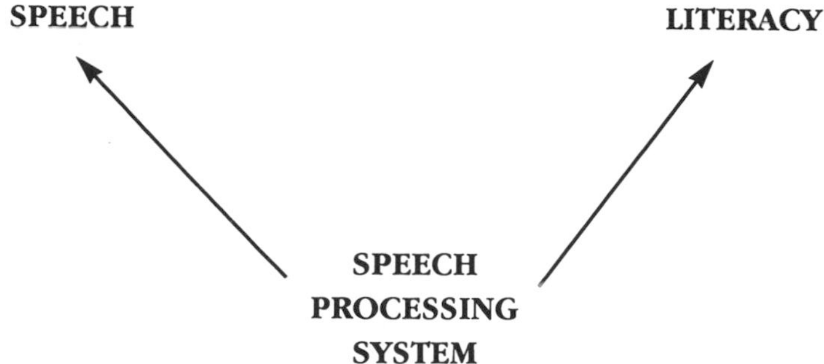

Figure 1.1: The relationship between speech and literacy development

But what is this speech processing system? How does it develop? How can it be investigated? We will attempt to address these questions in this book by taking a psycholinguistic perspective on children's speech and literacy development and difficulties. In this chapter we will begin to define the psycholinguistic approach by examining the different ways in which speech problems have been classified. Then, with reference to a simple processing model we will explore further the co-occurrence of spoken and written language development and difficulties.

Classification of Speech Problems in Children

In order to understand the rationale behind the psycholinguistic approach it is helpful to examine other approaches and compare how speech problems have been classified from different perspectives. Three perspectives have been particularly influential in determining how practitioners conceptualize children's speech problems:

- medical;
- linguistic;
- psycholinguistic.

ACTIVITY 1.1

Aim: To reflect on how the terminology used to describe speech problems is rooted in classificatory systems derived from different academic disciplines.

Write down all the words you know that describe or label a speech difficulty.

See Key to Activity 1.1 at the end of this chapter for some of the words you may have written down, then read the following account of the different ways of classifying speech problems.

The medical perspective

From the medical perspective, speech and language problems are classified according to clinical entity (Crystal and Varley, 1993). Commonly used labels include: *dyspraxia* , described by Milloy and MorganBarry (1990, p.121) as a difficulty 'in initiating, in directing and in controlling the speed and duration of movements of articulation', which occurs in the absence of obvious neuromuscular abnormality; *dysarthria*, an 'impairment of movement and co-ordination of the muscles required for speech, due to abnormal muscle tone' (Milloy and MorganBarry, 1990, p.109); and *stuttering,* nonfluent speech (see Rustin, 1991 for an introduction to this topic). You may also have written down some common causes of speech difficulties such as *cleft palate* (a congenital abnormality of the oral structure; see Stengelhofen, 1989 for further information), *hearing loss* or *environmental deprivation*; or some medical conditions associated with speech difficulties, e.g. *autism*, *learning difficulties*, *Down's syndrome, psychiatric disorder*.

Viewing speech and language disorders from a medical perspective can be helpful in various ways. Firstly, through the medical procedure of differential diagnosis, a condition may be defined through the identification of commonly occurring symptoms (for example, Stackhouse, 1992b discusses the cluster of symptoms commonly used to identify developmental verbal dyspraxia under four headings: clinical, speech, language and cognitive). Secondly, for some conditions, such as hearing loss or cleft palate, medical management can contribute significantly to the prevention or remediation of the speech or language difficulty, e.g. by cochlear implant or surgical repair. Thirdly, the medical perspective may be helpful when considering the prognosis for the child's speech and language development; for example, it is important to know if a child has a progressive neurological condition (see Lees, 1993 for discussion of acquired speech and language disorders in children).

However, the medical approach has major limitations as a basis for the principled remediation of speech problems in individual children. Firstly, a medical diagnosis cannot always be made. Often the term 'specific speech and/or language impairment' is used once all the other possible medical labels have been ruled out, for example hearing loss, abnormality of the oral structure, learning difficulty (Bishop and Rosenbloom, 1987). The aetiology of children's speech difficulties is thus not always clear. Secondly, even if a neuroanatomical correlate or genetic basis for a speech and language impairment can be identified, the medical diagnosis does not predict with any precision the speech and language difficulties that an individual child will experience, so the diagnosis will not significantly affect the detail of day-to-day teaching and therapy programmes. Two children diagnosed as having the same condition in medical terms may present with a different profile of speech and language problems. Dyspraxia is a good example. Stackhouse and Snowling (1992a) report two case studies of children diagnosed as having developmental verbal dyspraxia, who differed with regard to their abilities in auditory processing, articulation and literacy skills (see also Chapter 8, this volume). In order to further our understanding of children's speech and language problems, and to plan appropriate therapy, the medical perspective needs to be supplemented by the linguistic approach.

The linguistic perspective

The linguistic perspective is primarily concerned with the description of language behaviour at different levels of analysis. If a child is said to have a *phonetic* difficulty, the implication is that s/he has problems with pronouncing the speech sounds used in the ambient language. For example, an English-speaking child who uses a voiceless lateral fricative [ɬ] (like the first sound in the Welsh place name LLANDUDNO) instead of [s] in a word like SEA could be described as having a phonetic difficulty. Such a child may also be described as having an *articulatory* difficulty. Both of these terms emphasize that the child's difficulty is with the *production* of sounds.

You may also have written down *phonological* in your list of words. This refers not to the children's ability to produce speech sounds, but to their ability to *use* sounds appropriately to convey meaning. For example, if a child uses [t] for [s] at the beginning of words (even though s/he can produce a [s] sound in isolation perfectly well) both SEA and TEA will be produced as "tea" [ti] and SEW and TOE as "toe" [təʊ]. Thus, the child fails to distinguish between target words and is likely to be misunderstood by the listener. This failure to signal contrast between words is known as a phonological problem. Speech and language therapists tend to use the term 'phonological' in a linguistic sense to describe speech difficulties that involve this loss of contrastivity (e.g. PIN and BIN both produced as "bin" [bɪn]; TEA and KEY both produced as "tea" [ti]), thus reducing the child's intelligibility. Such children may be referred to as having a phonological *delay* if their pattern of speech development is behind but following normal lines, or a *disorder* if the problem is severe in terms of being very delayed or somehow different from the normal pattern of development. The term disorder is still used but has become less popular because it implies that the speech system of children with speech difficulties is disorganized in some way. This is not in fact true. Even children who are unintelligible because of severe speech difficulties have some order in their speech system. For this reason, phonological *impairment* or *disability* is often used instead of *disorder*.

These terms can be used irrespective of the causation (which may not be apparent anyway) or medical condition associated with the speech problem. Some authors and speech and language therapists use the term *phonological disorder* or *phonological disability* as a medical diagnosis by exclusion, much in the way that the term *dyslalia* was used in the past, to refer exclusively to a speech disorder that has no known origin, as opposed to speech disorders resulting from cleft palate, hearing loss, dyspraxia, dysarthria etc. In our view, any child, regardless of the anatomical or neurological causation of the speech difficulty, is correctly described as having a phonological problem if their speech is unintelligible to the listener because of a loss of contrastivity. Used in this way, *phonological* is unequivocally a linguistic term (like *semantic, syntactic, pragmatic, phonetic*) rather than a medical, or indeed psycholinguistic, term. This issue is returned to later in this chapter.

Possibly, you also wrote *prosodic* in your list. 'Prosody' and the adjective 'prosodic' are used to refer to features of speech such as rhythm, stress and intonation, as opposed to the consonants and vowels (the latter are sometimes also referred to collectively as *segments* or *phones*). Prosodic problems can co-occur with segmental phonetic and/or phonological problems. Sometimes they manifest as residual difficulties in children who have resolved their segmental problems (i.e. with consonants and/or vowels) but are left with jerky or staccato utterances. If a child's speech sounds 'odd' and specific segmental problems cannot be pinpointed, s/he may have prosodic problems which are particularly evident in connected speech. Children with prosodic problems can have difficulties with many aspects of speech and need careful investigation by a speech and language therapist. Like segmental problems, prosodic problems can be described as phonetic or phonological, according to how they impact on the linguistic system and thus the child's intelligibility (see Wells, Peppé and Vance, 1995 for further discussion of this topic).

If you extended your list to include language as well as speech, you may have mentioned disability or impairment of *grammar* (sentence structure), *morphology* (word structure), *semantics* (word and sentence meaning) and *pragmatics* (interactional and contextual aspects of linguistic organization). You will note that we have not included phonology in this list of language terms even though some authors refer to phonology as a level of language rather than of speech. Phonology is in fact the interface between speech and language: it refers to the way we convey meaning through speech for the purposes of communication. Placing phonology under a heading of speech rather than language is a somewhat arbitrary decision.

All these terms have been derived from the linguistic sciences (linguistics and phonetics) which have provided us with an indispensable foundation for the assessment of speech and language difficulties.

Phonetic and phonological analyses, for example, are used to identify patterns in the speech data, and it is now widely agreed that such a systematic linguistic description of the child's speech is a precondition for appropriate remediation (Grunwell, 1992). However, the linguistic model has its limitations as well. Although a systematic phonological description can provide the basis from which hypotheses can be generated about the nature of a child's speech disorder, it is still a *description* and not an *explanation* of the disorder. Specifically, a linguistic analysis focuses on the child's speech output, but does not take account of underlying cognitive processes. For this we need a psycholinguistic approach.

The psycholinguistic perspective

The psycholinguistic approach attempts to make good some of the shortcomings of the other approaches by viewing the children's speech problems as being derived from a breakdown at one or more levels of input, stored linguistic knowledge, or output. This involves the use of a theoretical model of speech processing from which hypotheses are generated about the level of breakdown that gives rise to disordered speech output. These hypotheses are then tested systematically. If you have written in your list of terms any of the following, then you are already adopting a psycholinguistic perpective: *auditory discrimination/memory/sequencing*; *word store* or *lexicon, phonological awareness, motor programming/planning* or *execution*.

The adjective 'phonological' in the context of psycholinguistic studies is often used differently from the same term in linguistics. For example, 'phonological' as in *phonological memory codes* has little to do with the contrastive use of speech sounds. So-called 'phonological memory' has been investigated via digit (number) span, rhyme and speech repetition tasks. The results have been interpreted as indicating that children with specific speech or language impairment have a phonological working memory deficit (Raine, Hulme, Chadderton, et al., 1991; Gathercole 1993) though this conclusion has been disputed (van der Lely and Howard, 1995; Vance, Donlan and Stackhouse, 1996).

A related use of the term 'phonological' may be more familiar to teachers working with literacy development, where training in *phonological awareness* has been found to facilitate literacy development (Bradley and Bryant, 1983; Wise, Olson and Treiman, 1990; Hatcher, Hulme and Ellis, 1994, Hatcher, 1996). Phonological awareness involves a child reflecting on the sound structure of an utterance rather than its meaning. Typical activities include: segmenting (dividing) sentences up into words; words into syllables (the beats of the word) and phonemes (the individual speech sounds in the word); and rhyme games (see Goswami and Bryant, 1990 for a general discussion of research carried out into phonological awareness and literacy development and Chapter 3 of this volume for discussion of phonological awareness tasks). In concepts such as *phonological awareness* and *phonological memory*, the adjective 'phonological' is used to refer quite broadly to the sound structure of words, in relation to the child's ability to reflect on and make use of this sound structure in order to perform cognitive tasks.

It is therefore important to distinguish a *phonological problem* – a term used to describe children's speech output difficulties in a linguistic sense – from a *phonological processing problem* – a psycholinguistic term used to refer to the specific underlying cognitive deficits that may give rise to speech and/or literacy difficulties. Very often *speech processing* and *phonological processing* are used interchangeably. In this book, we will adopt the general term *speech processing* to refer to all the skills included in understanding and producing speech, including peripheral skills such as articulatory ability and hearing. Phonological processing should be used to refer only to the cognitive skills underlying the processing and production of speech.

In summary, the essence of the psycholinguistic approach is the assumption that the child receives information of different kinds (e.g. auditory, visual) about an utterance, remembers it and stores it in a variety of *lexical representations* (a means for keeping information about words) within the *lexicon* (a store of words), then selects and produces spoken and written words. Figure 1.2 illustrates the basic essentials of a psycholinguistic model of speech processing. On the left there is a channel for the input of information via the ear and on the right a channel for the output of information through the mouth. At the top of the model there are the lexical representations which store previously processed information, while at the bottom there is no such store. In psycholinguistic terms, *top-down* (T–D) processing refers to an activity whereby previously stored information (i.e. in the lexical representations) is helpful and used. A *bottom-up* (B–U) processing activity requires no such prior knowledge and can be completed without accessing stored linguistic knowledge from the lexical representations. This notion will be developed more fully in subsequent chapters. For now, remember the four key anchor points of the model:

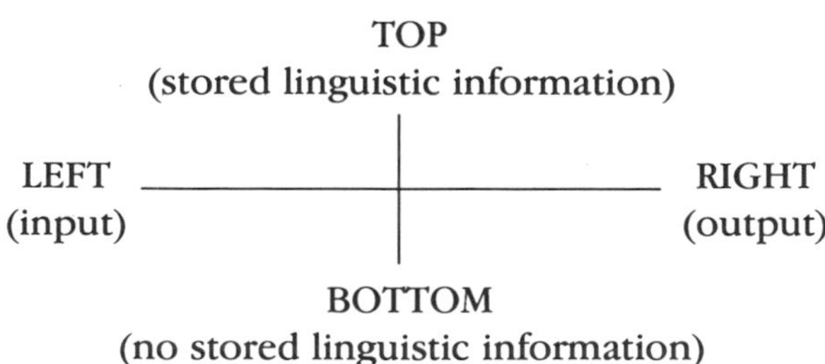

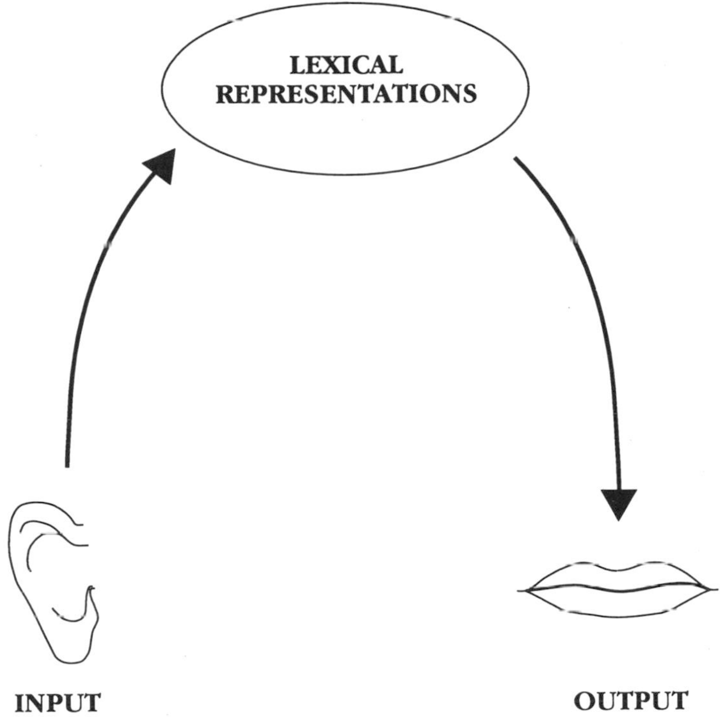

Figure 1.2: The basic structure of the speech processing system

Children with speech difficulties have one or more problems somewhere in the speech processing system depicted in Figure 1.2. The aim of the psycholinguistic approach is to find out exactly where on this model the child's speech processing skills are breaking down and how this might be affecting speech and literacy development.

At this point, we will consider a little further what happens at the top of the model. What exactly is the stored linguistic information that we can draw on when processing speech?

ACTIVITY 1.2

Aim: To consider what information is stored at the top of Figure1.2 in the lexical representations.

Think about the word CAT.
Write down all the things you know about this word.

Check your response with Key to Activity 1.2 at the end of this chapter then read the following.

Perhaps the first thing you noted was that you know what the word means – you have a *semantic representation* for this word which stores information about the attributes of a CAT (e.g. small furry domestic animal with whiskers) and may have classified it along with similar animals, e.g. DOG. You can discriminate the spoken word from other similarly sounding words, e.g. CAT vs CAP, and can detect speech errors made in that word, e.g. "tat" [tæt] for CAT. You therefore have a *phonological representation* for CAT, which stores enough information to allow a word to be identified on the basis of auditory and visual (e.g. lip reading) cues; the phonological representation may thus be regarded as the sensory gateway to the semantic representation or meaning of the word. You also know how to say the word CAT: you do not have to work this out every time you want to produce the word. This stored set of instructions for the pronunciation of the word will be referred to as the *motor program*. However, you do not produce this word in isolation very often. It is more likely to be put into a sentence structure, e.g. "Have you fed the CAT?" Part of your knowledge of CAT is that it belongs to a certain class of word (i.e. nouns), which can be used in some positions in the sentence but not others, and which has a plural form (i.e. CATS) that can be derived by rule. Such knowledge is stored in your *grammatical representation* for the word CAT. Finally, you have no trouble recognizing the printed form of this word and do not have to assemble letters one by one when you want to spell it. You have therefore stored information about what this word looks like in its printed form and this is held in your *orthographic representation.* In summary, information about a word is stored in the following representations within the lexicon:

- semantic representation;
- phonological representation;
- motor program;
- grammatical representation;
- orthographic representation.

A Psycholinguistic Approach to Speech Problems in Children

The psycholinguistic approach draws attention to both input and output channels as being possible sources of difficulty for children with speech problems. A child whose speech difficulties arise from a hearing impairment, for example, has a fault at the bottom left of the model in Figure 1.2 – in the ear. A problem here affects not only how words are heard but also how they are classified and stored. Children use their knowledge of a word – stored in the representations within the lexicon – as a basis for their production of spoken language. Imprecise storage therefore affects speech output even in the absence of faulty mechanisms along the output channel between the lexicon and the mouth on the right-hand side of the model. (In this and the next two chapters 'ear' should be taken as shorthand for the auditory system and 'mouth' for the vocal tract, i.e. the organs involved in articulating speech.)

A similar situation arises for children who in spite of normal peripheral hearing have problems processing spoken information, i.e. deficits located above the ear on the left-hand side of the model. These might include difficulties discriminating between similar sounding words or a limited memory for spoken words. Any problems on the input side of the model – between the ear and the lexicon – are likely to lead to inaccurate or imprecise representations of words, which will be reflected in the speech output derived from these representations. In summary, contrary to a common assumption, speech difficulties are not always the result of problems on the *output* side of the model.

Of course, some speech problems do arise directly from output difficulties. An obvious example of this is a physical abnormality in the mouth (i.e. at the bottom right-hand side of the model) which affects the ability to execute sounds and words clearly, for example as in the case of children with a cleft lip and palate. Articulatory difficulties are also typical of children with cerebral palsy, whose speech may be dysarthric (e.g. slurred or jerky) because of muscular weakness or spasticity.

Speech output difficulties do not only result from problems at the bottom right of the model, however. In order to produce a word, the child needs to have the components of the word assembled into the correct sequence. This *motor program* is a set of instructions for the pronunciation of the word that is sent on to the mouth. Assembling new motor programs is particularly difficult for children described as having articulatory or verbal dyspraxia. These children's speech is characterized by inconsistent productions of familiar words, for example, CATERPILLAR /'katəˌpɪlə/ → "capertillar" ['kapəˌtɪlə], "taperkiller" ['tapəˌkɪlə], "takerpillar" ['takəˌpɪlə]. It is as though these children have an impression of what they want to say but cannot get the bits in the right order. As one 14-year-old boy with dyspraxia said:

> "My mouth won't cooperate with my brain!"
>
> Stackhouse, (1992a)

The psycholinguistic approach allows us to locate a speech processing difficulty at the level of input, representation or output. Some children may only have problems at the output side of the model. However, many children with serious and persisting speech and literacy problems will have pervasive speech processing problems affecting input, output and representations. It can no longer be assumed that children described as verbally dyspraxic, for example, have only one locus of breakdown, at the level of motor programming, i.e. on the output side of the model. Psycholinguistic investigations have shown that children diagnosed as having developmental verbal dyspraxia often have more than one level of output difficulty which accounts for the persisting nature of this speech difficulty (Stackhouse and Snowling, 1992b; Ozanne, 1995).

The effect of such a complex output difficulty on a child's developing speech processing system should also be considered. Spoken output also forms input to the speaker, since normally-developing children as well as adults monitor their own speech. Further, when rehearsing new words for speech or spelling it is usual to repeat them. An inconsistent or distorted output may therefore have a knock-back effect on to auditory processing skills and the developing lexicon. Even if there is not a primary deficit in the auditory processing system, inconsistent speech output characteristic of the child with developmental verbal dyspraxia may interfere with successful rehearsal of new and complex words. It is therefore not surprising that children with dyspraxic speech difficulties often have associated input difficulties (Bridgeman and Snowling, 1988).

Psycholinguistic research into developmental speech disorders has shown that different children can be unintelligible for different reasons and that different facets of unintelligibility can be related to different underlying processing deficits (Chiat, 1983, 1989; Stackhouse and Wells, 1993 and Chapter 9 of this volume). Thus, psycholinguistic assessment allows us to differentiate between children in terms of their psycholinguistic profile of input, representation and output skills. The individual child's psycholinguistic profile provides a basis for planning a systematic remediation programme. For example, the type of activities chosen for a child will depend on whether there are problems on the input or output side or both, or whether the representations are accurate. Allocation of children to different kinds of therapy and teaching groups can be made on the basis of such information; adopting a psycholinguistic approach to the assessment of speech and literacy skills can thus lead to a rethinking of teaching and therapy service delivery (Popple and Wellington, 1996).

So far, we have focused on spoken language processing. However, one of the strengths of the psycholinguistic approach is that it can also be used to study children's reading and spelling difficulties, and thus enables the connections between spoken and written language to become apparent. In order to begin to understand the relationship between spoken and written language in children, it is important to examine how reading and spelling develop.

Reading and Spelling Development

In 1985, Uta Frith presented a three-phase model of literacy development in which the child moves from an initial *logographic* or visual whole word recognition strategy of reading, on to an *alphabetic* phase utilizing letter–sound correspondences and finally to an *orthographic* phase dependent on segmentation of larger units: morphemes.

In the first phase, children's reading is limited by the extent of their orthographic lexicon (their store of written words). They can only recognize words that they know and they are not able to decode unfamiliar words. When spelling, children may have some learnt programs for familiar words such as their own name but, in general, spelling is *non-phonetic* in this phase and does not show sound–letter correspondences. For example, a normally-developing 5-year-old spelt ORANGE as ‹oearasrie›. This was quite typical for children of her age. She had segmented the first sound of the word correctly and shown an awareness of letter forms and word length. The incidence of this type of spelling soon diminishes in young normally-developing children (Stackhouse, 1989) but it persists in children with a history of speech difficulties (Clarke-Klein and Hodson, 1995; Dodd, Gillon, Oerlemans, et al., 1995).

Breakthrough to the alphabetic phase occurs when the child can apply letter–sound rules to decode new words. When reading, the child may sound out letters in the word and then blend them together to produce the target, e.g. [f - ɪ - ʃ] → FISH. At the beginning of this phase, *semiphonetic* spelling occurs. Vowels are often not transcribed, and letter sounds might be used to represent syllables, e.g. BURGLAR → ‹bgl›, sounded out as [bəgələ] to represent the three segmented syllables in the word. Gradually, the child learns how to fill in the gaps. Vowel names are helpful, e.g. BOAT → ‹bot› where the letter ‹o› is used to represent the sound used for the letter name, i.e. [əʊ], and spelling becomes more logical or *phonetic*. Targets are recognizable even if the spelling is not conventionally correct, e.g. ORANGE → ‹orinj›, indicating that phonological awareness skills are developing normally. The child is segmenting the word successfully and applying letter knowledge, but has not yet learned (or been taught) the conventions of English spelling.

Finally, in the orthographic phase, the child is able to recognize larger chunks of words such as prefixes and suffixes (e.g. ADDITION) and to read more efficiently by analogy with known words. Once the child has the skills to perform at each phase, the most appropriate strategy for the task can be adopted depending on the different kinds of words presented for reading or spelling.

Frith (1985) suggested that it is the failure to progress through these phases that is characteristic of children with literacy problems. Children with *delayed* development may progress through these phases albeit at a slower rate than their peer group. Children with *specific* literacy difficulties, however, (i.e.unexpected reading and spelling problems given their cognitive abilities), may be unable to progress through the normal phases outlined above and need to develop compensatory strategies or ways round barriers to their literacy development. These children are often called *dyslexic.* Although a contentious term (see Stanovich, 1994), there is overwhelming evidence that such a condition exists, that it is often inherited, and that it is characterized by phonological processing difficulties (Snowling, 1996).

A particularly severe form of dyslexia which occurs when a child's development is arrested at the logographic phase of literacy development is known as *phonological dyslexia.* This is characterized by a particular difficulty with applying speech processing skills to literacy. Children with phonological dyslexia have poor phonological awareness skills, limited memory for phonological information, and poor verbal repetition and naming skills. A consequence of these deficits is that they are unable to break through to the alphabetic phase of literacy development. They are unable to read new words because they cannot decode letters into sounds and blend them together to produce the word. Further, their spellings may be predominantly nonphonetic, particularly in longer and more complex words (Snowling, Goulandris and Stackhouse, 1994). Goulandris (1996) discusses in more detail how to assess spelling skills.

A modified version of Frith's phase account of literacy development is presented in Figure 1.3. A list of the skills necessary to progress from phase to phase has been added on the right-hand side of the figure; the majority of these skills involve spoken language.

ACTIVITY 1.3

Aim: To investigate the relationship between speech processing and the development of reading and spelling.

Look at the skills necessary to break through from the logographic to the alphabetic phase, listed in Figure 1.3. Then look back at Figure 1.2. Consider how reading and spelling development might be affected by a speech processing problem arising:

(a) on the input side (between the ear and the representation);
(b) within the phonological representations (i.e. in the word store itself);
(c) on the output side (between the representations and the mouth).

Compare your ideas with the following account.

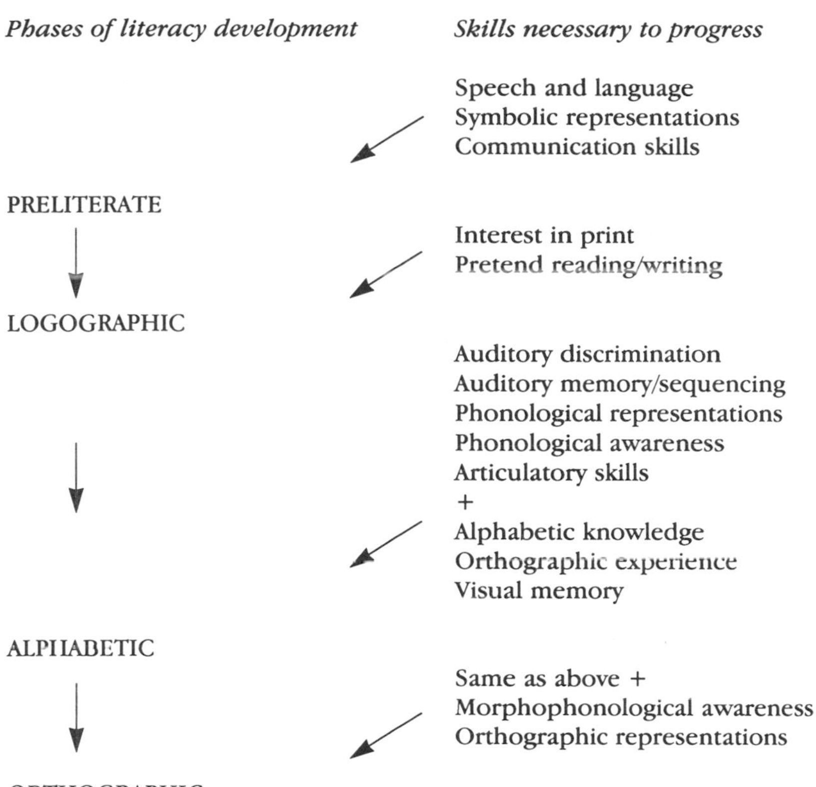

Figure 1.3: The prerequisite skills for each stage of Frith's (1985) model of literacy development (adapted from Stackhouse, 1992c)

It is clear that speech processing skills play a major role in the development of reading and spelling. Without intact *input* skills children cannot process what they hear. If minimal pairs of words such as PIN/BIN or LOST/LOTS are not differentiated at the level of auditory discrimination and sequencing, they may not be stored as separate lexical items with distinct phonological representations. This auditory processing problem will therefore have a knock-on effect on how words are stored in the child's lexicon. An inaccurate or imprecise *phonological representation* of a word will be particularly problematic when the child wants to spell or name that word, since the phonological representation is the basis for spontaneous written or spoken production. Consistently accurate *output* skills are particularly important for rehearsing verbal material in memory and for reflecting on the structure of words in preparation for speech and spelling. Without this verbal rehearsal children find it difficult to segment utterances into their components – a necessary prerequisite for allocating letters to sounds to form spellings of new words. Literacy success is therefore dependent on coupling speech processing skills at the input, representation and output levels with alphabetic knowledge gained through orthographic experience.

Working from the premise that speech processing is the basis for speech and literacy development and difficulties (see Figure 1.1), it could be assumed that any child with speech difficulties will also have literacy difficulties – but is this true?

Reading and Spelling Problems in Children with Speech Disorders

Given the current emphasis on phonological processing deficits in children with literacy problems (Snowling and Hulme, 1994), it would be easy to assume that all children with speech and language difficulties will have reading and spelling problems. However, this is not the case. Research indicates that children whose speech problems are the result of a more peripheral output difficulty, such as structural abnormality or cerebral palsy, are no more likely than their normally developing peers to have *specific* reading and spelling problems, e.g. dyslexia (Stackhouse, 1982; Bishop, 1985; Bishop and Adams, 1990). They may, however, be susceptible to delayed reading and spelling development because of associated hearing or health problems resulting in time away from school. Associated dyslexic difficulties are most likely to occur when the speech difficulty is specific and persisting rather than a more general speech delay or isolated articulatory difficulty (Dodd, Gillon, Oerlemans, et al., 1995). Indeed, it is the children who are described as having a phonological impairment or developmental verbal dyspraxia who seem guaranteed to have associated literacy problems (Stackhouse, 1982; Snowling and Stackhouse, 1983; Stackhouse and Snowling, 1992a).

It is therefore not surprising that a recent study found that children with persisting speech problems were particularly at risk for literacy problems. Bird, Bishop and Freeman (1995) investigated a group of 31 boys in the age range of 5 to 7 years with phonological disability to see if (a) the severity of the speech problem, and (b) the presence of additional language impairments were significant prognostic factors for literacy development. Their performance on a range of phonological awareness tasks (such as rhyme, phoneme matching and segmentation) and reading and spelling tasks (including nonword reading and spelling) was compared to a group of normally developing boys matched on chronological age and nonverbal ability. The boys with speech problems had particular difficulty with the phonological awareness tasks even when no spoken response was required. The majority of the boys had significant literacy problems when followed up at around 7;6. The presence of additional language impairments did not significantly affect the child's literacy outcome in this study. However, the severity and persistence of the speech problem did. This supports the ***critical age hypothesis*** put forward by Bishop and Adams (1990). As long as a child's speech difficulty has resolved by around 5;6, then reading and spelling may progress normally; if not, associated literacy problems are often found.

Sometimes a speech problem may seem to have resolved in terms of the outward signs of improved intelligibility but the underlying phonological processing problem persists and interferes with later literacy development. This may manifest in subtle speech errors such as /f - θ/ confusion, e.g. FIN for THIN or vice versa; or /r - w/ confusion, e.g. WHITE for RIGHT or vice versa; reduced clusters (e.g. CRISPS → [kɪps]), metathesis that may result in spoonerisms (e.g. CAR PARK → "par cark" [pɑ kɑk]); or unclear connected speech (Stackhouse, 1996 gives examples of speech errors to look out for in older children). Even adults with developmental dyslexia who appear to have normal speech can exhibit speech difficulties on specific articulatory tests (Lewis and Freebairn, 1992).

One of the strengths of psycholinguistic assessment is that it taps the underlying speech processing deficits in children who have not been considered to have speech and language difficulties. It is therefore particularly useful in uncovering the hidden verbal deficits in children with dyslexia (Stackhouse and Wells, 1991). Further, it can reveal that, like speech problems, reading and spelling difficulties can be related to specific levels of breakdown in speech processing. This will become clearer if we now examine literacy from a speech processing perspective.

A Speech Processing Perspective on Literacy

First, let us consider what is meant by literacy from a psycholinguistic point of view.

To do this we can redraw our simple speech processing model, portrayed in Figure 1.2, adding a visual input channel – the eye – and a written output channel – the hand (see Figure 1.4). The principles of the model, remain the same (left vs right; top vs bottom). Just as in spoken language, written language has an input channel (represented by the eye) which conveys information to the top of the model where it can be stored in linguistic and visual forms (the representations) and processed for meaning.

Reading comprehension is underpinned by the child's existing verbal language comprehension skills (Stothard, 1996). When reading, however, processing words for meaning does not always happen. It is quite possible to read text silently or out loud perfectly well but have no recollection or understanding of what has been read. This happens to us all, particularly when tired or when grappling with new topics in

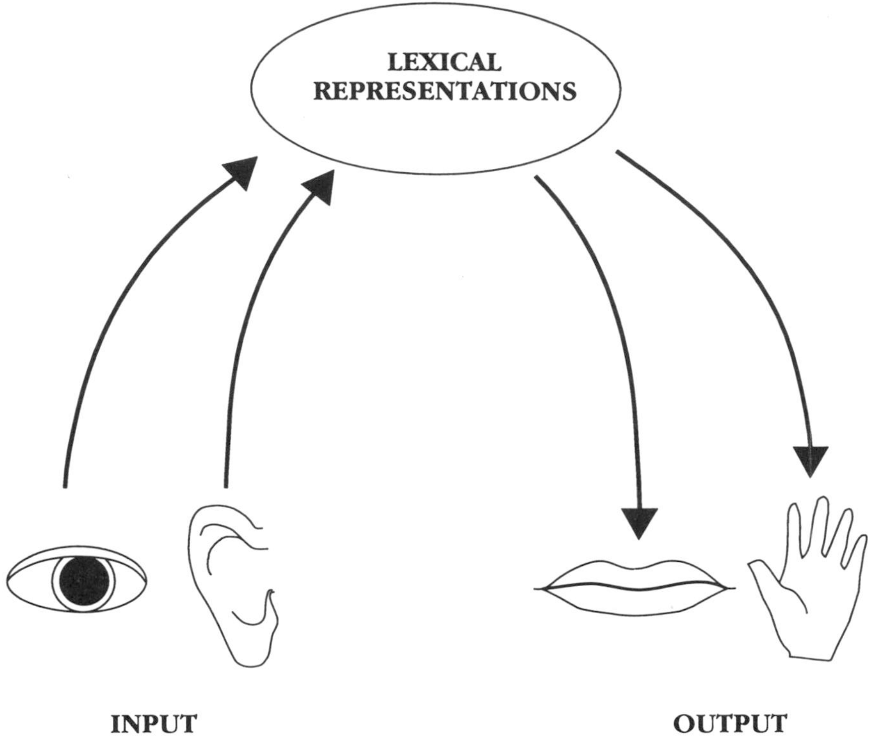

Figure 1.4: The basic structure of the speech processing and literacy system

text books! It is also typical of young readers who have learned how to decode words written on a page into a spoken form but may not understand the vocabulary or sentence structure being used in the text. This is not construed as a problem since it is through reading that children can develop their vocabulary and grammatical knowledge. In normal development, T-D and B-U skills are associated. However, in atypical development a *hyperlexic* condition arises where language comprehension – a T-D processing skill – is not developing in line with B-U reading decoding skill (i.e. converting the written form to spoken words) and a *dissociation* or lack of connection occurs between B-U decoding skill and T-D comprehension skills. Hyperlexia has been reported in children with autism who may read aloud perfectly well and be able to decode unfamiliar words but who do not have any understanding of what they have read (Snowling and Frith, 1986).

On the output side of the model, correct spelling requires knowledge of the conventions for how words are formed in a particular language. When spelling familiar words children draw on stored spellings in their orthographic representations. This T-D approach to spelling may be described as 'automatic' spelling in that children can output quickly words with which they are familiar and for which they already have a stored spelling program.

Sometimes a child will be asked or will want to write familiar words (i.e. words already in his/her vocabulary) for which s/he has not yet developed an orthographic representation. If the word is in the child's *spoken* vocabulary, there will be a stored motor program for speaking the word that can be used as a basis for spelling. If the word is in the child's *receptive* vocabulary only, i.e. the child can recognize it as distinct from other words but does not use it in speech output, then there will be a stored phonological representation from which a motor program can be derived and used to support spelling.

However, a child may be asked to spell a word that s/he has never heard or seen before. In this case there are no stored representations to draw on. The child will therefore need to hold on to the word in a temporary store in order to segment it into its components and allocate appropriate letters. One way of doing this is to assemble a new motor program from the temporary auditory image so that the word can be rehearsed verbally (this may be subvocally, i.e. not necessarily out loud) which gives the child an opportunity to reflect on the word's structure. For example, a common strategy children use when they are trying to work out the components of a word is to elongate it or emphasize different aspects of it, such as its beginning or end. Once the child has worked out the segments that make up the new word, s/he is in a good position to assign corresponding letters. Spelling can therefore take place by decoding the word heard into its segments and allocating the appropriate graphemes. This B-U approach to spelling is typical of beginner spellers who may be quite happy to output clearly segmented units that are incorrect in terms of conventional spelling rules but logical in terms of their components, (e.g. the spelling of GIRAFFE as ‹jrarf›, from a child with a Southern British English accent). However, experienced spellers will use T-D processing as well, checking their output for spelling conventions or making analogies with the spellings of known similar words stored in their orthographic representations.

Adopting this speech processing perspective on spelling illustrates why children with speech difficulties are particulary vulnerable to spelling problems (Robinson, Beresford and Dodd, 1982; Stackhouse and Snowling, 1992a). In each of the spelling scenarios above, the child is dependent on intact motor programming skills and/or accurate phonological representations. The lack of either or both of these may account for a child's speech problems as well as their spelling difficulty. In some cases both input and output speech processing deficits are present in children with specific literacy problems who do not have obvious or severe speech difficulties. For example, Robert, a 9-year-old boy with dyslexia spelt TRAFFIC as ‹trathic› and FINGER as ‹thinger›. On an auditory discrimination test he was unable to distinguish between pairs of words which contrasted /f/ and /θ/ (e.g. FIN vs THIN). Failure on this input test suggested that words containing /f/ and /θ/ were not fully specified in his phonological representations. Further, in his speech output, he produced /θ/ as [f], and /ð/ as [v], so that spellings based on his stored phonological representations or on his speech output were almost certain to be wrong.

Spellings are often executed via handwriting, though other mediums can be used, e.g. plastic or cardboard letters, rubber stamping, or typing on a computer keyboard. The form used for written expression can be quite independent of spelling ability. It is possible to practise handwriting as a purely motor or aesthetic skill as in the art of calligraphy. Similarly, letter rubber stamps using different coloured ink pads or computer printouts of letters in different fonts and typescripts can be created by children as part of an art and design curriculum. The form literacy output takes will not be dealt with any further in this text. Handwriting in particular, however, is a very important skill to develop and can be quite problematic for some children with speech and literacy problems because of associated visuo-motor difficulties (see Taylor, 1996 for further discussion and for useful guidelines on how to help children with handwriting difficulties).

ACTIVITY 1.4

Aim: To investigate the psycholinguistic processing involved in written language by examining reading and spelling along the top / bottom dimension of the speech processing model.

Look at the following aspects of literacy skill and mark beside each one whether it is a T-D activity, i.e. reliant on stored linguistic knowledge in the lexical representations, or a B-U activity, i.e. it can be performed without accessing the lexical representations. For some aspects you may want to put both T-D and B-U – explain why.

Reading Aloud

Continuous text

Single words – familiar

new

Reading Comprehension

Continuous text

Single words

Spelling

Spontaneous writing

To command – familiar single words

new single words

Handwriting

Check your response against Key to Activity 1.1 at the end of this chapter and then read the following.

Reading aloud continuous text would normally be a T-D activity. However, it is quite possible to read text via B-U (decoding) skills, particularly when T-D information is not available. This happens when a normal reader is asked to read a text comprising nonwords, or an unfamiliar language in a familiar script. It is also possible for a normal skilled reader to read a text while thinking about something completely different and thus not accessing stored knowledge within the semantic system that would be relevant to the text. B-U skills may also be better than T-D skills in some children with language difficulties, such as in the condition of autism where hyperlexia may be a feature (as discussed previously).

Reading aloud single familiar words is normally a T-D activity because the child can utilize stored orthographic representations and read words 'automatically'. Reading aloud new and therefore unfamiliar words is a B-U activity because there is no stored orthographic representation and therefore the word needs to be decoded by using letter-to-sound conversion rules (e.g. the letter ‹b› is pronounced [b]). When these sounds have been abstracted from the letters they can be blended together to form the new word. However, an alternative strategy for reading new words which is both B-U and T-D is to read the word by analogy with a known and similar word (T-D) but then make the necessary changes via applying B-U skills. For example, if a child can read the word CAT and is asked to read a new word: MAT, s/he can recognize that the new word has AT as in CAT (T-D) but that the new word has a different first letter, i.e. M. By decoding (B-U) this as the sound [m] and attaching it to the segmented and familiar AT s/he can produce the new word MAT.

When reading for comprehension, whether it be continuous text or single words, T-D processing has to be involved because prior linguistic knowledge is necessary for understanding; this prior knowledge is stored in the semantic and grammatical representations.

Spontaneous writing is normally a T-D activity because its function is usually to convey meaning through writing. Spelling familiar single words to command is normally via T-D skills as the child can utilize stored orthographic representations and may already have a motor program for how the word is written. In contrast, spelling new single words is achieved by B-U skills; the word is segmented into its components and the appropriate letters are attached to each segment. If this spelling is checked for spelling conventions or rules against familiar words for which the spelling is known, however, then the child is also utilizing T-D skill.

Handwriting is a B-U skill when it is purely a motor activity produced independent of meaning of the written form. However, when stored motor programs for familiar words and phrases are used this may be described as a more T-D activity.

By analysing the various aspects of literacy in this way, it is clear that both T-D and B-U skills are necessary for reading and spelling to develop normally. Deficits in T-D or B-U processing or both will impact on a child's literacy development in different ways. Identification of a child's T-D and B-U processing skills is therefore necessary for understanding literacy difficulties and for targeting intervention appropriately. The process of identifying these skills constitutes our psycholinguistic investigation.

Speech Processing Deficits in Children with Literacy Problems

Having ascertained that the basic model we used in Figure 1.2 to locate speech difficulties can also be used to describe different aspects of literacy performance, the next question to address is what happens to literacy performance when there is a deficit at some point in the speech processing model.

Snowling, Stackhouse and Rack (1986) investigated the underlying speech processing skills in seven cases of developmental dyslexia (six children age range 8–13 years and one adult). The cases were selected on the basis of (a) specific reading and spelling difficulties in the context of normal IQ and (b) poor nonword reading compared to real word reading. None had serious speech difficulties at the time of testing but three of them had received speech and language therapy in the past. Tests of reading, spelling, and speech processing were administered. The results showed that all of the cases, regardless of their reading age, (range 7;5 to 12 years), adopted a visual/T-D rather than a sound/B-U approach to their literacy development.

Despite this similarity in general reading performance, qualitative analysis revealed individual differences in the nature of the underlying speech processing deficit and its effect on spelling in particular. For example, Tina had input problems evident on her performance on *Wepman's Auditory Discrimination Test* (Wepman and Reynolds,

1987) on which she could not discriminate between minimal pairs such as MAP/NAP or COPE/COKE. In contrast, John performed well on tests of input processing but had obvious, though not severe, speech output difficulties, for example when making a distinction between voiceless consonants /p, t, k, θ, f, s / and the corresponding voiced consonants /b, d, g, ð, v, z/.

ACTIVITY 1.5

Aim: To illustrate how spelling errors may result from problems with input and output speech processing skills (i.e. the left/right dimension of the speech processing model).

Compare and contrast the following spellings from John and Tina described above. Write down your first impressions and any comments on specific spelling errors. Consider how their errors might be related to their speech processing difficulties.

John (output problems)

Target		*Spelling*
POLISH	→	‹bols›
SACK	→	‹sag›
CAP	→	‹gab›
MEMBERSHIP	→	‹meaofe›
ADVENTURE	→	‹afvoerl›

Tina (input problems)

Target		*Spelling*
LIP	→	‹persye›
TULIP	→	‹peper›
TRAP	→	‹mupter›
NEST	→	‹teryes›
BANK	→	‹capuny›
CATALOGUE	→	‹catofleg›
REFRESHMENT	→	‹threesleling›

Check your response with the following account.

John was able to transcribe the initial segment of words on most occasions. However, he had difficulties transcribing particular sounds that he could not pronounce even though he could distinguish them perfectly well on an auditory discrimination test. For example, his difficulties in speech with the voice/voiceless contrast, e.g. /p/~/b/, /k/~/g/, were reflected in his spelling: POLISH → ‹bols›, SACK → ‹sag› and CAP → ‹gab›. He had great difficulty when spelling longer words which became unrecognizable, for example MEMBERSHIP spelt as ‹meaofe›, and ADVENTURE as ‹afvoerl›. John's speech output problem prevented successful verbal rehearsal of these longer words and thus interfered with his syllabification of them prior to spelling.

Tina often failed to represent the initial segment in her spelling. She had a tendency to write the last sound of the target first, for example LIP spelt as ‹persye›, and TULIP as ‹peper›. She appeared to be relying on lip reading and therefore confused sounds made in the same place of articulation (e.g. /p/ and /m/). When these two errors were combined, her spelling was difficult to interpret, e.g. TRAP → ‹mupter›. Sound/letter order seemed unimportant to her (NEST → ‹teryes› BANK → ‹capuny›). On three syllable spellings she showed an awareness of increased word length but often substituted words that she knew for individual syllables (CATALOGUE → ‹catofleg›, REFRESHMENT → ‹threesleling›).

A comparison of these two children's spelling performances suggests that the level at which speech processing breaks down will determine not only the nature of *spoken* language problems as discussed earlier, but also the nature of *written* language problems. Identifying the underlying processing relationship between spoken and written language performance enables appropriate remediation to be carried out. Some children may have a very specific level of breakdown that might be targeted in remediation and to some extent compensated for by other strengths. John is a well documented example of this (Snowling and Hulme, 1989; Snowling, Hulme, Wells, et al., 1992).

It is not the intention to imply that *only* the psycholinguistic approach is necessary when investigating children with speech and literacy problems. In particular, the other two approaches discussed earlier in this chapter, the medical and linguistic, are equally important if a balanced view of a child's development is to be obtained. However, it is the aim of this book to focus on the psycholinguistic approach and examine how this approach can be put into practice.

So What Is Psycholinguistics?

Psycholinguistics is the study of the relationship between language in its different forms (e.g. spoken, written, or signed) and the mind. Its aim is to 'find out about the structures and processes which underlie a human's ability to speak and understand language' (Aitchison, 1989). The focus is usually on what is happening within the individual rather than between individuals in groups.

Psycholinguistics is not new as an academic discipline. In 1953 at the Summer Seminar on Psycholinguistics, it was viewed as a 'confluence of three compatible fields, linguistics, learning theory and information theory' (Jenkins, 1966). It has clearly developed since that time and the importance of learning theory may now not be so obvious. It is a very wide ranging discipline but its main concern is summed up by the two questions posed by Garman (1990) at the beginning of his textbook on psycholinguistics:

1. How does a listener recognize words in the stream of speech, or in patterns on the page, and arrive at an understanding of utterances?
2. How does the speaker go about putting ideas into forms that can be expressed as patterns of articulatory, or manual, movements?

When psycholinguistics is viewed in this way, we can see that all practitioners working in the area of speech, language and literacy draw on psycholinguistics in some way every day of their working life. However, many feel that this application is at a tacit level only and thus somewhat piecemeal. This book aims to show how principles of psycholinguistics can be used when investigating children's speech and literacy development. It will define terms within a single systematic framework to allow comparisons to be made between children with speech and literacy problems. The focus will be on profiling individual children's speech processing capabilities and deficits as a basis for remediation.

The psycholinguistic approach to assessment is therefore about investigating underlying processing skills. This is not limited to clinical populations but is just as useful for investigating speech and language skills in normally-developing children. Neither is it restricted to children. Psycholinguistic investigation of adults with acquired speech and language difficulties, for example following a stroke, is common practice and well-established in the literature (e.g. Kay, Lesser and Coltheart, 1992).

Summary

The main reasons for adopting a psycholinguistic approach as a major part of our investigation of speech and literacy problems in children can be summarized as follows:

- Its application is not confined to a particular group of children or dependent on any particular diagnosis. It can be used even when there is no medical diagnosis.
- It can be applied equally well to the study of normally-developing children, thereby enhancing understanding of the normal develop-

mental process. Normal control data can be collected for comparative purposes.
- It has led to a greater appreciation of the complex nature of speech disorders in children. In particular, it has highlighted individual differences in groups of children given the same diagnosis, e.g. dyspraxia, phonological disability.
- It can help identify different types of speech and literacy errors and suggest explanations for them.
- It allows exploration of the relationship between spoken and written language problems by identifying processing deficits that underlie both.
- It can uncover hidden speech and language processing problems in children who have not been considered to have speech and language difficulties, e.g. children with dyslexia.
- It draws attention to the importance for the child of developing precise representations within the lexicon, as a basis for both speech and literacy performance.
- It offers the possibility of a systematic framework for the investigation of children with speech and literacy problems.
- The identification of the child's processing strengths and weaknesses allows a more accurate targeting of therapy and teaching.
- It can provide common theoretical ground for professionals working with children with speech and literacy problems, e.g. speech and language therapists, teachers, educational psychologists and thereby foster collaborative working.

KEY TO ACTIVITY 1.1

Terminology used to describe speech problems.

You may have written down some of the following words to describe or label a speech difficulty:

> dyspraxia, dysarthria, stuttering, lisp, cleft palate, hearing loss/deafness, tongue-tied;
>
> phonological delay, phonological disorder, phonetic problem, articulation, prosodic disorder;
>
> delayed/immature, disorder, defects;
>
> environmental, accent, bilingualism.

n.b. Although environmental factors may contribute to delayed speech development, a child's *accent* should not be placed in a list of speech *difficulties*. Similarly, *bilingualism* is not in itself a speech problem – rather the opposite in fact: a great skill to have. However, some children with speech and language difficulties may find exposure to more than one language problematic (see Duncan, 1990 for further discussion).

KEY TO ACTIVITY 1.2

What you know about the word CAT?

What the word means.
How it sounds when spoken.
How to say it as an isolated word.
How and when to use it in sentences.
What it looks like when written down.

KEY TO ACTIVITY 1.4

A top-down (T-D) and bottom-up (B-U) view of reading and spelling

Reading aloud`
Continuous text – normally T-D but could be B-U.
Single words
familiar – normally T-D but could be B-U.
new – B-U if decoded. T-D and B-U if by analogy.

Reading comprehension
Continuous text – T-D.
Single words – T-D.

Spelling
Spontaneous writing – normally T-D.
To command
familiar single words – normally T-D.
new single words – B-U. T-D if spelling compared with known words by analogy.

Handwriting
B-U.

Chapter 2
What Do Tests Really Test?
I – Auditory Discrimination and Speech

Speech and language therapists, teachers and psychologists have for many years made use of a range of procedures in order to assess children's speech and literacy skills. These procedures take the form of published tests, techniques found in research studies and also methods that derive from accumulated clinical and teaching experience. Most of these procedures have not been designed with a psycholinguistic model or framework in mind: articulation tests such as the *Edinburgh Articulation Test* (Anthony, Bogle, Ingram, et al., 1971) or the *Test of Articulation* (Goldman and Fristoe, 1969) are clear examples. Nevertheless, traditional tools of assessment can be viewed from a psycholinguistic perspective. In Chapter 1, the essence of the psycholinguistic approach was characterized as the assumption that the child receives information of different kinds (e.g. auditory, visual), remembers it and stores it in a variety of representations within the lexicon, (e.g. phonological, semantic, orthographic), then selects and produces spoken and written words. If with this definition in mind, we consider the kinds of assessment traditionally used to assess speech and literacy skills, we can see that they all make psycholinguistic demands upon the child being tested, requiring him or her to receive linguistic information, remember it, store it, or retrieve it. Popular assessment procedures of this kind in effect tap different levels of psycholinguistic processing in the child. If analysed and classified appropriately, they can form the basis for a comprehensive psycholinguistic investigation of developmental speech and literacy disorders.

In this chapter, we will analyse the psycholinguistic properties of tests of speech and auditory skills through a series of activities. These activities are designed to heighten awareness of what tests are *really* testing from a psycholinguistic perspective regardless of what they might be called in their titles. It is not our aim to provide a comprehensive review of all materials currently available. The tests exemplify the procedures most often used.

Auditory Discrimination

Hearing is one of the first areas checked when a child presents with a speech problem. However, normal performance on a hearing threshold test does not guarantee that the child has normally functioning input skills. A child with auditory processing difficulties may pass a routine hearing test but be unable to detect differences between certain speech sounds or pitch changes. Some children with specific language disorder and dyslexia have difficulties at this level of functioning (Tallal, Stark and Mellits, 1985; Merzenich, Jenkins, Johnston, et al., 1996). Thus, input skills are not an all or nothing phenomenon: an individual child with speech difficulties may be able to discriminate some sound contrasts perfectly well and others not at all (Stackhouse and Wells, 1993). An auditory processing difficulty is one of the strongest hypotheses put forward by Bishop (1992) as a cause of language disorder in children. Some written language difficulties may also be rooted in problems with auditory processing skills (Tallal, 1980; Masterson, Hazan and Wijayatilake, 1995).

Tests of auditory discrimination should therefore be carried out routinely when investigating children with speech and literacy skills. There are a number of procedures available (see Locke, 1980a and b for a comprehensive review). A popular paradigm for testing children's auditory discrimination is illustrated in *Wepman's Auditory Discrimination Test* (Wepman and Reynolds, 1987), and the auditory discrimination subtest of the *Aston Index* (Newton and Thomson, 1982). In both of these, the tester presents two spoken words, e.g. WEB~WED, LACK~LACK (from *Wepman's Auditory Discrimination Test*), LET~NET, BUN~BUN (from the *Aston Index*) and the child has to say if the two words sound the same or different.

This procedure has also been adopted in auditory discrimination tests using nonwords, i.e. words which do not exist in the language but conform to its phonological patterns and are therefore potential words. An example of an English nonword is BUP. The child therefore listens to pairs of *unfamilar* spoken words and has to say if the items in the pair are the same or different e.g. DUP~BUP, BUP~BUP.

Such testing can be at different levels of difficulty. When testing older children with speech and literacy problems, for example, it is important to challenge their auditory skills at an appropriate level for their age. A child may be able to perform perfectly well on auditory tasks comprising short simple Consonant Vowel Consonant (CVC) words and nonwords, as in the examples given above, but not when the task comprises more complex words. For this reason, Stackhouse (1989) devised a test involving more complex nonwords. In this test the child is presented with pairs of words in which the order of the elements of a consonant cluster has been manipulated, e.g. WESP~WEPS, DASK~DAKS, or with pairs of longer words in which the initial consonants of two of the syllables are transposed, e.g. 'IBIKUS~'IKIBUS, 'BIKUT~'BITUK. Children with phonological processing difficulties often find auditory discrimination of sound sequences particularly difficult even though they can discriminate between simple words perfectly well (Stackhouse and Snowling, 1992a).

Bridgeman and Snowling (1988) combined real and nonwords in their test designed to investigate the perception of sound sequences in children with verbal dyspraxia. The procedure was the same as for *Wepman's Auditory Discrimination Test* – the children had to decide if a pair of words spoken by the tester were the same or different. However, half of the items were simple CVC combinations while the other half comprised words with clusters. There were therefore four sets of stimuli words:

	CVC	*CVCC*
Real words	LOSS~LOT	LOST~LOTS
Nonwords	VOSS~VOT	VOST~VOTS

A number of 'same' items were also included in each condition (e.g. LOSS~LOSS; LOST~LOST; VOSS~VOSS; VOTS~VOTS). Twelve children with developmental verbal dyspraxia ranging in age from 7;2 to 11 years were tested using these materials and their performance was compared to reading-age matched control children. There was no difference between the two groups of children when they were asked to discriminate words without clusters. Indeed, all of the children were at ceiling on this task. However, the children with speech problems performed less well on the cluster reversal condition, particularly on nonword items (VOST~VOTS). This suggests that children described as having verbal dyspraxia may have a specific difficulty processing sound sequences even though they can discriminate simple minimal pairs such as DIS~DIT, TOT~TOSS perfectly well.

A difficulty with sound sequence discrimination may not always be apparent in conversation. A child may be able to detect the meaning of similar sounding words (e.g. GHOST~GOATS, MIST~MITTS) from the context in which they occur. This is more difficult, however, if either of the words in a pair could be appropriate. For example, insert GOAT or COAT as appropriate in the following sentences taken from Cassidy (1994):

(a) I like the _______ with the long fur.
(b) Mum put her _______ in the cupboard.

Sentence (a) is an ambiguous sentence: either COAT or GOAT could be inserted. A child with problems discriminating [k]–[g] at the beginning of words would not be able to detect the target word in such a sentence. In contrast, the semantic context will enable the child to select the appropriate target in sentence (b). This illustrates the subtle interaction between auditory discrimination difficulties and comprehension problems (see Vance, 1994 for further discussion).

If children do not develop distinct representations of items involving similar sounding segments, e.g. /s/ ~/ʃ/ (s~sh), /f/~/θ/ (f~th), or if they have stored imprecisely the sequence of sounds within the cluster, e.g. [ts]~[st], then they may experience particular problems when trying to use these words in speech and spelling. For example, Stackhouse (1996) reports the case of an 8-year-old boy, Thomas, who was unable to sort words according to their intial or final sounds, for example he thought that CHEAP and CHAIR began with /ʃ/ (sh) and that MASH ended with /ʧ/ (ch). This confusion was reflected in his spelling, e.g. SHADOW was written as ‹chadow› and MEMBERSHIP as ‹memberchip›. An objective of testing auditory discrimination is therefore to establish if the child has enough input processing skills to distinguish between similar sounding words and to store precise representations of those words in the lexicon. Intact input processing skills are therefore necessary for developing phonological representations as a basis for speech production and spelling.

All the tests described so far have used stimuli presented verbally. Auditory discrimination tests can also include picture material, e.g. when the child looks at a pair of pictures PEAR and BEAR, and has to decide if they sound the same or different. The *Auditory Discrimination and Attention Test* (MorganBarry, 1988), for children in the age range of 3;6 – 12 years, is based on this procedure. Having checked that the items are in the child's vocabulary first, the tester presents the child with separate pairs of pictures covering a range of different sound contrasts and clusters, e.g. COAT~GOAT, SUM~SUN, CROWN~CLOWN. The tester names each item in the pair in random order on six occasions (fewer at the lower end of the age range). The child is asked to identify which item the tester has named by posting a counter underneath the appropriate picture.

An alternative to this picture choice procedure is to present the child with one picture, for example of a SOCK, and to ask the child: (a)"Is this a SOCK?", (b)"Is this a TOCK?," (c)"Is this a SOT?". To which the child responds "yes" or "no" after each question as appropriate (Locke, 1980b). This allows a wider range of items to be tested since only one picture is required. It is also a useful way of confronting the child with his/her own production of a target. The above example of SOCK could be used if a child produces [t] for [s] (see (b) above), or [t]for [k] (see (c) above). This test procedure confirms if a child can recognize the correct form even if s/he is unable to produce it.

This procedure was used in an investigation of Michael, a 7-year-old boy with word-finding difficulties (Constable, Stackhouse and Wells, in press). To explore the relationship between Michael's phonological representations (i.e. his knowledge of the sound structure of words), and his word-finding skills, a more complex series of test items was developed. For example, he was presented with a picture of a HOSPITAL, and was asked: "Is this a HOSPITAL?"; "Is this a HOSPIPAL (/ˈhɒspɪpəl/)"? "Is this a HOSTIPAL (/ˈhɒstɪpəl/)?" It was found that items on which he accepted the incorrect production (e.g. "Is this a HOSTIPAL?" – Response: "yes") were also the items which he had difficulties accessing in his speech production. The findings therefore suggested a direct relationship between the precision of his phonological representations and his word-finding skills.

The procedure used in this investigation is known as an ***auditory lexical task*** since it is checking not only if the child can detect differences between words at an auditory level but also how those words have been stored in the representations. If the child accepts for example the tester's production of /ˈhɒstɪpəl/ or /ˈhɒspɪpəl/ as correct for HOSPITAL, then it suggests that the stored form of the target HOSPITAL is imprecise, i.e. lacking some important phonological information. This will lead to difficulties when the child wants to produce that word in speech or spelling.

This whistle-stop tour of auditory discrimination tests reveals that there is a range of procedures available for use, but are they all testing the same thing?

ACTIVITY 2.1

Aim: To compare and contrast a range of auditory discrimination tasks and to consider where they may be placed on the simple speech processing model introduced in Chapter 1 (See Figure 2.1).

Copy Figure 2.1 on to a sheet of A4 paper. Take each of the auditory discrimination tasks listed below and mark by a cross on your copy of Figure 2.1 the level at which the optimum processing occurs for each task, i.e. the furthest point you have to go from the 'ear' for the task to be achieved. For example, if you feel that a task can be completed without any reference to the child's lexical representations (i.e. their stored knowledge of words, e.g. information about semantics or phonology) then you will put your cross at a point nearer to the bottom than the top of the model. If completing a task is dependent on the child having stored representations of the test items then your cross will appear nearer to the top than the bottom of the model. For the purpose of this activity, assume that your model has normal peripheral hearing and therefore no cross should appear in the ear itself.

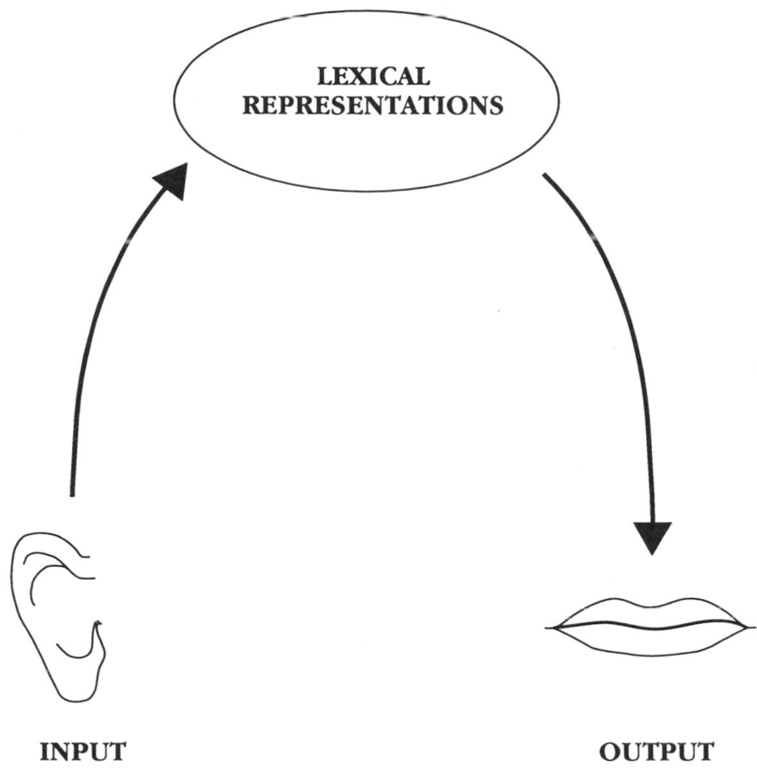

Figure 2.1: Copy of the speech processing model from Chapter 1

In this activity, all the tasks are *input* tasks. Therefore, all of your crosses should be on the line between the ear and the lexical representations and no crosses should appear on the output side of the model, i.e. between the representations and the mouth. Even though some of the tasks require a verbal response (e.g. to say "same" or "different"), this response could equally be replaced by a nonverbal response (e.g. shaking or nodding head, pointing to symbols) without changing the nature of the task. It is therefore not counted as an output response for the purposes of this activity. For simplicity's sake, we have not included the eye in this model even though some of the tasks involve pictures. Normal visual processing can be assumed.

Remember that the model has two dimensions: left/right and top/bottom (see Chapter 1). However, these dimensions are not organized in terms of difficulty. Tasks placed lower down on the model are not necessarily easier than tasks placed higher up. Similarly, tasks placed on the left-hand side of the model are not necessarily easier than those placed on the right-hand side.

Helpful Questions to Ask

Answering the following questions about each of the tasks will help you to make a decision about where to put your crosses:

1. Does the child have lexical representations for the stimuli used in this task?
   If the answer to this question is *No*, then your cross will be low down on the model. If the answer is *Yes*, then you need to answer question 2.
2. Does the child have to access these lexical representations in order to complete the task?
   If the answer to this question is *Yes*, then your cross will be high up on the model.
   If the answer is *No*, then your cross will be lower down on the model.

With these questions in mind, work through the following tasks placing a cross for each of the tasks at an appropriate point on your copy of Figure 2.1.You should write the abbreviated labels given for each of the tasks by the side of your cross, e.g. RWDisc for real word discrimination or NWDisc for nonword discrimination. This will help later when we collate a range of different tasks.

The Tasks

1. Real word auditory discrimination (RWDisc) – the child is given pairs of words spoken by the tester to decide if they sound the same or different, e.g. PIN~BIN, BIN~BIN, TEA~KEY, SEW~TOE.
2. Nonword auditory discrimination (NWDisc) – the child is given pairs of nonwords spoken by the tester to decide if they are the same or different, e.g. KES~KET, VIS~VIT, FOS~FOS.
3. Complex nonword auditory discrimination (CompNWDisc) – the child is given more complex nonwords spoken by the tester to decide if they are the same or different, e.g. IBIKUS~IKIBUS, BIKUT~BITUK, STEMP~STEMP.
4. Noise discrimination (N/Disc) – the child hears two musical instruments or two shakers from behind a screen and is asked if the two noises presented sound the same or not.
5. Picture choice auditory discrimination (PicChoice/Aud) – the child listens to the tester naming one of two pictures and points to the one being named, e.g. KEY~TEA, WATCH~WASH.
6. Picture Yes/No auditory discrimination (PicY/N) – child looks at one picture and has to respond "yes" or "no" to the tester's question "Is this a ------", e.g. target picture of a FISH, tester asks: "Is this a FISH?"; "Is this a PISH?"; "Is this a TISH?"; "Is this a FIT?"; "Is this a FIS?".

When you have completed this activity, check your responses against Key to Activity 2.1 at the end of this chapter, then read the following.

Auditory discrimination: real words

As pairs of common real words were used to test auditory discrimination in Task 1 (RWDisc), it is likely that a child performing this test would have the lexical representations for these items. It is therefore possible for a child to use T-D processing to confirm their suspicion that a pair of words presented are not the same. For example, a child may respond "different" because s/he knows the test items are semantically different. This still counts as an auditory discrimination task since the child must be able to detect the difference between the beginning of the words in the first place in order to have classified them as having different semantic associations.

Detecting that a pair of words sound different, however, can be done as a B-U activity through auditory processing, i.e. the child does not *necessarily* have to access the representations. Your cross for this task should therefore be around halfway between the ear and the lexical representations.

This test raises an interesting issue about what is a real word. The items in this example were high frequency words, i.e words commonly understood by young children. However, sometimes what looks like a real word to the tester may be a nonword for the child because it is not yet in his/her vocabulary. After all, real words are all nonwords until we have learned what they mean. To ensure that the test administered really is a *real* word auditory discrimination test, a vocabulary check of the items should be carried out first.

Auditory discrimination: nonwords

In contrast, nonword auditory discrimination (Task 2 – NWDisc) cannot be helped by existing semantic knowledge since the test items by definition are unfamiliar and not previously stored. You should therefore have the cross for this task about halfway between the ear and the cross for real word discrimination (Task 1– RWDisc). We make the distinction between real and nonword discrimination on our model because children *can* use T-D information (e.g. semantic knowledge) when dealing with real words, even if they do not have to. However, it is quite possible to complete the real word auditory discrimination task as though it comprised nonwords. Normally-developing children perform equally well on both real and nonword discrimination tasks, i.e. real word presentation is not an advantage to them. When assessing children with speech and literacy problems, however, there may be a discrepancy between performance on these two tasks. For example, a child who has B-U processing difficulties, i.e. trouble with auditory processing, may perform significantly better on an auditory discrimination task comprising real words compared to nonwords, because they are able to draw on their semantic knowledge for support. It would be wrong to assume, however, that the opposite pattern (i.e. better nonword than real word performance) will diagnose T-D processing problems. If children with T-D processing problems have intact auditory processing skills, they may complete both of these tasks in a B-U way and perform equally well on both real and nonword tests (as do normal controls). However, this in itself is an important finding since it indicates a processing strength that can be utilized in the child's intervention programme.

Task 3 – complex nonword auditory discrimination (CompNWDisc) – is a trick task. You may have put the cross higher than the one for the more simple nonword discrimination task (Task 2 – NWDisc) because you felt it was a more difficult task. Indeed it is; but the difference is in terms of the *task demand* rather than the *level of processing* required. It is still a nonword task but with longer words. It should therefore be located at the same level as Task 2 (NWDisc) but we have put it to the side to show that it is more demanding on children's processing skills. This separation of task demand from processing level is important because it allows a range of tasks to be developed for each level of processing that will be suitable for children of different ages.

Thus, at each level in the model you can increase the demand a task makes by increasing (a) the articulatory complexity of the test items and/or (b) the memory load. Very often, a more demanding task involves more than one level in the model. For example, auditory discrimination of complex nonwords (Task 3 – CompNWDisc) may be helped by successful spoken rehearsal of the test items in order to make a decision about whether the items are the same or different. This ostensibly auditory discrimination task may therefore require some output skill. Certainly, children with speech output difficulties have found this task very difficult (Stackhouse and Snowling, 1992a).

This test raises two important issues. First, a test may not always be as straightforward as it appears. Second, when interpreting test results, it is important to take into account not only the accuracy score but also *how* the child has performed the test. For example, on Task 3 (CompNWDisc): Did the child rehearse the test items? If so, could s/he do so accurately? If rehearsal was inaccurate or inconsistent in terms of output, did this interfere with performance on the test? Answers to these questions will reveal whether spoken rehearsal should or should not be encouraged in therapy and teaching activities.

Auditory discrimination: noises

Task 4 – noise discrimination (N/Disc)— is probably the easiest one to locate on the model. Your cross should be just above the ear for this since it is not a hearing threshold test (for this, the cross would be in the ear) but it is below the level of the other crosses for tasks involving spoken words. Task 4 (NDisc) is a much more peripheral skill than the others and young normally-developing children perform well on this task. Children with poor listening and attention skills, however, may perform badly on it. For some children, poor performance on such lower level tasks are indicative of more serious auditory processing problems such as found in specific language disorders (Tallal, Stark and Mellits, 1985; Bishop, 1992) or acquired language disorders (Vance, 1991; Lees, 1993).

Auditory discrimination: picture choice

The two tasks involving pictures (Tasks 5 – PicChoice/Aud and 6 – PicY/N) should have their crosses at the top left-hand side of the model. For both of these tasks children *have* to access their representations. Tasks 5 and 6 are therefore put at the same level. However, it is debatable which is the more difficult of the two. In Task 5 – picture choice auditory discrimination (PicChoice/Aud), the child has to use the phonetic information heard to access a word which then has to be matched to one of the two pictures presented. If the tester says KEY but the child perceives it as TEA, then the wrong item will be accessed in the lexicon and the child will respond by pointing to the picture of TEA instead of KEY. By definition, this is testing a phonological contrast since the items are all real minimal pair words.

Auditory lexical decision: real / nonwords with picture

Task 6 (PicY/N) is tapping the same level as Task 5: if the child accepts TAT ([taet]) as correct for a picture of a CAT, it suggests that there is a 'fuzzy' representation of the initial consonant of that item. However, as the administration of Task 6 (PicY/N) does not require minimal pairs of words that can both be easily represented in picture form, it allows a more challenging assessment of the child's representations since finer phonetic distinctions between target sounds can be made. For example, with a picture of a SHOP, the tester can ask: "Is this a SHOP [ʃɒp]?"; "Is this a SOP [sɒp]?"; "Is this a SYOP [sjɒp]?"; "Is this a [ɕɒp]?"; "Is this a [çɒp]?"; etc. (cf. the HOSPITAL example mentioned earlier). Test 6 (PicY/N) can therefore be designed to be more challenging than Task 5 – the picture choice auditory discrimination test (PicChoice/Aud) – though both are still targeting the same level. For this reason they are put side by side, with Test 6 (PicY/N) to the right of Test 5 (PicChoice/Aud).

This activity illustrates an important application of psycholinguistics to practice. It allows us to be more aware of what we are testing. Although all of the tests in this section can be labelled as *Auditory Discrimination Tests*, they clearly tap a range of different skills. It is no longer sufficient to say that the child has passed or failed an auditory discrimination test. There needs to be an explanation of what level of processing the test targeted as well as what strategies the child used to complete the task. It is quite possible for a child to take two tests of auditory discrimination and pass one and fail the other! Such a pattern of results may seem puzzling if not interpreted from a psycholinguistic perspective (e.g. superior performance on a real word vs a nonword auditory discrimination test suggests that a child is relying on T-D processing skills to compensate for weaker B-U processing skills).

Activity 2.1 has raised some basic principles about psycholinguistic assessment. The following key points have arisen from the analysis of auditory discrimination tests:

- Real word tasks may be completed without accessing the representations.
- Real words not in the child's vocabulary are effectively nonwords and will be processed as such.
- Nonwords do not have lexical representations and therefore have to be processed at a lower level on the model.
- Tasks involving pictures tap the child's lexical representations and are therefore placed at or near the top of the model.
- A task involving complex stimuli is not necessarily processed at a *higher* level than the same task presented with simple stimuli. It does, however, make more *processing demands*.
- A task is made more demanding by increasing articulatory complexity of the stimuli, memory load, and the number of processing levels involved.
- A child can perform well on one test of auditory discrimination and poorly on another depending on his/her processing strengths and weaknesses.
- An isolated single test result may be misleading. More than one test can be administered for comparison to check B-U (e.g. nonword auditory discrimination) versus T-D processing skills (e.g. picture choice auditory discrimination).
- The tasks administered need to be appropriate for the child's age and stage of development.

Speech

In Chapter 1, we discussed a number of reasons why a child may have speech difficulties. The aim of a psycholinguistic assessment is to establish not only what processing level or levels of breakdown are giving rise to the child's difficulties but also which levels are intact. The first two levels to check on the psycholinguistic model are the ears and the mouth; i.e. does the child have normal hearing and oral movement for speech. An oral examination can examine both structure and function (Huskie, 1989; Ozanne, 1992; Henry, 1990). A number of procedures are available which incorporate measures of articulatory skills such as rate of movement and sound production in isolation and in sequences of nonsense syllables, e.g. the *Nuffield Dyspraxia Programme* (Connery, 1992), the *Paediatric Oral Skills Package:POSP* (Brindley, Cave, Crane, et al., 1996) and the *Time-By-Count Test of Diadochokinetic Syllable Rate* (Fletcher, 1978).

A range of speech tasks can be included in your psycholinguistic assessement. *Picture naming* (often also referred to as confrontation naming) is one common technique. For this, one can use published test material or the traditional flashcard assessment favoured by many speech and language therapists. The *Edinburgh Articulation Test – EAT* (Anthony, Bogle, Ingram, et al., 1971) is one of the few standardized tests of articulatory maturity (age range 3-6 years). As it gives an articulation age and standard score it offers the possibility of an objective cut-off point below which further investigation of a child's speech development is indicated (i.e. when the standard score is <85). It can therefore be used for screening children with speech disorders and also in research projects to match individuals or groups of children on articulation age.

Other procedures have slightly different aims. For example, to cover a wide range of sounds in different positions in the words (Grunwell, 1985), or to include material for eliciting connected speech (e.g. Goldman and Fristoe, 1969) or specific phonological processes (e.g. Weiner, 1979). These tests and procedures are not new. Tests and materials used for psycholinguistic assessment do not have to be recent. Tests are only materials – it is the way the tester uses and interprets the results that is important.

Speech repetition tasks provide valuable diagnostic information and can be a routine part of speech assessments. Repetition tasks can include real and nonword repetition as well as sentence repetition. Spontaneous speech can also be collected and analysed since this provides evidence of the child's spoken abilities function 'on-line'.

Let us now examine from a psycholinguistic perspective some popular ways of testing speech production.

ACTIVITY 2.2

Aim: To compare and contrast a range of speech output tasks by plotting them on your copy of the speech processing model used in Activity 2.1 (presented in Figure 2.1).

Take each of the speech tasks listed below and mark by a cross on your copy of Figure 2.1 the level of processing that each task is tapping. For example, if you feel that a task can be completed without any reference to the child's lexical representations (i.e. their stored knowledge of words, e.g. information about semantics or phonology) then you will put your cross at a point nearer to the bottom than the top of the model. If completing a task is dependent on the child having stored representations of the test items then your cross will appear nearer to the top than the bottom of the model.

In this activity, all the tasks are *output* tasks. Therefore, all of your crosses should be on the line between the lexical representations and the mouth. No crosses should appear on the input side of the model, i.e. between the ear and the lexical representations, even though the tasks also involve input processing (we will return to this issue in Chapter 6). For the purpose of this activity, you can assume that your model has normal input processing up to the level of the lexical representations.

Remember that the model has two dimensions: left/right and top/bottom (see Chapter 1). However, these dimensions are not organized in terms of difficulty. Tasks placed lower down on the model are not necessarily easier than tasks placed higher up. Similarly, tasks placed on the left-hand side of the model are not necessarily easier than those placed on the right-hand side and vice versa. Remember also, that for simplicity's sake, we have not included the eye in this model even though some of the tasks involve pictures. Normal visual processing can be assumed.

Helpful Questions to Ask

Answering the following questions about each of the tasks will help you to make a decision about where to put your crosses:

1. Does the child have lexical representations for the stimuli used in this task?
   If the answer to this question is *No*, then your cross will be low down on the model. If the answer is *Yes*, then you need to answer question 2.
2. Does the child have to access these lexical representations in order to complete the task?
   If the answer to this question is *Yes*, then your cross will be high up on the model.
   If the answer is *No*, then your cross will be lower down on the model.

With these questions in mind, work through the following tasks placing a cross for each of the tasks at an appropriate point on the output side of your model copied from Figure 2.1. You should write the abbreviated labels given for each of the tasks by the side of your cross (e.g. Nam for naming, and NWRep for nonword repetition). This will help later when we collate a range of different tasks.

The Tasks

1. Real word repetition (RWRep) – say this word after me: GLOVE; TRACTOR; UMBRELLA (from Vance, Stackhouse and Wells, 1995).
2. Nonword repetition (NWRep) – say these after me: GLEV /glɛv/; TRECTEE /ˈtrɛkti/; AMBRAHLLI /æmˈbrɑli/. (These nonwords are matched to and pronounced with the same stress pattern as in the real words in 1. above, taken from Vance, Stackhouse and Wells, 1995).
3. Picture naming (Nam) – look at these pictures and tell me what they are, e.g. ELEPHANT, CHIMNEY, PENCIL (from the *Edinburgh Articulation Test*, Anthony, Bogle, ingram, et al., 1971).
4. Oral examination of function (OE) – move your tongue from side to side as quickly as you can. Push your lips forward then spread them in a big smile – do this three times as quickly as you can (based on the assessment from the *Nuffield Dyspraxia Programme*, Connery, 1992).
5. Repetition of syllables (SyllRep) – e.g. [pə] [pə] [pə]; [tə] [tə] [tə] (Fletcher, 1978).
6. Sentence repetition (SentRep) – say this sentence after me: e.g. HIS UMBRELLA IS YELLOW; THE LADDER IS BY THE HOUSE (from Vance, Stackhouse and Wells, 1995).

When you have completed the above, check your responses against Key to Activity 2.2, then read the following.

Real word repetition

When the stimulus is a real word, as in Task 1 (RWRep), the child is likely to have a motor program for that word (i.e. instructions for the pronunciation of the word) as part of the lexical representation. The child may access this stored motor program to perform real word repetition. However, real word repetition does not have to go via the stored representations since the child can merely ‘parrot’ the word back to you, treating it like an unfamiliar word (see later). Your cross for real word repetition should therefore be just around halfway between the representations and the mouth.

Nonword repetition

Nonword repetition, as in Task 2 (NWRep), does not go via the representations since the word is unfamiliar. The child therefore has to assemble a new motor program in order to produce the novel item (perhaps using the stored programs for similar known words to assist this process, cf. Dollaghan, Biber and Campbell, 1995). Your cross for nonword repetition should therefore be halfway between real word repetition and the mouth to denote that different strategies are possible. Children who have B-U processing difficulties have problems with nonword repetition. One way this may be manifested is by a larger number of *lexicalizations* of the nonwords in a child's responses, i.e. similarly sounding real words are produced instead of the unfamiliar nonword, e.g. NUST /nʌst/ repeated as "nest" (Stackhouse, 1993; and see Chapter 4 this volume, for further discussion).

Naming

Naming pictures (Task 3 – Nam) does require the child to access his/her own representations of the word. The child has to identify a picture and verbally produce its name without having heard it spoken by the tester. Naming is a complex cross-modal task. In order to convert a visual stimulus into a spoken form the child has to identify the picture semantically before accessing the existing motor program for that word (see Figure 2.2). If it is a word that is present in his/her receptive vocabulary, i.e. one with which the child is familiar but for which s/he does not have an existing motor program, s/he may have to reflect on the phonological representation of that word in order to create the motor program for it (see Figure 2.3). Your cross for the naming task should therefore be the highest one for your speech tasks and occur on the top right of your model – above real word repetition and close to the lexical representations.

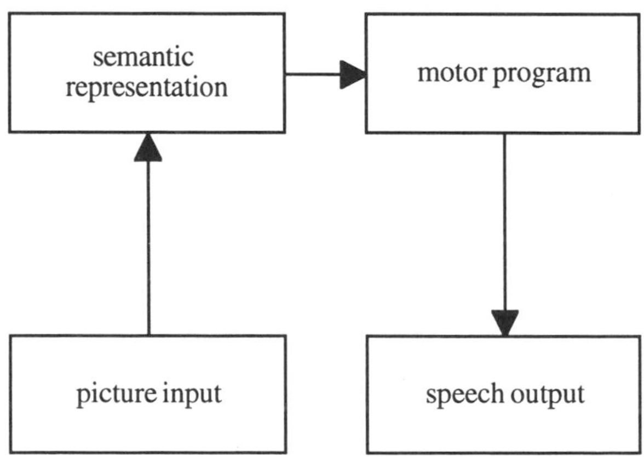

Figure 2.2: Naming a word already in the child's spoken vocabulary

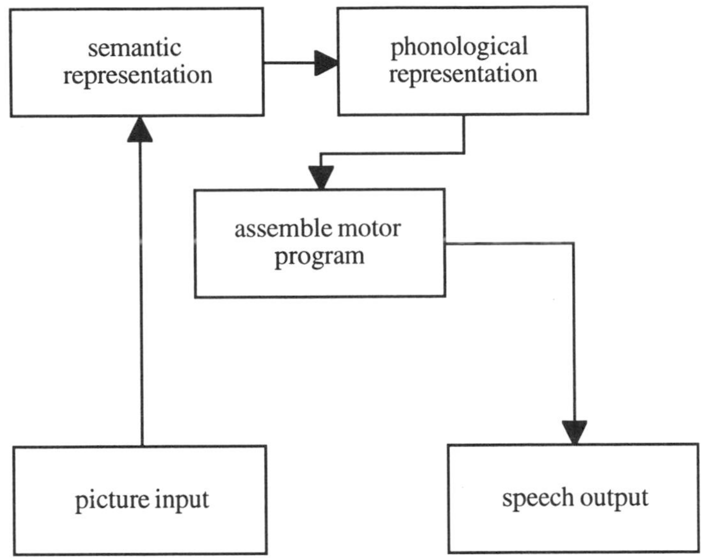

Figure 2.3: Naming a word for which the child has no stored motor program

Oral examination

Your cross for oral examination (Task 4 – OE) will be at the lowest point on the right-hand side of the model – in the mouth if you like! Oral examination has nothing to do with a child's stored linguistic knowledge. It involves examining the movements required for normal function of feeding, facial expression and to some extent speech. Similarly, even when you add the repetition of speech sounds to this assessment as in syllable repetition (Task 5 – SyllRep), it is not a linguistic activity – the child does not even have to recognize that the sounds you are making are anything to do with speech. However, because there is a link between oral movements and speech sound production, we have placed the cross for syllable repetition (Task 5 – SyllRep) to the side of the one for oral examination (Task 4 – OE). It is still near the periphery of the output side of the model.

Sentence repetition

Finally, sentence repetition (Task 6 – SentRep) has been placed along with word repetition. Although the child has to repeat more words, this task does not require the child to understand the sentence or spontaneously produce the grammatical construction themselves. Spontaneous production of that kind (as in conversation or picture description) would be a higher level task alongside naming since the child would need to draw on previously stored grammatical knowledge. It is arguable however, that if the child does have the grammatical knowledge to produce similar sentences spontaneously then the sentence repetition task will be easier. It is important to distinguish between testing children's grammar and testing speech skills when using sentence repetition. Sentence repetition tasks in which the sentences have been graded for grammatical complexity and length are used to investigate children's grammatical knowledge, e.g. the Sentence Repetition subtest of the *CELF-R – Clinical Evaluation of Language Fundamentals – Revised* (Semel, Wiig and Secord, 1987; UK version: Klein, Constable, Goulandris, et al., 1994). Task 6 (SentRep) above, however, has been specifically designed to investigate children's connected speech production. For this purpose, the length and grammatical complexity of the sentences used for the repetition task have been controlled. Task 6 (SentRep) has therefore been placed at the same level as word repetition but to the left side to indicate that it has a greater processing load. Thus, in Key to Activity 2.2 tasks located on the inside of the model but at the same level as another task are more challenging tests of that particular level.

Having completed this speech task analysis, the next step is to consider how performance on one task might relate to performance on others. By comparing a child's performance on a range of speech tasks his/her speech profile can be drawn. This profile will indicate the nature of the child's speech processing difficulty and will therefore provide useful information on which intervention can be based.

Speech Profiles

Investigations applying a range of speech tasks to children with speech and literacy problems have revealed that different profiles of performance on the tasks reflect different levels of breakdown in speech processing. Stackhouse and Snowling (1992b) presented tasks of single-word naming and repetition, nonword repetition and connected speech to two 11-year-old children, Michael and Caroline, with severe speech and literacy problems (see also Chapter 8 of this volume). The target words increased in syllable length, e.g. KITE, ROCKET, CARAVAN, TELEVISION, and also included clusters (teachers may refer to these as blends as in ST, SP etc), e.g. NEST, SPIDER, STAMP. A control group matched on articulation age on the *Edinburgh Articulation Test* (Anthony, Bogle, Ingram, et al., 1971) was also included in this study (articulation age range: 3 years to 5;6, chronological age range: 3;3 to 5;6). Compared to these normally-developing children, the performance of Michael and Caroline on the speech tasks was much more variable. Interestingly, their psycholinguistic speech profiles were also different from each other even though they had been given the same diagnostic labels of dyspraxia and dyslexia. Caroline performed poorly across all of the tasks but found the connected speech condition particulary difficult. Michael had a much more uneven profile. He performed as well as the normal controls on real word repetition and naming but had specific difficulty with repeating nonwords. This highlights the importance of using normal control data for comparison purposes when working with children with difficulties (see Vance, Stackhouse and Wells, 1995 for a discussion of the speech profiles of normally-developing children). Without this comparison, these different profiles would not have been detected. For example, Michael would have appeared to be poor across all of the tasks and his specific lexical difficulty in dealing with new words would not have been detected. A rather different speech profile emerged from DF: the 5-year-old boy with speech difficulties described by Bryan and Howard (1992). He was much better at imitating nonwords than real words. In the next activity, we explore the reasons why children with speech difficulties might present with different profiles.

ACTIVITY 2.3

Aim: To interpret contrasting speech profiles.

Consider the following scenarios taken from different children's performances on speech tasks. What do they suggest about the psycholinguistic nature of the child's speech difficulties? With reference to the speech processing model described in Figure 2.1, write down your hypotheses about where the level of breakdown is or is not for each of the following:

1. Real word repetition better than naming.
2. Naming better than real word repetition.
3. Real word repetition better than nonword repetition.
4. Nonword repetition better than real word repetition.
5. Real and nonword repetition equally poor.
6. Real (single) word repetition better than sentence repetition.

When you have completed this activity check your responses against Key to Activity 2.3 at the end of the chapter, then read the following.

Real word repetition better than naming

If naming a word is worse than repeating it (Scenario 1), it suggests that the child has the articulatory ability to produce the word (since s/he could repeat it) and therefore lower level articulatory skills are intact. In Scenario 1, the child is having difficulty producing the word from his/her own representations (naming). This may be because of imprecise phonological representations, or an incomplete stored motor program, or because of poor links between the semantic and phonological representations and/or motor program. All of these possible deficits make the word difficult to access and result in word-finding difficulties (Constable, Stackhouse and Wells, in press).

Naming better than real word repetition

If the opposite occurs, as in Scenario 2, where naming is better than real word repetition, then input skills should be investigated since the child can name familiar words from his/her own stored representations but does not process items presented auditorily for repetition.

Real word repetition better than nonword repetition

If nonword repetition is worse than real word repetition (Scenario 3) – this may be quite normal! In a study of 100 normally-developing children aged between 3 and 7 years, Vance, Stackhouse and Wells (1995) found that older children scored less well on nonword repetition than on real word repetition. This is an important finding because it illustrates again the necessity of having normal controls for comparison purposes. A test without such controls is of very limited value. On all the tasks presented, it is the degree to which a child's performance differs from the control group that determines whether there is a specific difficulty or not. Children with specific speech difficulties and literacy problems often perform significantly more poorly than normal controls on nonword repetition compared to real word repetition, i.e. the difference between real word and nonword repetition is greater than expected. This suggests difficulties with creating a motor program for a new word.

Nonword repetition better than real word repetition

The finding that some children are better at nonword repetition than real word repetition may therefore seem unlikely (Scenario 4). However, as mentioned earlier this was just the profile of DF (Bryan and Howard, 1992). In fact, this is not unusual; it occurs in early normal development and is often labelled as a 'habit'. For example, one of the first words learned by a child might be CAR. This might have been learned at a time when the child pronounced [k] as [t]. The production of CAR as [ta] may become the fixed motor program for that item. Subsequently, the child learns to pronounce [k], and learns new words in which this sound is produced accurately (e.g. CARPET, CARROT) but fails to update the original stored motor program for the lexical item CAR which has become a 'frozen' item. In DF's case, which is discussed further in Chapter 7, therapy was successfully targeted at increasing his awareness of contrasts which he could pronounce but did not make in spontaneous speech. This resulted in the 'frozen' form being 'thawed' with accurate pronunciation ensuing.

Real and nonword repetition equally poor

If real and nonword repetition are equally poor (Scenario 5), it suggests that the child may have more generalized articulatory difficulties that affect all speech tasks. This might be the pattern seen in children with structural abnormality or dysarthria arising from cerebral palsy. This pattern of equal difficulty across tasks may also be indicative of very pervasive phonological processing difficulties where more than one level is involved. Caroline aged 11 years, for example, was equally poor across the range of speech tasks. She had noticeable vocal tract incoordination involving resonance problems (poor control of air flow) which suggested lower level articulatory dificulties in addition to her motor programming problems (Stackhouse and Snowling, 1992b).

Real (single) word repetition better than sentence repetition

It is not uncommon for sentence repetition to be worse than single word repetition in children with speech and literacy difficulties (Scenario 6). Such children may not be able to repeat word sequences as a result of poor auditory memory. Children will also perform poorly on sentence repetition as a result of grammatical difficulties. This may be particularly apparent in spontaneous sentence production in conversation or in picture descriptions.

Key to Activity 2.3 is a summary of the diagnostic implications of the different patterns of performance on the speech tasks presented here. A word of caution, however. This table only summarizes the *hypotheses* about the child's difficulties that can be derived from their performance on the speech tasks. Before we can be sure of our basis for intervention, these hypotheses need to be checked out against our observations and testing of other areas, for example auditory processing or articulatory skills. This will be discussed further in Chapter 5.

One further scenario – real word repetition better than spontaneous production of a word – was reported recently in the following extract from a letter written by a speech and language therapist who has been using a psycholinguistic approach :

> '.......I have a lovely example on tape of a child with both speech and language problems trying to say the word PUPPETEER with all the sort of groping I used to say was typically dyspraxic struggle, but when he couldn't access the word at all and I supplied it, he could imitate it with no problems'

Bridget Tempest, Dawn House School, Nottinghamshire

The superiority of word repetition over spontaneous production suggests a specific word-finding difficulty. It is not uncommon for such a difficulty to be masked by what appears to be dyspraxic speech errors such as groping for targets and incomplete utterances. Indeed, speech and word-finding difficulties often co-occur.

That quotation captures the essence of psycholinguistic speech assessment. It illustrates the diagnostic power of speech profiling and also how quick and easy psycholinguistic assessment can be! We do not have to administer any specific test to be doing a psycholinguistic assessment. Neither do we need a number of sessions in which to do it. We can formulate hypotheses about a child's difficulties from observations of a spontaneous conversation in the classroom or a clip of video/audio tape. The psycholinguistic approach is in the head of the user and not in a case of tests. Clearly, we will need to test out our hypotheses if they are the basis for a child's remediation programme and this will normally involve administering some specific tasks. However, it would be wrong to assume that we *must* have new and specifically designed tests in order to carry out a psycholinguistic assessment.

Summary

This chapter does not provide an exhaustive list of test materials. Tasks typical of different types of test procedures have been described in order to illustrate the psycholinguistic properties of popular tests that are used. The aim of the activities is to heighten awareness of the psycholinguistic nature of tasks which can then be applied to current and future materials that may be encountered.

The identification of the child's speech processing strengths and weaknesses is essential for planning and delivering appropriate therapy. It is not helpful to match a teaching or therapy programme to a label of a disorder, e.g. dyspraxia, phonological disability, dyslexia, because children who have been given the same label can present with different speech processing profiles. Different teaching and therapy approaches are needed to deal with these different profiles which represent the balance of processing strengths and weaknesses in individual children.

This chapter has illustrated how flexible the psycholinguistic approach can be; because it is a way of thinking, it can be used in any situation to formulate hypotheses about a child's strengths and weaknesses and to monitor progress. Testing out these hypotheses can be done through a range of materials that are already familar. To refine our hypotheses, however, comparisons need to be made between tests, and with this in mind some specifically designed tests may be helpful.

Scoring children's performance on tests in a right/wrong fashion is an important step in a psycholinguistic assessment. However, noting how the child deals with the test material is equally important and most informative when planning teaching and therapy, e.g. is verbal rehearsal used and if so is it helpful? Noting the child's error responses is particularly revealing. A child's responses on a test may indicate associated difficulties in other areas, e.g. word-finding problems on a picture naming test designed to assess articulation, auditory-lexical problems on a nonword repetition test designed to test motor programming skills, memory problems on a sentence repetition test designed to assess articulation of connected speech. It is not difficult to generate hypotheses about a child's speech and literacy difficulties – the challenge is to test them out in a systematic way.

We can now extend our list of principles of psycholinguistic assessment by adding the following:

- Psycholinguistic assessment is an approach carried in the head of the user and not in a case of tests.
- A psycholinguistic assessment can take a few minutes or extend over long periods of time.
- Psycholinguistic screening and monitoring need not involve tests; listening and observing are equally important.
- The types of errors produced on a test give an insight into the child's processing strengths and weaknesses.
- Observing the strategies adopted by the child in order to complete the task are as important as scoring accuracy on the task.
- A child's response on one test may reveal associated problems in other areas.
- Most materials have the potential to be used in a psycholinguistic way; they do not have to be specifically designed or new.
- A test administered in isolation will result in more questions than answers. Results from different tests need to be compared in order to establish a child's processing capabilities.
- Specifically designed tests are useful for testing and refining hypotheses about a child's processing strengths and weaknesses.
- A target presented in a picture form cannot be converted to an auditory form without going via the child's semantic system.
- Tests used for psycholinguistic profiling should have normal control data for comparison purposes.

KEY TO ACTIVITY 2.1

Location of auditory discrimination tasks on the speech processing model

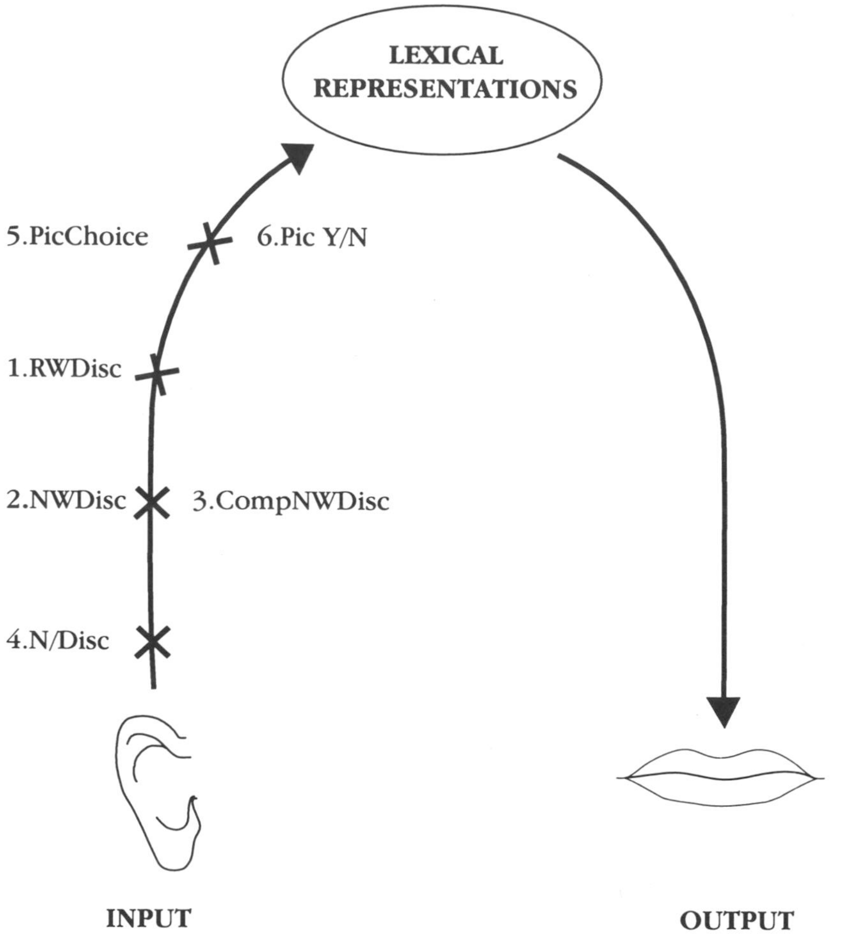

KEY TO ACTIVITY 2.2
Location of speech tasks on the speech processing model

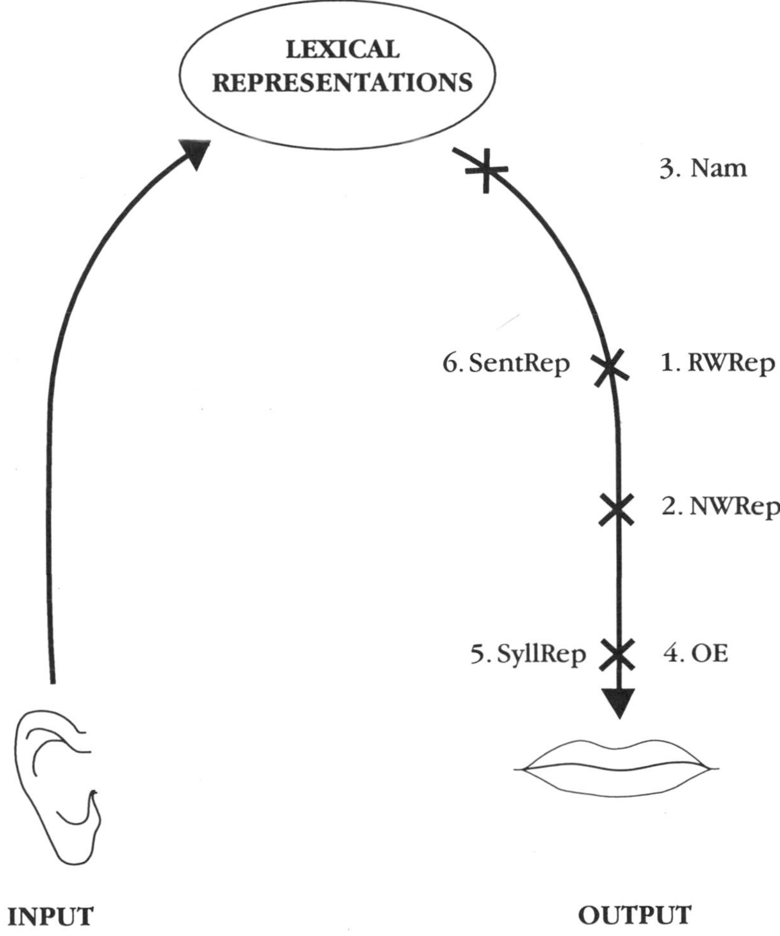

KEY TO ACTIVITY 2.3
Hypotheses to account for a child's performance on speech tasks

1. Real word repetition better than naming
   check: lexical representations and retrieval

2. Naming better than real word repetition
   check: auditory processing

3. Real word repetition better than nonword repetition
   check: motor programme assembly

4. Nonword better than real word repetition
   check: lexical updating

5. Real and nonword repetition equally poor
   check: articulatory skills

6. Real (single) word repetition better than sentence repetition
   check: grammar and auditory memory

Chapter 3
What Do Tests Really Test? II – Phonological Awareness

Phonological awareness refers to the ability to reflect on and manipulate the structure of an utterance as distinct from its meaning. It is tested by a range of tasks which include rhyme knowledge, blending and segmentation and manipulation of syllables, clusters and phonemes (Lewkowicz, 1980). Children need to develop this awareness in order to make sense of an alphabetic script, such as English, when learning to read and to spell. For example, children have to learn that the segments (the consonants and vowels) in a word can be represented by a written form – letters. When spelling a new word, children have to be able to segment the word into its constituent parts before they can attach the appropriate letters. When reading an unfamiliar word, they have to be able to decode the printed letters back to segments and blend them together to form the word. Environmental exposure to nursery rhymes, sound games and the printed word helps children to distinguish form from meaning and facilitates the sound play and literacy development typical of normally-developing children.

Normally-developing children learn not only how to perform phonological awareness tasks but incorporate phonological awareness skills into their everyday lives, for example rhyme games are very common in the play of young children (Chukovsky, 1963). In contrast, children with speech and literacy problems can find such tasks extraordinarily difficult (Hulme and Snowling, 1992; Snowling, Hulme, Wells, et al., 1992; Snowling, Goulandris, and Stackhouse, 1994). Further, the severity of the speech problem, when measured by speech intelligibility, may be a significant predictor of performance on phonological awareness tasks (Webster and Plante, 1992).

The Relationship Between Phonological Awareness and Literacy Development

Phonological awareness as a predictor of literacy development

Phonological awareness has been found to be a strong predictor of literacy development. Among the various phonological awareness tasks available, however, some have proved to be better predictors than others. In general, early phonological awareness skills such as syllable segmentation (Liberman, Shankweiler, Fischer, et al., 1974) and knowledge of nursery rhymes (MacLean, Bryant, and Bradley, 1987) are not such powerful predictors of literacy outcome as later developing phonological awareness skills, such as phoneme segmentation and manipulation (Adams, 1990). This does not mean that rhyme is not a useful skill. A longitudinal study by Bryant, MacLean, Bradley, et al., (1989) monitored the rhyme awareness and literacy progress of 65 children from the ages of 4;7 to 6;7. Their data suggested that sensitivity to rhyme is a prerequisite for phoneme segmentation which in turn plays an important role in learning to read.

The development of proficient rhyme skills may also be a precursor of children's abilities to read by analogy with similar words (Goswami, 1990). Recognizing the similarities in sound and appearance within rhyme families (e.g. CAT, HAT, SAT, FAT) allows children to use efficient reading and spelling strategies (see section on rhyme later in this chapter). Phoneme segmentation skills and letter knowledge, on the other hand, may be more predictive of children's ability to read unfamiliar words by a sounding out strategy, e.g., [kə] – [æ] – [tə] → "cat" (Muter, 1996).

Phonological awareness: a prerequisite or consequence of literacy development?

During the 1970s and 1980s, there was much debate about whether phonological awareness was a prerequisite or consequence of literacy development (Mann, 1986; Read, Yun-Fei, Hong-Yin, et al., 1986). It is now clear that the relationship is a reciprocal one, and that children's phonological awareness develops from a tacit to more explicit level through increased orthographic experience. For example, Zhurova (1963) reported that when a young child called IGOR was asked if his name was "Gor", he confidently replied that it was not, but he was unable to supply the missing initial vowel. Instead, Igor responded by elongating the initial vowel without segmenting it from the rest of the word: "*Eeeee*gor". This suggests that although Igor had developed some phonological awareness, he did not have the skills necessary to complete the task. To become really efficient at more advanced phonological awareness tasks, children are aided by their orthographic knowledge. Adolescents who were good spellers, for example, performed better on a spoonerism test than adolescents who were poor spellers (Perin, 1983). The good spellers were able to conjure up the orthographic forms of the words and use this to help them transpose the appropriate letters / phonemes in order to produce a spoonerism on popular singers' names, e.g. BOB DYLAN → "Dob Bylan" (see section on spoonerisms later in this chapter for further discussion of how this task is performed).

Not all phonological awareness tasks, however, are dependent on literacy skill. Liberman *et al.* (1974), for example, demonstrated that normally-developing preschool children could perform syllable segmentation tasks. Young children can also identify initial phonemes in words before they can read, often by reflecting on their speech production. Orthographic experience, however, sharpens children's phonological awareness skills and allows them to make finer distinctions, such as identifying phonemes *within* words, or the components of clusters which are not distinct from each other when spoken (e.g., SPL, SCR). For example, a normally-developing prereader, aged 4:6, was able to say that STRAWBERRIES began with "str", but could not identify what segments were in the cluster STR. To do this, children are aided by seeing the written form which helps them identify the components.

Figure 3.1 illustrates how a child's phonological awareness develops along a continuum of tacit to explicit awareness (see 'level of awareness'), and is the cumulative result of auditory, articulatory and reading experience (see 'feedback'). Popular phonological awareness tasks are presented in a developmental progression from left to right (see 'level of analysis') which relates to children's increasing experience of auditory, articulatory and visual feedback. The phonological awareness tasks become progressively more dependent on literacy experience to the right of the figure. Orthographic experience shows the child how words are structured (e.g. word/syllable boundaries, vowels, clusters), and thus, facilitates a more explicit level of phonological awareness. The effect of orthography on phonological awareness was demonstrated by Ehri and Wilce (1980). They presented 24 9-year-old children with counters to mark the number of phonemes detected in a series of single words that they then had to spell. Half of the words contained hidden

FEEDBACK Auditory Articulatory Orthographic
Lip reading

LEVEL OF ANALYSIS
Syllable segmentation
Rhyme
Blending
Sound segmentation
Sound manipulation
Cluster segmentation

LEVEL OF AWARENESS Tacit ——————————————————> Explicit

Figure 3.1: The development of phonological awareness skills (from Stackhouse, 1989)

letters (e.g. PITCH / RICH, COMB / HOME). The results indicated that those children who could spell the words also marked with a counter the hidden letters as additional *sounds* in their segmentation of the word.

Training studies

Findings from training studies, in particular, have contributed to our understanding of the relationship between phonological awareness and literacy development. Bradley and Bryant (1983) studied 65 children who were non-readers and below average on phonological awareness tasks when starting school. The group was divided into four subgroups as follows:

Experimental groups

(a) Trained in sound categorization tasks involving listening for shared sounds in words (e.g. HEN~HAT; HEN~MAN) or odd one out tasks (e.g. CAT, SAT, LEG, HAT).

(b) Trained as in (a) but the children were shown how each sound was represented in the alphabet by the presentation of plastic letters.

Control groups

(c) Trained in semantic categorization involving listening for words that were associated in meaning (e.g. HEN~PIG are both farm animals) or odd one out tasks (HORSE, COW, LION, SHEEP).

(d) Received no training.

Training took place in 40 individual sessions over 2 years. At the end of this time group (a) who had received sound categorization training was no different from control group (c) who had received semantic categorization training. In contrast, the children in group (b) were significantly better than controls on reading and spelling measures. The findings from this study suggest that phonological awareness training needs to be linked with explicit letter knowledge teaching for gains to be made in children's literacy development.

Similar results were obtained in a more recent training study targeting 7-year-old children who were reading around the 5;9 year level. Hatcher, Hulme and Ellis (1994) divided 128 poor readers matched on IQ and Reading Age into the following training groups:

Experimental groups

(a) Phonological awareness alone.

(b) Reading alone.
(c) Phonological awareness plus reading.

Control group

(d) No training other than routine classroom experience.

Each of the experimental groups received 40 30-minute sessions over a 20-week period. A range of reading, spelling and phonological awareness measures were taken before and after the training period. The results showed that group (c), who had received both phonological awareness training and reading instruction, was the only group to make significantly more progress than the controls on reading and spelling measures. Group (b) – reading alone – was significantly better than the controls on one measure only: early word reading (a reading recognition task). Group (a) – phonology alone – although better on the phonological awareness tasks at the end of the study was no better than the controls on any of the reading and spelling measures. The results of this study support the earlier findings of Bradley and Bryant (1983), that phonological awareness training alone does not necessarily facilitate literacy development. Literacy development is dependent on children's ability to link their phonological awareness skills to letter knowledge and reading experience. Hatcher *et al.* (1994) termed this the *phonological linkage hypothesis.*

Connecting Phonological Awareness with Speech and Literacy Development

It was argued in Chapter 1 that both speech and literacy development are dependent on an underlying speech processing system comprising input / output channels and stored representations (see Figure 1.1 in Chapter 1). An intact speech processing system is also necessary for the development of phonological awareness. However, phonological awareness is often assessed in isolation through various phonological awareness test batteries and is rarely related to children's underlying speech processing skills. Figure 3.2 attempts to illustrate the relationship between speech, literacy and phonological awareness and how all three are dependent on the speech processing system described in Chapter 1.

Through developing the speech processing system for the purpose of spoken communication, children develop awareness of the sounds and structure of their language. This allows them to match spoken output with the written form, e.g. through letter knowledge and orthographic experience. Tests of phonological awareness are really tapping

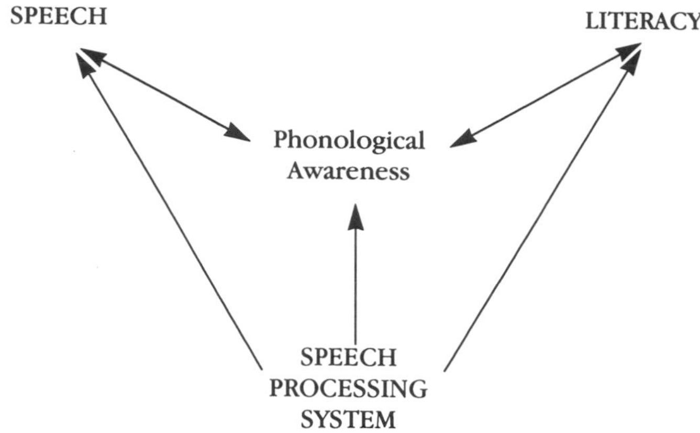

Figure 3.2: The connection between speech and literacy development

the integrity of this underlying speech processing system and are therefore an essential part of a child's psycholinguistic assessment. Not only do phonological awareness tasks identify a child's processing strengths and weaknesses by uncovering different levels of difficulty or limitations on processing capacity, they can also be used to identify children at risk for literacy problems. Children with poor phonological awareness have a faulty or immature speech processing system. Consequently they have a faulty or weak foundation for the development of literacy skills. It is therefore not surprising that children with phonological awareness problems often have associated speech and literacy problems since all may be derived from the child's speech processing system (Stackhouse, 1997).

This chapter examines popular phonological awareness tasks (rhyme, segmentation, blending and spoonerisms) from a speech processing perspective. As in Chapter 2, we do not aim to be comprehensive in our discussion of test materials. Instead, we focus on tests that exemplify common assessment procedures.

Rhyme

Rhyme tasks are widely used in assessment and teaching (Bradley and Bryant, 1983; Stackhouse, 1992c; Catts and Vartiainen, 1993; Hatcher, 1994; Layton and Deeney, 1996). Rhyme ability is an important measure of a child's speech processing skills and can be observed at quite a young age. To understand the concept of rhyme, children need to detect what it is that rhyming words have in common and also how they differ from each other. For example, the words CAT, MAT, BRAT, SPLAT all have the same *rhyme*: i.e. the vowel and any consonant(s) following the vowel (in this case: AT). They differ in their *onsets*, i.e. any consonant(s) preceding the vowel (in this case: C, M, BR, SPL). Rhyme skills therefore reflect an understanding of the major constituents of the syllable, i.e. onset and rhyme.

Children begin to develop their rhyme knowledge through exposure to nursery rhymes and songs. This experience can then be mapped on to increasing exposure to letters and the printed word. Having developed the ability to segment onsets from rhymes (e.g.C/AT, M/AT, BR/AT, SPL/AT), children are in a good position to match what they see in the written form to what they hear spoken. The ability to segment onset and rhyme in words facilitates reading and spelling by analogy with known words (Goswami, 1994; Muter, 1996). For example, when confronted by the printed word HAT for the first time, a child who can already read (or spell) CAT and MAT will recognize the rhyme AT as a chunk [æt] from known words but detect that the new word has a different onset. Through letter knowledge, the child can read the onset as [h] and then blends [h] + [æt] to read the new word HAT. When spelling, s/he may already have a motor program for writing AT which can be utilized. This is much more economical than having to segment every bit of a new word and blend it together, as in [h] + [æ] + [t] → HAT when reading, or allocating letters to each bit when spelling.

Without the understanding that syllables can be divided into an onset/rhyme structure, each word in the rhyme string CAT, MAT, HAT, FAT, SAT, RAT, BAT, FLAT, BRAT, SPLAT, SPRAT would have to be learned as a separate item rather than being incorporated into an existing sound family of -AT words. Children with speech and literacy problems, however, have specific difficulties developing these rhyme connections and are consequently very disadvantaged when learning to read and spell (Bird and Bishop, 1992; Marion, Sussman and Marquardt, 1993; Wells, Stackhouse and Vance, 1996). It is therefore important to assess rhyme skills routinely as part of a psycholinguistic investigation since this assessment can uncover speech processing problems that may be underlying a child's speech difficulties and alert us to potential literacy problems.

There is a range of rhyme tasks available which can be used to tap different levels of phonological processing in children. Broadly, these can be divided into (a) *rhyme judgement* – deciding whether two items rhyme or not, e.g. FAN~VAN, FAN~FIN; (b) *rhyme detection* – deciding which items in a sequence of items rhyme and which do not, e.g. FAN VAN PIN and c) *rhyme production* – spoken production of a word or a string of words that rhyme with a given target. Stimulus items can be presented or spoken by the tester via pictures. If a picture presentation is used for (a) and (b) above, the child can respond silently by pointing to the picture(s) they believe to be the correct response or by naming the correct picture. If a spoken presentation is given, nonword test items can be used as well as real word stimuli.

Appropriately classified, this range of rhyme tasks is particularly suited to psycholinguistic investigation, since between them they tap both input and output channels and also representations.

ACTIVITY 3.1

Aim: To compare and contrast different types of rhyme tasks and consider where they may be placed on the simple processing model used in the last chapter (see Figure 2.1).

Make a copy of Figure 2.1 on a sheet of A4 paper.

Take each of the rhyme tasks listed below and mark by a cross on your copy of Figure 2.1 the level at which the optimum processing occurs for each task, i.e. the furthest point you have to go from the 'ear' for the task to be achievable. In this activity, you will need to use both the input and output sides of the model. For example, if you feel that an input task can be completed without any reference to the child's lexical representations (i.e. their stored knowledge of words including information about semantics or phonology) and without spoken output, then you will put your cross on the left side of the model at a point nearer to the bottom than the top. If a task involves a spoken response and you feel that it can only be completed by accessing the lexical representations, then the cross will occur higher up on the output side (between the representations and the mouth) than a task which requires a spoken output but not access to previously stored linguistic knowledge.

Remember that the model has two dimensions: left/right and top/bottom. However, these dimensions are not organized in terms of difficulty. Tasks placed lower down on the model are not necessarily easier than tasks placed higher up. Similarly, tasks placed on the left side of the model are not necessarily easier than those placed on the right side. Remember also that for simplicity's sake, we have not included the eye in this model even though some of the tasks involve pictures. Normal visual processing can be assumed. Assume also that your model has normal peripheral hearing and normal speech production skills. None of the tasks are tapping peripheral skills only, and therefore no cross should appear in the ear or in the mouth.

Helpful Questions to Ask

Answering the following questions about each of the tasks will help you to make a decision about where to put your crosses:

1. Is this an input or output task?
   Answer this question by asking another: Was the response expected spoken or silent? If the answer to this question is *spoken* then it is an

output task and the cross should be on the right side of the model (unless the spoken response is merely "yes" or "no" and could be equally indicated by a nonverbal response, e.g. nodding or shaking head or pointing. In this case, the task would be classified as an input one). If the answer to this question is *silent*, then the task is an input task and the cross should be on the left side of the model.

2. Does the child have lexical representations for the stimuli used in this task?
   If the answer to this question is *No*, then your cross will be low down on the model. If the answer is *Yes*, then you need to answer question 3.
3. Does the child *have* to access these lexical representations in order to complete the task?
   If the answer to this question is *Yes*, then your cross will be high up on the model. If the answer is *No*, then your cross will be lower down on the model.

With these questions in mind, work through the following tasks placing a cross for each of the tasks at an appropriate point on a model copied from Figure 2.1.You should write the abbreviated labels for each of the tasks by the side of your cross, e.g. RDet/Aud – Rhyme detection / auditory presentation; RDet/Pic – Rhyme detection / picture presentation. This will help later when we collate a range of different tasks.

The Tasks

1. Rhyme judgement of real words (spoken/auditory presentation and no pictures) (RJment/RW), e.g. do these rhyme?: CAT HAT; do these rhyme? CAT SHOE. The child has to respond "yes" or "no".
2. Rhyme judgement of nonwords (spoken/auditory presentation) (RJment/NW), e.g. do these rhyme?: LAT DAT,; do these rhyme? LAT FOO. The child responds "yes" or "no" as in Task 1.
3. Rhyme detection – spoken/auditory presentation and no pictures (RDet/Aud) e.g. tester presents three finger puppets. Each one says a word. The child points to the two puppets which said the rhyming words in the following: SHELL, BELL, SEA; BEAR, BOY, CHAIR.
4. Rhyme detection – picture presentation (no spoken/auditory presentation) (RDet/Pic), e.g. point to which two pictures rhyme: SPOON, MOON, KNIFE; HOUSE, HORSE, MOUSE.
5. Rhyme string production (RProd), e.g. tell me as many words as you can that rhyme with (a) CAT; (b) TEA; (c) GOAT.

When you have completed the activity, check your responses against Key to Activity 3.1 at the end of this chapter, then read the following.

Rhyme judgement: real words (spoken/auditory presentation, no pictures)

Task 1 is an input task since the verbal response required is minimal and could be replaced by a nod or shake of the head. In order to judge if two words rhyme or not, the child has to detect the difference in the onsets and the commonality of the rhyme. In this sense it is similar to the real word auditory discrimination task presented in Activity 2.1 and the same principles apply. The rhyme judgement task involving real words can be completed without reference to the representations, i.e. the child does not have to know the words already to succeed on this task. The child may, however, use T-D processing (from the semantic representations) to help them complete the task. Your cross should therefore be halfway between the ear and the representations, in the same place as the cross for auditory discrimination of real words in Activity 2.1.

Rhyme judgement: nonwords (spoken/auditory presentation)

Rhyme judgement of nonwords (Task 2) is also an input task but in contrast to Task 1 it cannot involve the representations. As the child could have completed both this task and the previous rhyme judgement task at the same level, you could have put your crosses at the same point for both. However, it is worth demarcating the two tasks because of the *possibility* of using T-D processing for judgement of real words. Your cross for nonword judgement should therefore appear around halfway between the ear and the cross for real word rhyme judgement. You will notice that this is in the same place as the cross for auditory discrimination of nonwords in Activity 2.1.

Rhyme detection: (auditory presentation, no pictures)

Rhyme detection of auditorily presented real words (e.g. Task 3) is another input task and involves the same skills as judging if two words rhyme or not (Tasks 1 and 2); the only difference is that there are more words to remember. A choice has to be made about which word is different from two other words on the basis of its rhyme. This is reminiscent of the discussion about where to place complex nonword auditory discrimination in Activity 2.1: the difference between the level of processing for the task and the processing load involved. For the same reasons we have placed rhyme detection of real words on the same level as rhyme judgement, but to the side, indicating it is a more challenging task. This distinction is important since a child who succeeds on rhyme judgement tasks is telling you that s/he understands what is involved in rhyme, even if unable to do rhyme detection. In the latter case, his/her capacity for doing the task may be overloaded so that performance will break down even though the child has the basic skills to perform the task. A child with this profile will need a different focus in their remediation programme from one who cannot perform tasks of either rhyme judgement or detection, to whom the concept of rhyme needs to be introduced and developed.

Rhyme detection: picture presentation only

Your cross for Task 4 – rhyme detection from a picture presentation – should be high up on the left side of the model. It is another input task but this time the presentation is through the visual modality. The tester is not naming any of the pictures for the child. The child therefore ***has*** to access his/her own representations in order to perform this task. First, the pictures have to be identified via the semantic representation before the child can conjure up the spoken form of the words to reflect on their structure and make a decision about which two rhyme or alternatively which is the odd one out. In this sense Task 4 is similar to the auditory discrimination tasks involving picture presentation in Activity 2.1 (discussed in Chapter 2).

Although Task 4 is meant to be 'silent' in that the child is not required to produce any rhyming words, normally-developing children often name the rhyme pictures out loud as a means of rehearsal when carrying out the task. The importance of this spoken rehearsal strategy for at least some children is evident in the following response from a normally-developing 4-year-old: when asked if two pictures rhymed she replied "I don't think so yet, cos I haven't talked!". Vance, Stackhouse and Wells (1994) reported a developmental trend in this use of verbal rehearsal in their investigation of rhyme skills in a group of 100 children in the age range of 3–7 years. Spoken rehearsal was particularly apparent in 4-, 5- and 6-year-olds but declined in the 7-year-olds, who were at ceiling (i.e. very successful) on the picture rhyme detection task. The smallest percentage of spoken rehearsal occurred in the group of 3-year-olds, who were struggling on this task and only performed at chance level (i.e. often just guessing the response). These findings suggest that spoken rehearsal is important when children are striving to achieve the task but that it declines once they have become proficient at the task.

Clearly, this has implications for children with speech output difficulties who could be disadvantaged in the use of this strategy. If accurate spoken rehearsal is, if not a prerequisite, at least a great help in learning to segment words in one's lexicon into onset and rhyme, then the inability to perform accurate rehearsal might be expected to have a negative effect on the development of onset-rhyme segmentation (Wells, Stackhouse and Vance, 1996 and see Chapter 10).

Rhyme production

Task 5, rhyme production, is clearly an output task and your cross should therefore appear between the lexical representations and the mouth – but where? It is not purely an articulatory performance task since awareness of the structure of words is needed. It would be easy to assume that children generate all their rhyme response from their lexicon by somehow connecting all the rhyming words they already know and producing them in a string. However, the finding that young normally-developing children produce a mixture of real word and nonword rhyme responses indicates that not all rhyme production responses are the result of such a lexical search (Vance Stackhouse and Wells, 1994). The nonwords that children produce cannot be stored in the representations, so must be being assembled at a lower level.

To generate rhymes there is a finite number of consonants that can go in the onset slot. Older children (and adults) can produce rhymes by changing the onsets by systematically working through the alphabet, dropping a different letter into the onset slot. For example, for what rhymes with CAT, they may respond: "At, Bat, Dat, Fat, Gat, Hat, Jat, Lat", rejecting items that do not rhyme, e.g. Eat, Oat. This rhyme string inevitably includes nonwords (Dat Gat Jat Lat) which the child may reject if only real words have been requested by the tester.

There may therefore be more than one strategy for producing rhyming words. One approach to the task is to generate a rhyme string that has been stored in the lexicon. Some words have a large rhyme pool and are popular targets for rhyme tasks (e.g CAT) while others have small rhyme pools (e.g. IRON) and therefore a restricted number of real word responses. However, even when dealing with words from large rhyme pools, the length of a child's rhyme production string will be restricted by the extent of his/her vocabulary development and how efficiently rhyming words have been linked together within the lexicon. Unfortunately, a child with speech and literacy difficulties may have trouble setting up such connections within the lexicon and may need to adopt an alternative strategy.

This alternative strategy may be to generate rhyming words by filling in the onset slot through a sound or letter strategy as described above. Children can check their responses against their own representations and reject any nonwords if only real words have been requested. Children with speech and literacy difficulties also have difficulty with this strategy, which may explain their persisting difficulty with rhyme production tasks (Stackhouse and Wells, 1991; Bird and Bishop, 1992; Stackhouse and Snowling, 1992a; Marion, Sussman and Marquardt, 1993). Both strategies normally employed to complete rhyme production tasks are problematic for them. In contrast, children without speech and literacy difficulties are able to employ both strategies. Rhyme production skills are typically in advance of rhyme detection skills in normally-developing children but are often a persisting source of difficulty for children with speech and literacy problems (Chaney, 1992; Reid, Grieve, Dean, et al., 1993; Vance, Stackhouse and Wells, 1994).

Your cross for rhyme production should occur high up on the right-hand side of your model but not as high as the one you had for the naming task in Activity 2.2. In that activity it was argued that naming could *only* be achieved via the representations. This is not the case for rhyme production, for which an alternative lower level strategy of mechanically filling in the onset slot is available. However, rhyme production is certainly facilitated by intact and well-connected lexical entries.

The activities in Chapters 2 and 3 illustrate that although tests may appear to be testing different areas, as reflected by their titles, e.g. auditory discrimination vs rhyme, they may in fact be tapping the same level of speech processing. The opposite is also true. Tests with the same title, e.g. 'auditory discrimination' or 'rhyme', can be tapping different levels of processing depending on how they are presented (e.g. auditory vs visual), what type of test stimuli are included (e.g. real vs nonword) and what response is required (e.g. silent vs spoken).

Breaking down tasks in this way leads to a shift of emphasis in our approach to assessment. Traditionally, assessments have been organized in terms of specific areas, e.g. memory, discrimination, speech, rhyme. This is often reflected in the sections and subheadings used by professionals in assessment reports written about children with speech and literacy problems. In the psycholinguistic approach to assessment, a collection of tests, regardless of their title or professed purpose, can be used as a vehicle for tapping different levels of processing. Memory, for example, is implicated at every level of processing and is not a separate testable entity (Vance, Donlan and Stackhouse, 1996). The aim of psycholinguistic assessment is to identify the profile of strengths and weaknesses in a child's processing skills, rather than to examine particular areas in isolation.

Onset / Coda Knowledge

The ability to detect the beginning and end of words and syllables is important when storing words and producing them in speech and spelling. Confusing consonants in these positions can lead to misunderstanding as well as speech and spelling errors. In the description of rhyme tasks, we described the *rhyme* as the part of the syllable that includes the vowel and any following consonants. The consonant(s) following the vowel are referred to as the *coda,* while the consonant(s) preceeding the rhyme are known as the *onset.* Thus, in the word CAT, the onset / rhyme division is C/AT, and the coda is T.

The popular 'I-Spy' game is a useful psycholinguistic assessment of onset knowledge. The child is asked to guess an item you have selected in the room, having been given a clue in the form of its first letter, or onset of the first syllable. The child's response can be very revealing. For example, a boy aged 7 years, referred because of his stammer, responded to "I spy with my little eye something in this room beginning with [d]," by looking around intently and suggesting "d-floor?, d-window?, d-telephone?". Further investigation revealed that his nonfluency was part of specific speech, language and literacy difficulties. This case is worth noting because the child's presenting stammer had been masking a speech processing impairment. In fact, there is a high incidence of phonological difficulties in young stammerers (Nippold, 1990; Wolk, Conture and Edwards, 1990; Boberg, 1993) and phonological awareness skills need to be assessed as a matter of routine (Forth, Stackhouse, Vance et al., 1996). The psycholinguistic approach to assessment is particularly useful in uncovering hidden speech and language processing difficulties whatever the presenting or obvious symptoms.

The I-Spy game as described above is clearly a production task since the child has to produce a series of spoken responses all beginning with the same onset: thus, it is conceptually similar to the rhyme production task described in the previous section. When the roles change and it is the child's turn to select an object in the room and supply an onset for the clue, then the task demands change too. Firstly, the child has to segment the onset from the word s/he has selected. It then becomes a detection task since the child has to listen to your responses and match them with his/her own stored representation of the selected item.

A specifically designed sound categorization task was devised by Lynette Bradley (1984). This comprises spotting the odd one out in a series of words. For example, in the following, which is the odd one out in each sequence and why?

(a)	SUN	GUN	RUB	FUN
(b)	HEN	PEG	LEG	BEG
(c)	BUD	BUN	BUS	RUG
(d)	PIP	PIN	HILL	PIG

Items (a) and (b) are tests of coda detection and (c) and (d) are tests of onset detection. However, it may have occurred to you that (a) and (b) could equally be called a rhyme detection task since changing the coda also changes the rhyme: the vowel, as well as the final consonant, is pronounced slightly differently (with more nasal escape of air) in FUN, SUN, GUN than in RUB, for example. This illustrates again the importance of analysing test items and deciding for yourself what is being tested – it may not always be what the title of the test suggests! Further, although often referred to as a detection test, this task does require the child to produce the word that is the odd one out.Within our framework, it would therefore be classed as a production task (see Chapter 5).

Clearly, sufficient memory is needed in order to hold on to four items while making an odd one out decision. Some children with specific speech and literacy difficulties have responded to each item on the Bradley test by repeating the last word in the item, having forgotten what came before, e.g. on (a)–(d): FUN, BEG, RUG, PIG. It is important to find out if the child really cannot detect onsets and codas or if there is a more generalized memory difficulty. This can be done by reducing the number of words in each item to three or incorporating pictures for memory support (compare the different rhyme tasks described in the previous section).

Blending

An assessment and teaching activity often used with school-age children is syllable and phoneme blending. This is when a child is presented with elements of a word, e.g. the syllables in COMPUTER (COM-PU-TER) or the phonemes in FISH (F-I-SH), and is asked to put them together to produce the word. The ability to do this correlates well with reading achievement and is a good predictor of reading performance (Fox and Routh, 1984; Perfetti, Beck, Bell, et al., 1987). The sound blending subtest of the *Aston Index* (Newton and Thomson, 1982) comprises both real and nonword test items, e.g. P – O – T; D – I – NN – ER; D – U – P; T – I – S – E – K. You may also see the same task referred to as auditory synthesis (cf. the *Fullerton Test of Adolescent Language*, Thorum, 1986), and find it in teaching programmes (e.g. Hatcher, 1994).

Children with speech and literacy problems have particular difficulties with production blending tasks. However, an isolated test result like this provides insufficient evidence to conclude that the child cannot blend the elements correctly; the problem may be that s/he is physically unable to produce the response. Another principle of psycholinguistic assessment is that a minimum of two tasks, normally one silent and one involving some production, need to be administered to identify with any precision the difficulty the child is having.

Silent blending tests have been devised where the child is asked to point to the picture (Goldman, Fristoe and Woodcock, 1976; Chaney, 1992; Counsel, 1993) or written word (Stackhouse, 1989) which represents the spoken target item. Here, unlike in production tasks, the child does not have to produce the spoken word. The finding that some children can succeed on such 'silent' tasks, even though they may have failed production blending tests, is encouraging and for such a child this strength can be used when planning a remediation programme.

Spoonerisms

Spoonerisms are fun for older children who enjoy metalinguistic games. The process involves transposing onsets of initial syllables, e.g. BILL WELLS → Will Bells; JOY STACKHOUSE → Stoy Jackhouse. The ability to perform spoonerisms is an advanced metalinguistic skill. Spoonerisms can therefore be a useful assessment tool for older children who can perform well on simpler phonological awareness tasks, such as rhyme or onset/coda tasks. Stackhouse (1992a) describes such a case in a longitudinal study of Keith, a boy with developmental verbal dyspraxia and dyslexia. By the age of 17 years, Keith could perform well on segmentation tasks involving rhyme and identification of segments at the beginning and end of words. However, more age-appropriate tasks revealed persisting high level segmentation difficulties.

One of the 'more age-appropriate tasks' used here was the spoonerism test devised by Perin (1983). Names of singers and pop groups were presented with the instruction to transpose the first sound of each word. For example, the spoonerism on CHUCK BERRY is "Buck Cherry". Keith found this difficult but persevered and scored 15/18 correct. Accuracy, however was at the expense of speed: reaction time was slow and there was normally a long pause between the first and second name. This raises an important general issue when assessing the psycholinguistic abilities of older children or children with hidden speech and language problems. A high accuracy score does not necessarily mean that the child has normally-developing speech or literacy skills. Speed of processing and responding is just as significant a diagnostic measure as accuracy of responses.

ACTIVITY 3.2

Aim: To analyse how spoonerism task are completed.

1. Try out Perin's spoonerism tasks on your colleagues and family. Ask them to reflect on how they have performed the task. Here are some of the items:

   Bob Dylan
   John Lennon
   Chuck Berry
   Led Zeppelin
   Johnnie Cash
   Four Seasons

2. Critically evaluate Perin's test items – summarize your points in note form.

Now read the following account.

It would seem that there are at least two general ways of tackling a spoonerism task. Feedback from normally-developing children and adults suggests that many conjure up the orthographic image of the word (its spelling) and then visually transpose the first letter of the two words in order to read back the response. It is therefore not surprising that Perin (1983) found in young teenagers a strong correlation between ability to perform well on her spoonerism task and spelling development. The second approach, as described by unimpaired adults, is to deal with the whole process auditorily without any recourse to the orthography.

If you tried out the above task on children you may have had a similar response to the following: BOB DYLAN – "Who?"; JOHN LENNON – "Was he in a group or something?". Apart from making the tester feel dated, there is an important psycholinguistic point here. If the material is unfamilar to the child then the stimuli in the item will be processed as nonwords even though they are real words for the tester. An important principle of designing material is to control for this possible confusion. One way of doing this is to avoid fashion or cult words. This will be discussed further in Chapter 11.

ACTIVITY 3.3

Aim: To compare and contrast a selection of phonological awareness tasks particularly useful for school-age children and to consider where they may be placed on the speech processing model.

Make another copy of Figure 2.1 from Chapter 2 – the simple speech processing model used in Activity 3.1.

For each of the following tasks, locate with a cross on your copy of Figure 2.1 the point of maximum processing demands, i.e. the furthest point you have to go from the 'ear' for the task to be achievable. In this activity, you will need to use both the input and output sides of the model. For example, if you feel that an input task can be completed without any reference to the child's lexical representations (i.e. their stored knowledge of words including information about semantics, phonology, and – in older children – orthography) and without spoken output, then you will put your cross on the left side of the model at a point nearer to the bottom than the top. If a task involves a spoken response and you feel that it can only be completed by accessing the lexical representations, then the cross will occur higher up on the output side (between the representations and the mouth) than a task which requires a spoken output but not access to previously stored linguistic knowledge.

Remember that the model has two dimensions: left/right and top/bottom. However, these dimensions are not organized in terms of difficulty. Tasks placed lower down on the model are not necessarily easier than tasks placed higher up. Similarly, tasks placed on the left side of the model are not necessarily easier than those placed on the right side. Remember also that for simplicity's sake we have not included the eye in this model even though some of the tasks involve pictures. Normal visual processing can be assumed. Assume also that your model has normal peripheral hearing and normal speech production skills. None of the tasks are tapping peripheral skills only, and therefore no cross should appear in the ear or in the mouth.

Helpful Questions to Ask

Answering the following questions about each of the tasks will help you to make a decision about where to put your crosses:

1. Is this an input or output task?
   Answer this question by asking another: was the response expected spoken or silent? If the answer to this question is *spoken* then it is an output task and the cross should be on the right side of the model (unless the spoken response is merely "yes" or "no" and could be equally indicated by a silent response, e.g. nodding or shaking head, or pointing. In this case, the task would be classified as an input one). If the answer to this question is *silent*, then the task is an input task and the cross should be on the left side of the model.
2. Does the child have lexical representations for the stimuli used in this task?
   If the answer to this question is *No*, then your cross will be low down on the model. If the answer is *Yes*, then you need to answer question 3.
3. Does the child *have* to access these lexical representations in order to complete the task?
   If the answer to this question is *Yes*, then your cross will be high up on the model. If the answer is *No*, then your cross will be lower down on the model.

With these questions in mind, work through the following tasks placing a cross for each of the tasks at an appropriate point on your model copied from Figure 2.1. You should write the abbreviated labels for each of the tasks by the side of your cross, e.g. Blend/RW (spoken blending of real words); Blend/NW (spoken blending of nonwords). This will help later when we collate a range of different tasks.

The Tasks

1. Silent coda detection (CDet) – point to the two pictures which end with the same sound: TAP, MOP, DISH; PEN, WATCH, SPOON.
2. Coda production (CProd) – tell me as may words as you can that end with [t].
3. Silent blending (Blend/Pic) – point to the picture of what I am saying: m-ou-se [m] - [aʊ] - [s]. Picture choice: HOUSE CAT MOUSE; the three pictures per item are not exposed to the child until the target word [m] – [aʊ] – [s] has been completed by the tester (Counsel, 1993).
4. Spoken blending of real words (Blend/RW). The child produces the target word from the segments spoken by the tester: SH-O-P, [ʃ] - [ɒ] - [p]; B-A-BY, [b] - [eɪ] - [bɪ] (from the *Aston Index*, Newton and Thomson, 1982).
5. Spoken blending of nonwords (Blend/NW) – procedure is the same as in Task 4. but the test items are: P-O-G [p] - [ɒ] - [g]; GL-E-B [gl] - [ɛ] - [b] (from the *Aston Index*, Newton and Thomson, 1982).
6. Spoonerisms – exchange the first sounds of the following: COLD TAP; FAT BEAR (from Vint, 1993).

When you have completed the above, check your responses against Key to Activity 3.3, then read the following.

Coda detection: pictures only

Your cross for coda detection (Task 1) should be on the top left side around the same place as the cross for rhyme detection (pictures). These cluster together because both rhyme detection from pictures and coda (or onset) detection from pictures are testing the child's awareness of the syllable structure of words they have had to access from their own representations, since they were not given the word by the tester.

Coda production

This is like rhyme production, except that the child needs to focus on the very end of the word, rather than the rhyme. Your cross should be at the same level as for rhyme production in Activity 3.1.

Silent blending

The cross for the silent blending task (Task 3) should be high up on the left-hand side, because it cannot be performed without accessing representations. The child has to take in the segments spoken and hold them in a temporary store while they are blended together to form a word. S/he then has to recognize the word and its meaning, which involves accessing both its phonological and semantic representations, in order to match it to a picture. We have placed it below Task 1, because the tester has helped the child to access the representation by producing the segments of the target.

Spoken blending: real words

Spoken blending of real words (Task 4) may not be such a high level task. Our cross for this is halfway between the representations and mouth on the output side since although it might help to access the representations for this task, the child does not have to access them in order to complete it. In fact, normally-developing children will often produce a correct response out loud and then show surprise that what they have said is a real word – one that they know. The opposite can occur in children with specific speech and literacy difficulties. When Michael, aged 14;6 years, was asked to produce the word PR-A-M, he was unable to do so. He replied "prom, promp.... we call it a pushchair!" (Stackhouse, 1993). Clearly, he had blended the segments sufficiently in his head to recognize and access the meaning of the word. His difficulty was in assembling the segment himself for production of the word. This was confirmed when he was 100 per cent correct on a silent test of blending (like Task 3 but using printed words instead of pictures) but scored zero on a blending production task (like Task 4). The case of Michael illustrates why one test result in isolation can be misleading and be a false premiss on which to base a remediation programme.

Spoken blending: nonwords

In contrast, there can be no help directly from the representations when producing nonword responses (Task 5) (but see Dollaghan,Biber and Campbell, 1995 for further discussion of this issue). Spoken nonword blending has therefore been put at a lower level on the ouput side than spoken real word blending. We continue to make the distinction that on tasks where real words are involved the child *can* draw on representations. The same point was made when discussing real and nonword rhyme detection and real and nonword auditory discrimination.

You will have noticed that the real and nonword spoken blending tasks are both taken from one test in the *Aston Index*. It is not uncommon to have this mix of real and nonwords in the same test and on some occasions it may be desirable – it depends what you want to test.

However, given that the child may treat these items differently, it is important to distinguish between a child's performance on the real and nonword items when scoring up the test and analysing the data.

Spoonerisms

Our cross for spoonerisms (Task 6) is near the top of the right-hand side. Accessing the orthographic representation of the word undoubtedly facilitates performance on this task. You may argue, however, from your experience of Activity 3.2, that this is not the case for those who report performing the task at an auditory level. For them it does not matter if the words are real or not: they merely move the segments around in a mechanical way. You may therefore want to have two crosses on your model – one top right and the other halfway down with the real word blending task. This reminds us that among normally-developing children there is evidence of more than one way to complete a task; there is no reason why this should not be the case in atypical development too. It also illustrates another important aspect of assessment – asking children to describe how they complete the task. This can reveal firstly whether the child has any insight into what they are doing at all ('meta' skills), and secondly what strategies they are finding helpful which might be incorporated more explicitly into their remediation programme. Conversely, they may have adopted strategies which limit their performance and which could usefully be eliminated or changed.

Summary

By completing the activities in Chapters 2 and 3, and mapping the findings on to a simple model of speech processing, we have worked out the essential structure and content of the psycholinguistic assessment framework that will be presented more formally in the next chapter.

The following principles of psycholinguistic assessment can be added to the list at the end of Chapter 2.

- Do not believe what you read in a test title or description.
- Tests of seemingly different skills (e.g. rhyme and blending) can tap the same level of processing.
- Tests of seemingly the same skill (e.g. rhyme tests) can tap different levels of processing (e.g. depending on if pictures are involved, if a spoken response is expected).
- Tests can be analysed in terms of (a) how they are presented, (b) the test stimuli involved and (c) the response required.

- Memory limitations will affect performance at each level and cannot be tested in isolation.
- Psycholinguistic assessment uncovers the underlying and sometimes hidden difficulties found in children presenting with a range of different symptoms.
- Popular children's games can be used for psycholinguistic assessment.
- A minimum of two tests need to be used to compare strengths and weaknesses in channels of processing (input/output) or levels of processing (bottom vs top).
- Speed of processing and response may be as important as accuracy of response when investigating a child's strengths and weaknesses.
- There may be more than one way of completing a task in terms of appropriate strategies to use.
- Tests involving 'fashion' words will quickly become dated and the stimuli will turn into nonwords.
- Real and nonwords should be dealt with separately when scoring results even if they occur within the same test.

KEY TO ACTIVITY 3.1

Location of rhyme tasks on the speech processing model

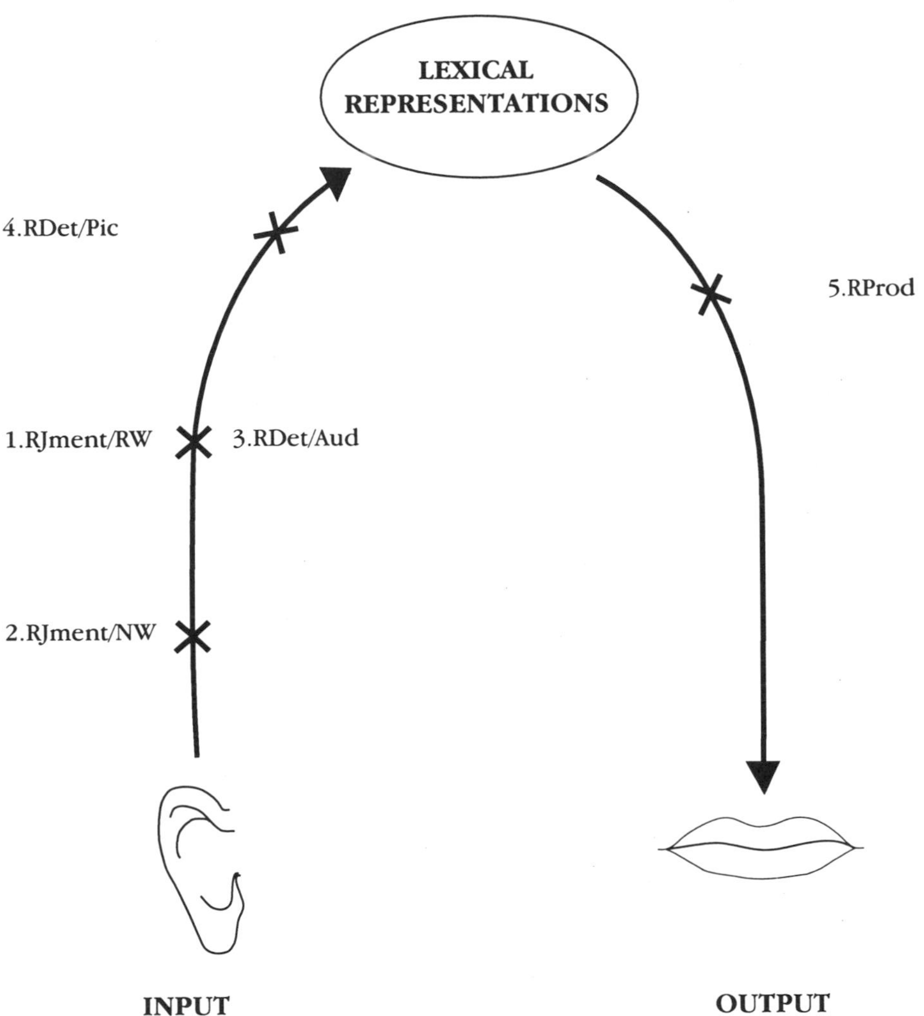

KEY TO ACTIVITY 3.3

Location of phonological awareness tasks on the speech processing model

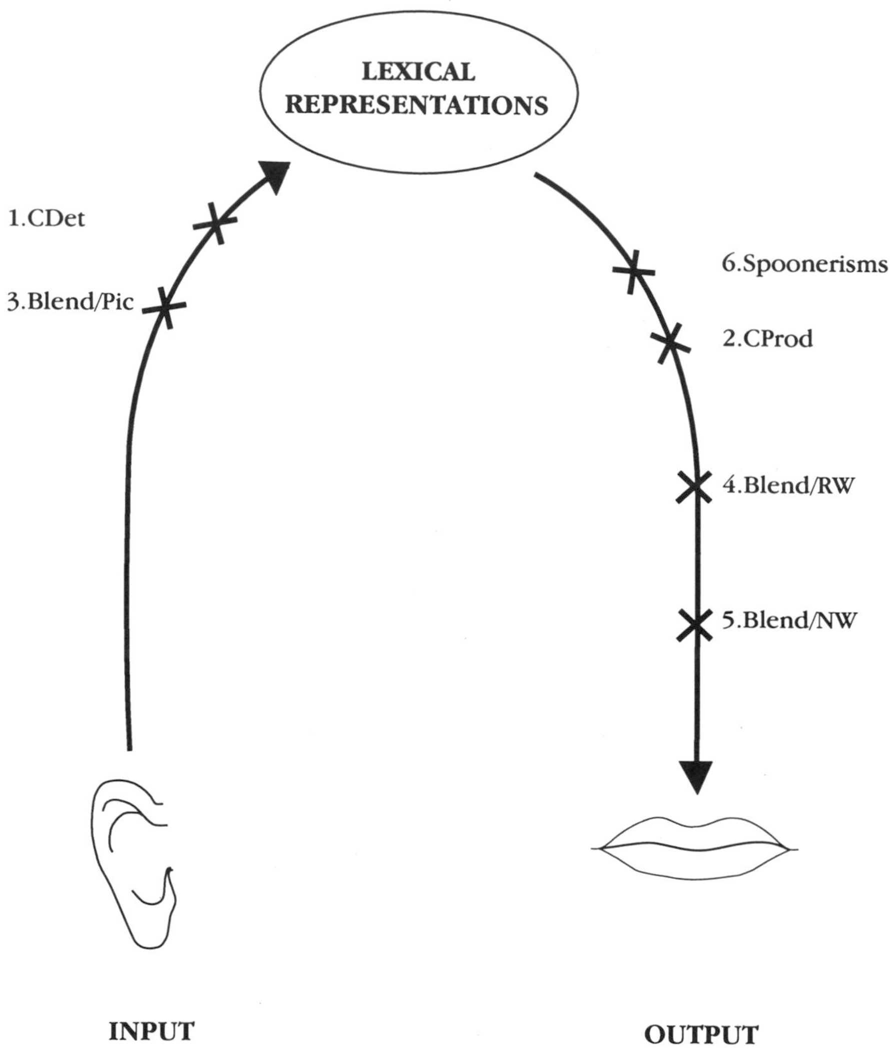

Chapter 4
The Assessment Framework

The framework presented in this chapter provides a structure for organizing a wide variety of assessment procedures in such a way that a child's performance on a range of tasks can be interpreted from a psycholinguistic perspective. It is grounded in psycholinguistic theory but the purpose is a practical one: to facilitate the planning of appropriate remediation for individual children. The individualized nature of this approach to assessment does not, however, preclude the subsequent therapy or teaching being carried out in groups.

The framework is based on the simple speech processing model presented in Chapter 1 (see Figure 1.2) and used for Activities in Chapters 2 and 3. It is organized in terms of a series of questions that can be posed about the levels of possible breakdown in processing that are giving rise to a child's speech and literacy difficulties. These questions distinguish between the child's *input* processing (the skills necessary for decoding the speech signal) and their *output* processing (for encoding and producing speech). It also posits *representations* for linguistic items, where linguistic information about words and other units (e.g. syllables) is stored. Input tasks appear on the left of the framework, output tasks on the right.

The framework also distinguishes between tasks which require prior linguistic knowledge for their completion (e.g. from stored representations as in a naming task); and those which require analysis and manipulation of sensory and physical phenomena, as in detection of acoustic signals and movement of the articulators. Tasks that are dependent on representations appear at the top of the framework and can be referred to as higher level tasks, while tasks that do not depend on representations appear further down towards the bottom of the framework, and as such are lower level tasks.

Assessment procedures are therefore defined within the framework along the two dimensions discussed in Chapter 1. First, tasks are classified according to the degree to which they are dependent on stored linguistic information in the lexical representations: top vs bottom; and second, tasks are classified as either input or output: left vs right (see Figure 4.1).

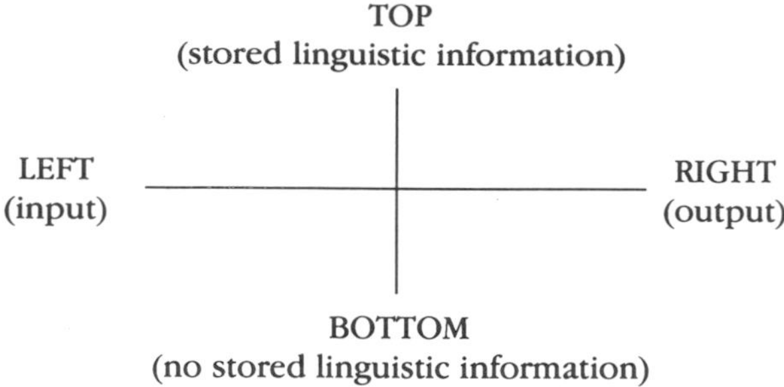

Figure 4.1: The two dimensions on which the assessment framework is based

Constructing an Assessment Framework

In the activities completed in Chapters 2 and 3, a range of tasks was analysed on the basis of the principles outlined above. These will now be integrated and presented on one sheet in order to see how the framework is constructed. The aim of the following activities is to construct this psycholinguistic assessment framework for practice.

ACTIVITY 4.1

Aim: To assemble the input side of the psycholinguistic framework.

Take your answer sheets from Activities 2.1, 2.2, 3.1 and 3.3 (showing your crosses for the different tasks). First list tasks from all four activities according to whether they were (a) on the input side of the simple model or (b) on the output side. Tasks that you located more in the representations should be allocated to 'input' or 'output' lists, according to whether or not the task requires a spoken response (remember that if the spoken response was merely "yes" or "no" then this did not constitute an output response since the child could replace this with a nonverbal gesture, e.g. nodding or shaking the head).

Look at Figure 4.2. It is a copy of the speech processing model used in the previous activities in Chapter 2 and 3. However, crosses have been added which indicate the levels at which related tests should cluster. These crosses are labelled A – F (C is missing, for reasons which will become apparent later in this chapter.).

Now transfer the tasks in your 'input' list to Figure 4.2, placing each task at the appropriate level (by one of the crosses) to reflect the processing level characteristic of each task as identified in the earlier activities. Compare your response with Key to Activity 4.1 at the end of this chapter, then read the following account.

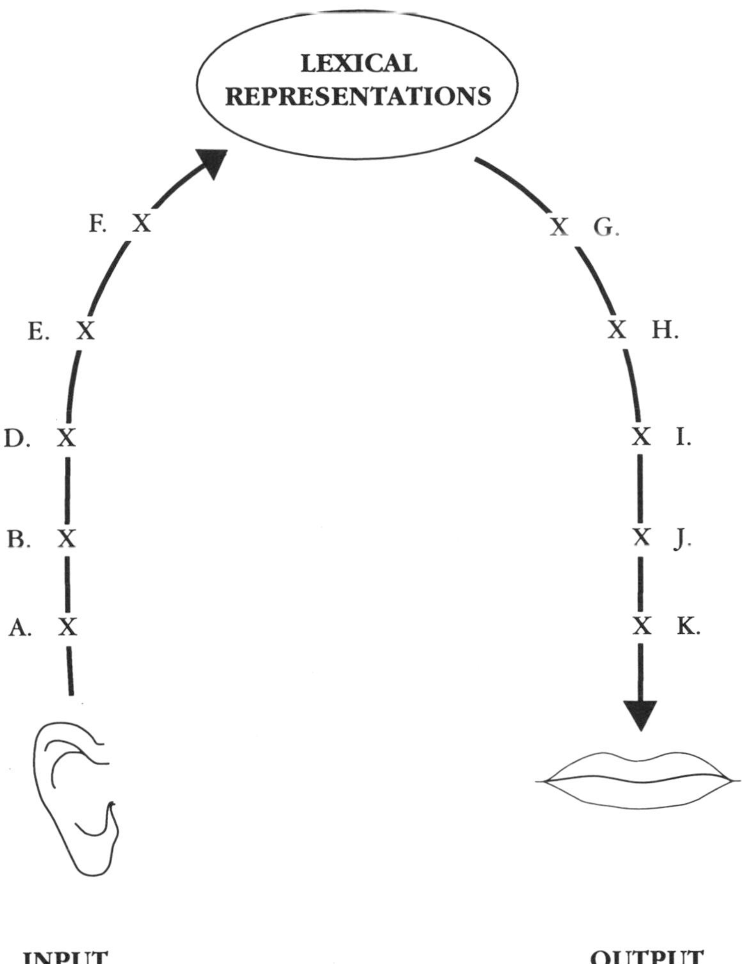

Figure 4.2: Crosses on the simple speech processing model to mark the levels at which tests cluster

Level A

Noise (nonspeech) discrimination has been placed at level A, just above the ear, since completing this task does not require any prior linguistic knowledge.

Level B

Complex nonword discrimination, simple nonword discrimination and rhyme judgement of nonwords, which all involve unfamiliar material, are placed at level B. This is because they involve verbal material rather than noise or other nonlinguistic sounds (and are therefore higher up than A) but do not involve lexical representations. They are thus at a low point on the input side.

Where there is more than one task at the same level, as at Level B, we can attempt to rank tasks in order of complexity, with the most complex tasks at the top of the list. Complex nonword discrimination is put at the top of level B because it requires the child to process more information (for each stimulus item) than in the other tasks. Rhyme judgement can be considered more difficult than simple nonword auditory discrimination since in general children can detect differences between simple words, such as BUP~DUP, more easily than identifying whether these two words rhyme, which requires some concept of rhyme in addition to the concept of same/different. For the purposes of this exercise, we have therefore placed the simple auditory discrimination task at the bottom of the list.

Note here that the same stimuli (e.g. BUP~DUP) could be used for either an auditory discrimination task or a rhyme task. The important difference between the two tasks is in the instructions given to the child. An auditory discrimination task requires a child to say if a pair of words are the same or different and focuses attention on the onset (first consonant). A rhyme judgement task requires a child to say if a pair of words rhyme or not and focuses attention on the nucleus and coda (vowel and final consonant) of the words.

Level D

Auditory discrimination of real words, and real word rhyme detection and judgement (auditory) can be performed at a purely auditory level, and to that extent resemble tasks at level B. For the real word tasks, however, T-D processing can be used as an alternative strategy: the child can draw on prior lexical knowledge for support. For this reason, the real word tasks are located higher up, clustering together at level D.

At Level D the same principles for the hierarchy of difficulty apply as at level B. Real word auditory discrimination is placed at the bottom of the set since it requires the child to make a more gross same/different judgement. Rhyme judgement and detection make more metalinguistic demands on the child and so are placed further up in the set. Rhyme detection is placed above rhyme judgement because of the greater memory load: three words have to be held in working memory, rather than two.

Level E

The tests at level E all involve a stimulus word spoken by the tester which is then matched to a picture. Although two of the tests are called auditory discrimination tasks (picture choice auditory discrimination test and the yes/no picture auditory discrimination test) they are both tapping a higher level than the auditory tasks clustering at B or D, since they require the child to draw on their own representations. In Chapter 2 these two tasks were described as ***auditory lexical tasks*** since they are a means of investigating the precision of a child's representations. The yes/no picture auditory discrimination task was placed above the picture-choice task because it can involve items that are phonetically closer to one another (see SHOP example in Chapter 2) and is therefore a more challenging investigation of the child's representations.

The picture-blending tasks involve a similar process. The child listens to the stimulus spoken by the tester and then selects the appropriate picture. The difference is that the stimulus spoken is fragmented into its phonetic constituents; the child has to blend these before knowing which word to select from the array of pictures. It thus involves an additional operation at the beginning of the process, and so is placed at the top of this level.

Level F

At the top of the input side at level F are tasks that require not only lexical access but also awareness of the phonological structure of the word presented. What makes this level distinct from level E is that none of the test items are spoken by the tester. All of the tasks involve picture identification and therefore lexical access prior to analysing the phonological structure of the word, for example in tests of onset/coda detection and rhyme detection from picture presentation. What sets this level apart from the others on the input side is that the phonological structure to be analysed is the one stored in the child's lexicon, not one given by the tester.

To achieve success on the tests at level F, the child has to first identify the picture correctly. This gives access to the semantic information that in turn provides access to stored phonological information about the word which the child needs in order to reflect on the word's phonological structure. If the child does not recognize the picture, or the word is not in their vocabulary, the phonological information cannot be retrieved. Very often in these tasks the child will say the word out loud or whisper it, indicating that they have accessed or assembled a motor program for the word. This gives them more insight into how the word is constructed, or at least allows them to hold on to the stimulus for longer while they reflect on its structure. In terms of task difficulty at level F, the rhyme task is placed below the coda detection task since children find this task easier than detecting differences between codas or vowel nuclei on their own (Kirtley, Bryant, MacLean, et al., 1989). This has been used as evidence for the importance of the onset–rhyme division in phonological development.

Having completed the input side of the framework, we can now turn to output tasks.

ACTIVITY 4.2

Aim: To assemble the output side of the psycholinguistic framework.

Take your list of 'output' tasks prepared at the beginning of Activity 4.1. Now transfer the tasks in the 'output' list to Figure 4.2, placing each task at the appropriate level to reflect the processing level characteristic of each task as identified in the earlier activities. The crosses provided on the model indicate the levels at which related tests should cluster. These crosses are labelled G – K.

Compare your response with Key to Activity 4.2 at the end of this chapter, then read the following account.

Level G

Naming (and spontaneous speech) is placed at level G because it involves spoken production based on the child's stored linguistic knowledge. Naming, for example, is a direct production of the child's representation of the test picture. There is no lower level support for this task; the child either can or cannot access the word for production. However, identifying why a child is having pronunciation errors when naming can only be achieved by comparing performance across speech tasks, as we did in Activity 2.3 (see Key 2.3), as words can be mispronounced for both T-D (e.g. inaccurate motor programs) and B-U reasons (e.g. oral structure abnormalities).

Level H

Although the sets of tasks at levels G and H are very close to each other, the levels are distinct for two reasons. First, in contrast to naming, the targets for the tasks at level H are provided by the tester. Second, it was argued in Chapter 3 that the ability to perform onset/coda production, spoonerisms and rhyme production tasks is not totally reliant on the child's representations. The tasks at level H are therefore *double level* tasks: (a) higher, because stored representations facilitate performance; plus (b) lower, because a more mechanical operation is also possible. For example, mechanically filling the onset slot with letters of the alphabet in order to produce a rhyme string to a given target CAT does not require the child to access their lexical representations. The result of using this strategy in isolation from the representations will be a rhyme string of nonword responses, as in "dat, lat, tat" with real words, e.g. "fat, sat", occurring by chance as different onsets are randomly chosen. On the other hand, if rhyme production is performed via the representations (i.e. by only producing previously stored words that are connected in terms of their rhyme) then only real words will be produced ("hat, mat, sat, fat"). The string will therefore be limited by the child's vocabulary development and knowledge of rhyming words. Young children, as well as older children with serious speech and literacy problems, may encounter difficulties at both of these levels: they are unable to perform the lower level mechanical operations, but at the same time their lexicon is not yet organized along phonological lines which allow connections between rhyming words to be made. The resulting attempted rhyme string may consist of real words only, often connected semantically rather than in terms of their phonological structure, e.g. CAT: dog, mouse, fish. Children who have difficulties with making semantic connections, for example some children with autism, may be able to produce a rhyme string perfectly well. Children who do not understand the task, as in the case of very young children or older children with pervasive language problems or learning difficulties may produce a random string of unrelated or idiosyncratically related words. These different possibilities illustrate the importance of a qualitative analysis of the child's responses to tasks: how the child responds can give insight into the strategy adopted, and thus into the processing level(s) they were (or were not) drawing on to perform the task.

While rhyme production could be carried out entirely successfully at a lower level, it remains as high as level H because it is more efficient if the child makes use of stored lexical knowledge about rhyming words and can access a ready-made rhyme string. Indeed, normally-developing children appear to make good use of both strategies and produce both real and nonwords in their rhyme strings (Vance, Stackhouse and Wells, 1994).

The coda production task is placed at level H because, in the same way as rhyme production, it can be performed directly from a stored network of representations organized appropriately. Alternatively, as with rhyme production, use can be made of a more mechanical slot filling routine. Onset production tasks could also be placed at this level and are normally easier than coda production tasks. This is because the onset task (like rhyme production) taps into the primary division of the syllable into onset and rhyme, whereas the coda task requires segmentation within the rhyme itself (Bradley, 1984; Treiman, 1993).

The possibility that the spoonerism task might be performed at different levels was discussed in Chapter 3. One can draw on stored orthographic knowledge, i.e. of the spelling of the two words presented. Alternatively, the stimuli can be processed without accessing lexical knowledge – at level I or level J depending on whether real words or nonwords are used as test items. Even if an orthographic representation is used to hold the two stimulus words, a mechanical transposition of the onsets still needs to be carried out so that the answer can then be 'read' back. If nonwords are presented, the orthographic representations can be assembled in a temporary orthographic loop while the second phase of the process is carried out. This obviously requires the alphabetic literacy skills necessary to assemble new words – skills which are not always available to children with speech and literacy problems. The alternative strategy available to the child is to hold the items in working memory, where they are maintained by oral rehearsal while the onsets are transposed and the spoken response is produced. This requires good auditory decoding and consistent speech output. By examining the spoonerism task in these ways it becomes clear why children with speech and literacy difficulties may find spoonerisms challenging – their inherent processing weaknesses affect the efficiency of both the orthographic and verbal strategies normally used.

The spoonerism task also demonstrates the importance of flexibility when interpreting the performance of individual children. Although the task (when real words are used) is located at level H for general classification purposes, one child might perform it completely at a high level via the orthographic representations, but another child at a lower level, i.e. without any recourse to representations. Locating the task at level H reminds us that performance on the spoonerism task does not have to depend on representations.

It seems then that normally-developing children (and adults) can use more than one strategy when carrying out the various segmentation tasks listed at level H. This may not be the case for all children with speech and literacy problems. The way the child tackles the tasks and the type of errors they make will reveal what strategy the child is using. These tasks are placed high on the output side because efficient performance is based on the conjunction of lexical skills with lower level verbal rehearsal skills.

Level I

Although blending a real word from its segments might seem similar to the tasks at level H, it was argued in Chapter 3 that it could be achieved without any recourse to the representations, i.e. the child does not have to know the meaning of the target in order to be able to produce it. Very often, the child does not realize that the target is a real word until s/he has spoken it. Further, in contrast to the other segmentation tasks at level H, the child does not have to generate new words, but merely to synthesize what is spoken by the tester. In this sense, blending has more in common with word repetition than with the tasks at level H, and so is properly located at level I. It is placed at the top of set of tasks at level I because of the processing load involved in synthesizing the word's phonological constituents in order to produce it, rather than just repeating a word.

Tasks at level I all have in common that they can be supported via the representations, but they do not have to be. (This is also true of the corresponding tasks on the input side at level D.) It was argued in Chapter 2 that sentence repetition and word repetition involve a similar level of processing, as they do not necessarily require access to linguistic knowledge. In sentence repetition, the child does not have to process the utterance grammatically in order to repeat it even though s/he may be assisted by doing so. Sentence repetition does, however, involve an increased memory load for the child, and so is placed above word repetition in the hierarchy of task difficulty.

Level J

Blending nonwords presented auditorily and repeating nonwords spoken by the tester need not involve T-D processing. They are therefore placed at level J. However, normally-developing children may be able to make use of output skills developed for similar sounding real words, and therefore by analogy have a head start on this task (Dollaghan, Biber and Campbell, 1995). For example, if there is already a motor program for the rhyme AT (as in CAT) it can be used to assemble the new word TAT. Some children may produce a similar sounding real word (e.g. CAT) instead of repeating the nonword TAT. They are using T-D processing to help them with this task but without completing the segmentation operation successfully, i.e. they identify that the word TAT sounds like a familiar word but do not change the onset. This type of error is known as a *lexicalization.* It can occur as a result of input difficulties, i.e. when the child believes that the tester produced a real rather than a nonword; or as a result of output difficulties, i.e. when in spite of perceiving the target as different from a similarly sounding real word, the child cannot produce the new motor program for that word.

A higher than average lexicalization response on nonword repetition tasks may therefore be indicative of auditory lexical processing problems. The child described by Stackhouse (1993) is a good example. Michael was an 11-year-old boy with developmental verbal dyspraxia and phonological dyslexia (see Chapter 1 for a discussion of these terms). Compared to a group of matched normal controls, Michael produced significantly more real words than nonwords on a nonword repetition test, e.g. SLEPPER → "slipper", and DACKS → "ducks". Out of the 30 items used on the test (from Stackhouse, 1989), the normal controls lexicalized on only 1.6 of the items (range 1–3). In contrast, Michael lexicalized on seven of the items. Further testing revealed that Michael had specific auditory processing difficulties. Auditory lexical difficulties were confirmed by his performance on input tasks. He was unable to detect nonwords embedded in a list of real words e.g. DISH, NIGHT, COAL, /brəʊl/ LADY, BOIL, /wɒɪl/. He accepted all nonwords as real words and went on to define them with confidence, e.g. for YITE he pointed to the *light* in the room, for TEED he gestured drinking a cup of *tea* and for HANE he touched his own *hair*. It was therefore not surprising that he performed less well than normal controls on complex nonword auditory discrimination. Fuzzy representations for lexical items meant that he was less able than controls to discriminate between similar sounding words.

Note here the use of normal controls. Even in normally-developing children some nonwords may be more readily lexicalized than others ; the general rule being the closer the nonword is to a real word the more likely the real word will be triggered. Lexicalization can therefore only be used as a diagnostic measure if information about normal controls is available. This is particularly important for identifying children with subtle auditory processing problems. Children with severe problems are likely to stand out by producing an obvious amount of lexicalizations in a test situation. Where norms are not available, clinical intuition has to suffice but this alone may not be sufficient to diagnose specific processing difficulties (Stackhouse and Wells, 1996; see Vance, 1996b, for further discussion of the importance of normal controls for auditory discrimination and speech tests).

Level K

Finally, syllable repetition and oral examination have been grouped together since they require no prior linguistic knowledge. They are therefore placed at the point nearest the mouth – level K. This corresponds to the nonlinguistic input task (discriminating between noises) at level A. Syllable repetition is placed above oral examination since it involves verbal production by the child, while structural examination does not.

We have now classified a collection of tests into sets on the basis of commonality of processing demands. Figure 4.3 shows the distribution of these sets of tests on both the input and output sides of the model. The next step is to identify what each set of tasks tells us about a child's processing skills.

ACTIVITY 4.3

Aim: To identify questions about a child's processing skills that need to be answered when investigating children with speech and literacy difficulties.

Each of the following 10 questions relates to a different level of processing. Select the question from the list below that corresponds to each of levels A–K in Figure 4.3. Write in the left column (under *Letter)* the letter of the level that corresponds to each question. You may find some questions easier to match to tasks than others. The less obvious ones include 2, 3, 8 and 9, where phonological representations and phonological units or constituents are implicated. When tackling this Activity, you may find it helpful to refer back to the analysis of tasks in Chapters 2 and 3, as well as to the earlier part of this chapter where you clustered groups of tests at the different levels (see Activities 4.1. and 4.2).

Letter

(1) Does the child have adequate sound production skills?
(2) Are the child's phonological representations accurate?
(3) Can the child manipulate phonological units?
(4) Can the child articulate speech without reference to lexical representations?
(5) Does the child have adequate auditory perception?
(6) Can the child discriminate between real words?
(7) Can the child articulate real words accurately?
(8) Can the child access accurate motor programs?
(9) Is the child aware of the internal structure of phonological representations?
(10) Can the child discriminate speech sounds without reference to lexical representations?

Check your response with Key to Activity 4.3 at the end of this chapter, then read the following.

Question 1 – Does the child have adequate sound production skills?

This refers to the bottom right of the model – level K. It asks if the child is capable of producing sounds and is not concerned about the meaningful context in which these sounds might occur. It is a fundamental question to address when dealing with any child with a speech difficulty. Some children will have obvious problems here, e.g. in the cases of structural abnormality or cerebral palsy, while other children may have more subtle oral motor difficulties, as in the case of developmental verbal dyspraxia or phonological impairments. Question 1 is answered by the set of tests at level K which examine the child's oral structure and function including the ability to produce sounds and sound sequences.

Question 2 – Are the child's phonological representations accurate?

This is answered by the tests clustering at level E on the input side and near (but not at) the top of the model. These auditory lexical decision tests involve discriminating pictures of minimal pair words or detecting the tester's accurate and inaccurate pronunciations of a target picture.

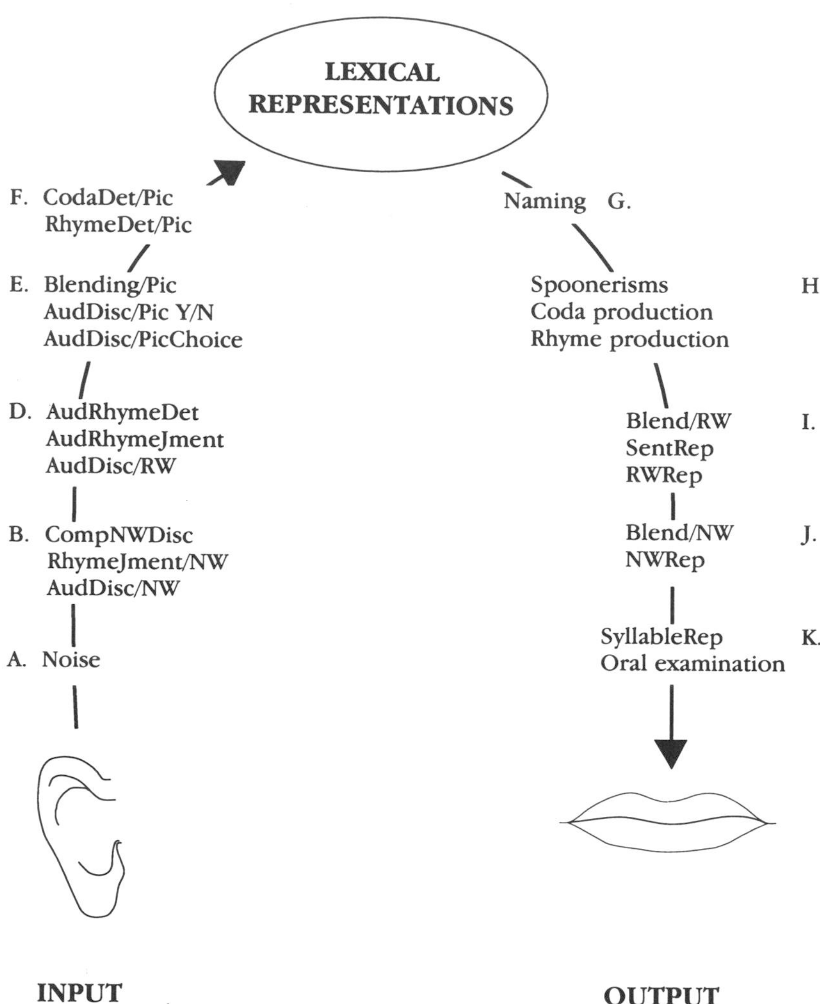

Figure 4.3: Classification of tests along the top/bottom and input/output dimensions of the simple speech processing model

The tests do not require the child to have any awareness of the constituents of phonological representations (as is required at level F – the top left-hand side of the model), but merely that the representations should be sufficiently specific to enable accurate word recognition.

Question 3 – Can the child manipulate phonological units?

This question is answered by the set of phonological awareness output tasks that cluster at level H. Each one of these tests (e.g. rhyme production, onset/coda production, and perhaps most obviously spoonerisms) involves the child in changing the targets given and then producing new words which incorporate these changes.

Question 4 – Can the child articulate speech without reference to lexical representations?

This refers to the child's ability to produce (and therefore this question must be on the output side of the model) nonwords (or new words) for which there are no lexical representations. It is answered by the nonword production tests clustering at level J.

Question 5 – Does the child have adequate auditory perception?

This refers to the bottom left of the model. Like question 1 (level K) above it is a fundamental question to ask about a child with speech difficulties, (e.g. are the difficulties related to a hearing impairment?). The routine test to be administered here would be a test of hearing threshold, e.g. through audiometry. Other tests discussed included discriminating environmental noises or other nonspeech sounds.

Question 6 – Can the child discriminate between real words?

This is typically answered by auditorily presented (i.e. spoken and without pictures) minimal pair auditory discrimination tasks (e.g. PIN~BIN) such as those in the set at level D. It is important to note that we have included rhyme judgement and rhyme detection tasks at this level too. Within our framework we do not sort tests on the basis of what they are called in their titles. Rather, we have analysed—through the activities so far—what processing levels the tests are tapping regardless of what they are called.

Question 7 – Can the child articulate real words accurately?

This clearly involves production and is therefore located on the right-hand side of the model. Because real words are specifically referred to, this question relates to a higher level than question (4) above, which involved nonwords (level J). Real word repetition would be the obvious test to answer this question since it examines articulation of real words specifically and does not make other demands on the child such as having to access the word for themselves as in naming or spontaneous speech. Question 7 therefore relates to the tests at level I.

Question 8 – Can the child access accurate motor programs?

This is located at the top right-hand side of the model since it refers to output and to accessing information stored in the lexical representations. When answering this question it is helpful first to consider if the child can access motor programs at all, and then to consider if the child can access *accurate* motor programs. Naming tests would be central in answering both parts of question 8. When analysing naming responses, it is important to differentiate between the children who cannot access the name of the picture and children who can access the name but who have difficulties pronouncing the name, e.g. "nocunars" [ˈnɒkjənəz] for BINOCULARS. Naming tests can be divided into two types. The first scores the child's ability to label pictures. An example of such a test is the *Word Finding Vocabulary Scales* (Renfrew, 1972) which clearly states in the instructions: 'Ignore articulation errors. Treat as correct for example, 'shoo' for 'screw'. But do not score as correct unless you are certain he is aiming at the right word'. If the child does not label the picture, s/he is encouraged to define the picture so that 'Don't Know Name' and 'Don't Know Picture' scores can be calculated. At no point does the tester provide the label of the picture for the child. In contrast, the second type of naming test is specifically concerned with how a child pronounces a word. An example of this type is the *Edinburgh Articulation Test* (Anthony, Bogle, Ingram, *et al.*, 1971) which accepts imitation of target words as a scorable response if the child does not spontaneously label the picture.

However, results from naming tests alone would not enable you to answer the second part of question 8, i.e. about the accuracy of the motor programs. This can only be answered by excluding other reasons for the child's speech errors since a number of other levels may affect the accuracy of a child's naming performance. For example, lower level speech output difficulties will affect how a child produces a word on a naming test, e.g. at level K. Further, the motor program may be inaccurate and based on a faulty phonological representation arising from input processing difficulties, e.g. at level E. This raises an important issue about this assessment framework. The questions set are best answered by comparing a child's performance across a range of tasks and can rarely be answered by a single test in isolation. This will be developed later in this chapter in the section Answering the Questions.

Question 9 – Is the child aware of the internal structure of phonological representations?

This is located at the top left-hand side of the model since it refers to information stored in the child's own lexical representations but does not require the child to produce a verbal response; only to be 'aware'. This awareness can be shown through nonverbal response such as gesture or picture pointing and is tested by the set of tasks at level F.

Question 10 – Can the child discriminate speech sounds without reference to lexical representations?

This is another input question since it refers to discrimination but not production. Unlike the question at level D, however, which asks about the child's ability to discriminate between real words, question 10 implies the use of nonwords (or new words) which have no lexical representation for the child to draw on. This question must therefore be located below level D – at level B (remember that we have left out level C in this activity).

The assessment framework is now organized on the basis of 10 different levels: A–K (but excluding C). A is equivalent to the ear on our basic speech processing model (see Figure 4.3) and K equivalent to the mouth. F and G are closest to the lexical representations at the top of the model. A question has been posed about each of these 10 levels in Activity 4.3. We can now re-order the questions from this activity giving each one its letter for reference as follows:

Input questions from top to bottom

F. Is the child aware of the internal structure of phonological representations?
E. Are the child's phonological representations accurate?
D. Can the child discriminate between real words?
B. Can the child discriminate speech sounds without reference to lexical representations?
A. Does the child have adequate auditory perception?

Output questions from top to bottom

G. Can the child access accurate motor programs?
H. Can the child manipulate phonological units?
I. Can the child articulate real words accurately?
J. Can the child articulate speech without reference to lexical representations?
K. Does the child have adequate sound production skills?

At each level, we have discussed examples of tests which tap that level and which will help to answer the question set. The tests have been chosen to illustrate the processing demands of each level and do not constitute an exhaustive list. The framework is not intended to have finite boundaries, and there are many more tests that can be incorporated into it which have not been mentioned. The framework thus provides a structure into which you can slot new assessments – published materials or ones you have designed for your own use. However, in order to incorporate new materials into the framework you may want to check that you have understood the principles that determine where a task is to be placed.

ACTIVITY 4.4

Aim: To check your understanding of the rationale behind the framework design.

With reference to Figure 4.2, where would you place these tests? You may find it helpful to look at the questions which go with each level. In the left hand column (under *Letter*), write the letter of the level at which you would place each of the following tests:

Letter

(1) The child is asked to repeat a word spoken by the tester three times as quickly as possible, e.g. CATERPILLAR.

(2) The child is presented with two pictures, e.g. GOAT and COAT. The tester inserts the target word into four spoken sentences. The child points to the picture of the word s/he hears in each sentence, (from Cassidy's, 1994 test of auditory discrimination in context), for example:

I like the COAT with long fur.
I like the GOAT with long fur.
Mum put her COAT in the cupboard.
Mum put her GOAT in the cupboard.

(3) Child looks at a picture, e.g. a FISH, but the tester does not name it. Child is asked to produce what the tester misses out when s/he produces the name of the picture, e.g. tester says "FI". The child should answer "sh" (from Stuart and Coltheart, 1988 and Muter, Snowling and Taylor, 1994).

(4) Child is presented with two puppets. The tester says "This puppet says BRISH. This puppet says BRIS. Which puppet said BRIS?". Child has to point to the appropriate puppet (from Vance, 1996a).

(5) The tester times how long it takes for a child to repeat the syllable sequence [pə tə kə], and compares this time with the norms for chronological age 6–13 years (from the *Time-by-Count Test of Diadochokinetic Syllable Rate*, Fletcher, 1978).

(6) The child is asked to produce as many words as they can that begin with /k/ (e.g. alliteration fluency subtest from the *Phonological Assessment Battery – PhAB*, Frederikson, 1995).

Check your responses with Key to Activity 4.4 at the end of this chapter, then read the following.

- early development of language skills in young normally-developing monolingual children,
- the language skills of multilingual speaking children with and without speech and language difficulties,
- auditory processing skills in children with specific and serious speech and language difficulties, e.g. children with acquired language disorder or persisting speech disorder.

The second and last question to address is a routine assessment, and relates to *output* skills.

Does the child reject his/her own erroneous forms?

ACTIVITY 4.5

Reflect for a moment on how you would answer the question above? Write down how you would assess this.
Now read the following.

One approach to addressing this question has been to play back the child's speech error for them to identify if their production was correct or not (Dodd, 1975; Locke, 1980a, b; Constable, Stackhouse and Wells, in press). For example, if the child is producing [p] for [f], the tester may show the child a picture of a FISH and ask "Is this a pish?", "Is this a fish?" This is an important procedure to follow but you will recognize that it has been classified as an input task at level E (auditory lexical tasks). There seems to be no equivalent output *test* for this last question since it requires an online measure. It can however be *assessed* by observing if children are uncomfortable about their output, i.e. they show signs of recognizing that what was said was not what was intended. This may be evident when a child rejects a spoken response as soon as it has been produced and then attempts to self-correct. This groping for a word can result from word-finding difficulties. Constable, Stackhouse and Wells (in press) described Michael aged 7;3 who produced the following for a picture of a MOUSTACHE: ['bɪjəʔ 'stɑʃ bʌ 'stɑʃ 'bɪjə 'bɪjəd 'stɑʃ 'stɑs bʌ'stɑs]. Here we can see that the word BEARD has also been activated and is interfering with his production of MOUSTACHE. Compare this with the following repeated attempts to articulate the word TREASURE by Caroline, a girl aged 11;9 with verbal dyspraxia : [s st 'stɛɾə 'stɛvə 'ʤɛvə 'stɛɪə 'ʤɛlɪʃ 'ʤɛdə] (from Stackhouse and Snowling, 1992b, see also Chapter 8 of this volume).

These examples illustrate the importance of a qualitative analysis of errors for revealing levels of difficulty encountered by the child. The groping for targets in an attempt to improve productions suggests that the child is not happy with what they have produced and therefore has self-monitoring skill. The type of errors produced can indicate the level of difficulty. In Michael's case, there was interference from two semantically related lexical items in his vocabulary, leading to word-finding difficulties. This was therefore a T-D problem. Caroline, on the other hand, had specific speech programming and articulatory (production) difficulties which suggested a B-U problem.

However, groping for targets is not always a sign of specific difficulties. Normally developing preschool children will try to correct their speech errors in this way and repeated attempts at a word should not necessarily be viewed negatively (see Chapter 7). Indeed, increased groping for words may result from therapy or teaching techniques aimed at increasing a child's awareness of a mismatch between their intention and their production. Unfortunately, however, unlike the normally developing child, the child with speech or lexical difficulties may not have the skills to make the necessary articulatory changes. Thus, instead of repeated attempts getting closer to the target, as happens in normal development, the attempts remain imprecise and sometimes get further away from the target. It is essential, therefore, that awareness training is coupled with work on speech production skills.

ACTIVITY 4.6

Aim: To place these last two questions in the assessment framework.

With reference to Figure 4.2, put two further crosses to mark the spot for these last two questions.

Write down in the following blank spaces the letters of the levels on either side of your new crosses.

Does the child have language specific representations of word structures?

goes between question letters —— and ——.

Does the child reject his/her own erroneous forms?

goes between letters —— and ——.

Check your response with Key to Activity 4.6 at the end of this chapter, then read the following.

The first question – *Does the child have language-specific representations?* becomes question C – the level omitted from Activity 4.1. It goes on the left-hand side of the model because it is answered through administering input tasks. It is placed above question B (*Can the child discriminate speech sounds without reference to lexical representations?*) because it involves accessing knowledge of language structure and cannot be performed as an auditory discrimination task comprising nonwords. It is placed below D (*Can the child discriminate between real words?*) because it involves nonword material.

The second question is a bit more tricky. You may have found that you wanted to put it in a number of places and were not fully convinced that it fitted with the other output tasks discussed. Strictly speaking, as the child is producing a spoken response, this question should go on the output side of the model. However, as the task used to answer this question is to observe how the child does or does not use self-monitoring skills to correct his/her speech errors, then it also involves input skills. Unlike the other tasks placed on the input side (particularly at B–E), however, these input skills involve *intra* auditory feedback (i.e. the child listening to his/her own speech) rather than *inter* auditory feedback (i.e. between speakers – the child listening to the tester's speech). The best place to put this question is therefore in a central position – between K and A – to mark a feedback loop between the output and input sides of the framework. It then becomes question L.

The assessment framework structure is now complete and is presented in Figure 4.4. Each question, referred to by a letter (A–L), marks a level on the simple speech processing model that we introduced in Chapter 1 and have used in the activities (see Figure 4.2). You can draw an ear by question A, a mouth by question K and an ellipse at the top centre of the framework to remind you of this. Remember also the two dimensions of this question framework: bottom-top and input-output (see Figure 4.1). In the activities in Chapters 2 and 3 you classified a number of tests along these dimensions. Appendix 2 lists a selection of popular procedures under the appropriate questions for easy reference. An attempt has been made to list tests underneath each question according to presumed degree of complexity. In general, the tests nearest the bottom of the list for each question are easier and therefore can be used with younger children, while those at the top are more suitable for older children.

It is not necessary or desirable to administer all of the tests to every child with speech and literacy problems. Neither is it necessary to assess every level, for example we do not do tasks at level C as a matter of routine. Tests should be selected that are the most appropriate for the child and in order to answer the questions relevant to that child.

INPUT	OUTPUT
F. Is the child aware of the internal structure of phonological representations?	G. Can the child access accurate motor programs?
E. Are the child's phonological representations accurate?	H. Can the child manipulate phonological units?
D. Can the child discriminate between real words?	I. Can the child articulate real words accurately?
C. Does the child have language-specific representations of word structures?	
B. Can the child discriminate speech sounds without reference to lexical representations?	J. Can the child articulate speech without reference to lexical representations?
A. Does the child have adequate auditory perception?	K. Does the child have adequate sound production skills?

L. Does the child reject his/her own erroneous forms?

Figure 4.4: The assessment framework

ACTIVITY 4.7

Aim: To personalize the assessment framework

Read through Appendix 2.
Highlight tests that are particularly relevant to your work.
Insert under the appropriate question additional tests that you use regularly.
Add new tests as you come across them.

We cannot provide the answers for this activity as this is where you can adapt the framework for your personal use. You may find it helpful to discuss with colleagues where tests should be placed within this framework.

Answering the Questions

Answering each question about a child's speech processing strengths and weaknesses will normally involve more than administering a single test from one level in the framework. Few single tests are objective enough to answer a question directly. The exceptions may be the more peripheral tests of hearing and oral structure and function. For these, objective instrumental measures are available, for example on the input side: tympanometry examines the efficiency of the ear drum and audiometry establishes hearing thresholds; on the output side, cineradiography (moving X-ray of the mouth when speaking) and nasal endoscopy (observation of the back of the mouth via the nose using fibre optics) examines the functioning of the soft palate.

These objective measures contribute towards a medical diagnosis such as hearing impairment or incompetent palatopharyngeal sphincter. They do not, however, determine how well the child will function at other processing levels. For example, children with hearing impairment can perform satisfactorily on tests higher up on the framework, e.g. on rhyme tasks (Campbell and Wright, 1988). On the output side, there is not always a direct relationship between nonlinguistic oral movements and the child's speech intelligibility (Ozanne, 1995; Williams, 1996). Some children with poor oral movements are surprisingly intelligible when compared to children with better oral movements but less intelligible speech (Evans, 1994).

Problems at one level of the framework therefore do not necessarily predict failure at a level further on. It is also important to remember that although sets of tests at each level were analysed in terms of their complexity, the levels themselves are not hierarchically ordered in terms of difficulty. It does not follow that the lower the level the easier it will be for the child. In fact, higher level tasks can be *easier* because the child can draw on prior knowledge. For example, a child with lower level input processing problems who cannot detect differences between nonwords may do better on tasks tapping higher levels which involve semantic knowledge. The opposite is also true. A child with a semantic deficit may be able to perform lower level auditory tasks perfectly well but not tasks higher up on the framework. In other words, when dealing with children with speech, lexical and literacy problems, the degree of difficulty is not at the levels in the framework but within the individual child, i.e. their processing strengths and weaknesses will determine which level(s) of tasks they find easy or hard.

Identifying specific deficits in speech processing skills can only be achieved by contrasting results from different tests *within* and *between* levels. Testing *within* levels establishes if the child cannot perform a task at all even if test items are simple and memory load reduced vs whether the child can complete a task but not when complex items are used or memory load is increased. For example, a child may be able to perform well on an auditory discrimination task comprising simple similar sounding nonwords, e.g. WEP~WEK but not on a similar task comprising multisyllabic complex words, e.g. IBIKUS~IKIBUS. This suggests that s/he does not have an auditory discrimination problem *per se* but may have an auditory memory and/or sequencing problem. Similarly, a child who can perform a rhyme judgement task (e.g. do these two pictures rhyme? – yes or no) but not a rhyme detection task (e.g. which two words rhyme when given a choice of three) understands the concept of rhyme but may not be able to remember the three items while a decision is made about which two words rhyme. This is different from the child who cannot perform either rhyme judgement or detection tasks, which implies that s/he has not developed a concept of rhyme. When working with older children in particular it is important to administer more complex tests, as appropriate for their age, since performance may be at ceiling on the more simple tests and the true extent of their difficulties can be missed.

Testing *between* levels is part of the diagnostic process of identifying the child's processing strengths and weaknesses. We discussed some possible scenarios of between level performance on speech tasks following Activity 2.3 (and see Key 2.3). However, we can now use the complete framework to extend these scenarios as a means of investigating speech difficulties. Naming is a good illustration of how to do this. If the child has errors on a picture-naming task it is important to ascertain if these are related to inaccuracies in the lexical representations, problems with assembling the word for speech, articulatory difficulties which affect pronunciation or all or any combination of these. The following steps illustrate how you might arrive at an understanding of the child's naming difficulties but they do not have to be taken in any prescribed order:

(a) Comparing performance at levels I (repetition of real words) and J (repetition of nonwords) will provide information about the child's motor programming skills (see discussion of Activity 2.3).
(b) Results from tests at level K (oral structure and function) will establish if the child has articulatory difficulties.
(c) Comparing performance at level G (naming pictures) with performance at level E (playing the child's naming errors back to him/her for identification of 'right' or 'wrong') will establish if the child's representations are or are not fully specified.
(d) Examining performance on tasks from levels B (auditory discrimination of nonwords) and D (auditory discrimination of real words) will identify any auditory discrimination problems that might result in lexical representations being underspecified.
(e) Finally, observing the child's self-monitoring skills (level L) and attempts (or not) to correct their own productions will indicate awareness of the output errors.

A qualitative analysis of these self-corrections observed at level L will confirm the test results taken from the other levels. For example, perhaps the corrections suggest a T-D semantic interference from within the lexicon (as in the BEARD/MOUSTACHE example above) or perhaps they are indicative of lower level articulatory struggle (as in the TREASURE example above). Although some children can be clearly identified as having T-D vs B-U problems, children with severe speech difficulties are unlikely to have such discrete levels of difficulty. It is quite possible for both T-D and B-U speech difficulties to co-occur within the same child, with different error types arising from different levels within the speech processing system (see Stackhouse and Wells, 1993 and Chapter 9 of this volume).

Summary

The principles of the assessment framework discussed in this chapter are summarized in the following list.

The framework

- The framework comprises a systematic approach to the assessment of children with speech, lexical and literacy problems.
- The framework focuses on speech processing skills which underpin speech, lexical and literacy development and difficulties.
- The framework provides a basis for principled remediation of speech and literacy difficulties.
- The framework can be applied to children learning more than one language.

- The framework does not constitute a complete assessment package.
- Problems at one level in the framework do not necessarily predict failure at a level further on in the framework.
- Higher levels in the framework are not necessarily more difficult than lower levels – it will depend on children's individual processing strengths and weaknesses as to which levels will prove easy or hard for them.
- Levels on the left (input) are not necessarily easier than levels on the right (output) – it will depend on children's individual processing strengths and weaknesses as to whether input or output tasks are more difficult.
- Questions A – L do not in themselves constitute a procedure, since they need not be taken in a prescribed order.

Tests

- Tests are used in the framework to illustrate the processing demands at each level.
- Tests sharing common processing demands can be collected together.
- Tests can be classified along a continuum according to how much demand is made on prior linguistic knowledge.
- There can be more than one way of tackling some of the tests in processing terms.
- Some flexibility is needed when interpreting test results within the framework to account for individual differences in how that test is performed.
- Normally-developing children as well as children with speech, lexical and literacy difficulties will perform the same test in different ways depending on their processing strengths and weaknesses.
- There is a hierarchy of difficulty within a set of tests at a given level, but not between the levels themselves.
- A single test result in isolation from others will not answer a question about a child's speech processing capabilities.
- Tests results need to be compared within and between levels in order to answer questions about a child's speech processing skills.
- Not all tests need to be administered to every child. Tests will be selected on the basis of observations, linguistic and educational assessments and medical information.
- Other tests can be slotted into the structure to suit the needs of the testers and their client groups.
- The complexity of the test and the instructions given will depend on the age or developmental stage of the child.

KEY TO ACTIVITY 4.1

Classification of input tests within the simple speech processing model

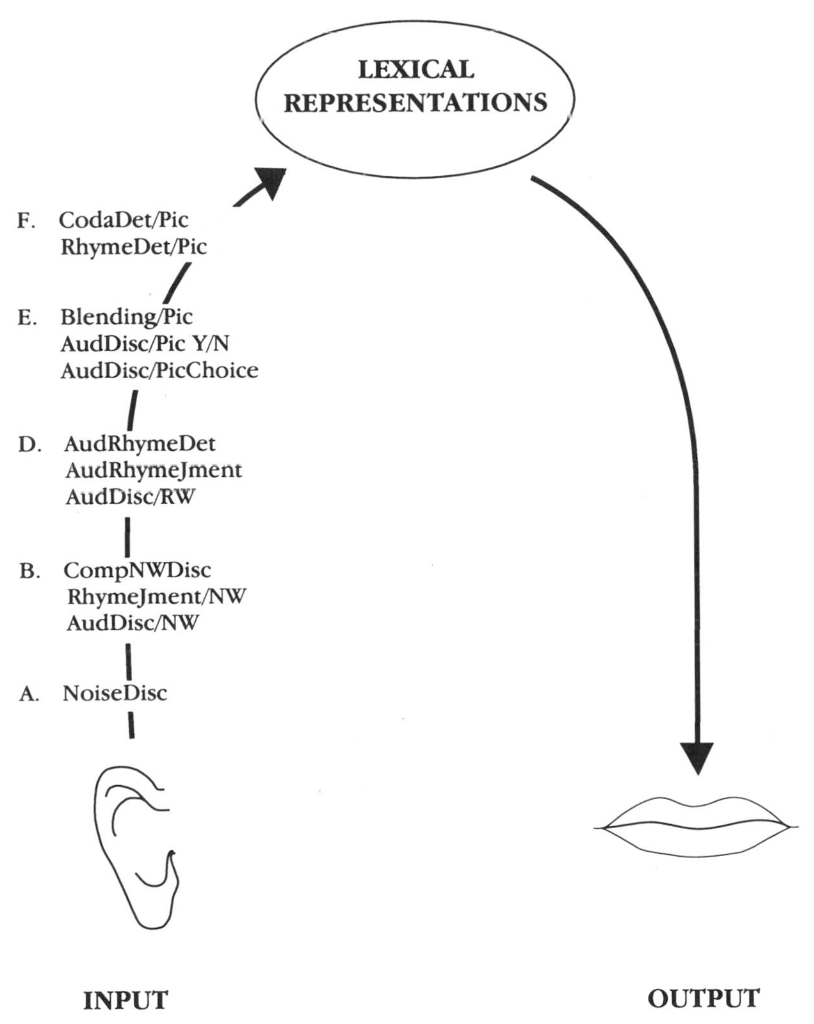

KEY TO ACTIVITY 4.2
Classification of output tests within the simple speech processing model

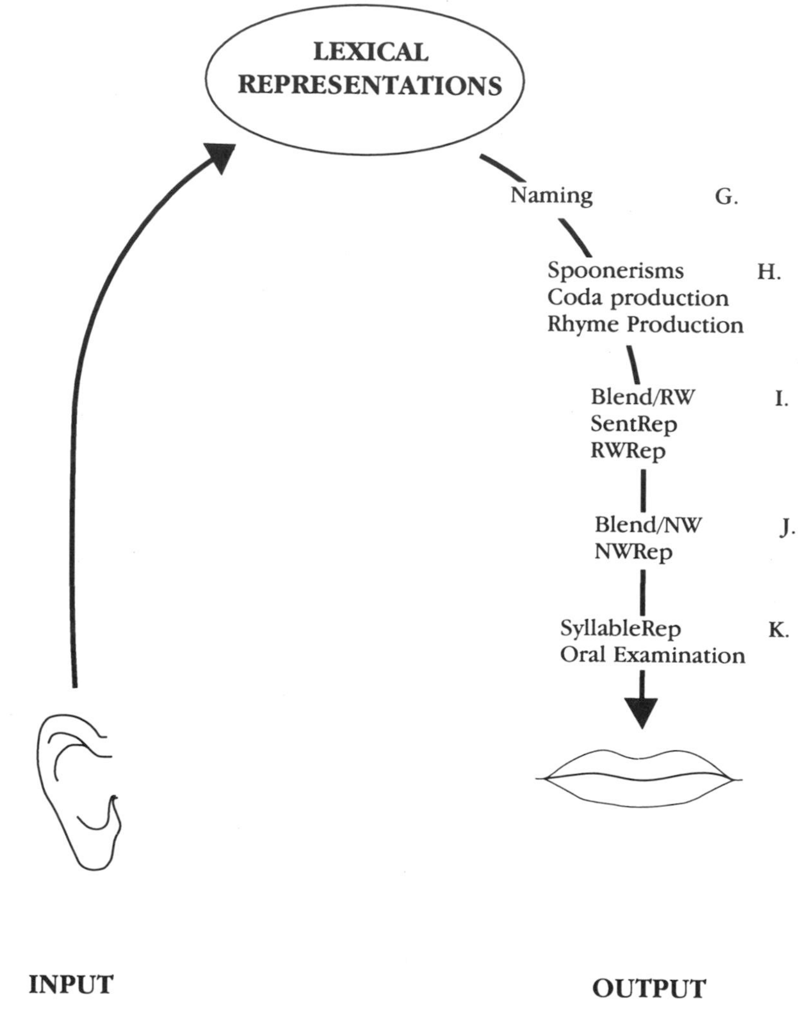

KEY TO ACTIVITY 4.3
Relating questions to levels on the speech processing model

Letter

K (1) Does the child have adequate sound production skills?

E (2) Are the child's phonological representations accurate?

H (3) Can the child manipulate phonological units?

J (4) Can the child articulate speech without reference to lexical representations?

A (5) Does the child have adequate auditory perception?

D (6) Can the child discriminate between real words?

I (7) Can the child articulate real words accurately?

G (8) Can the child access accurate motor programs?

F (9) Is the child aware of the internal structure of phonological representations?

B (10) Can the child discriminate speech sounds without reference to lexical representations?

KEY TO ACTIVITY 4.4
Classification of additional tests within the assessment framework

Letter

I (1) The child is asked to repeat a word spoken by the tester three times, as quickly as possible, e.g. CATERPILLAR.

E (2) The child is presented with two pictures, e.g. GOAT and COAT. The tester inserts the target word into four spoken sentences. The child points to the picture of the word s/he hears in each sentence, (from Cassidy's, 1994 test of auditory discrimination in context), for example:

I like the COAT with long fur.
I like the GOAT with long fur.
Mum put her COAT in the cupboard.
Mum put her GOAT in the cupboard.

G (3) Child looks at a picture, e.g. a FISH, but the tester does not name it. Child is asked to produce what the tester misses out when s/he produces the name of the picture, e.g. tester says "FI_". The child should answer "sh" [ʃ] (from Stuart and Coltheart, 1988 and Muter, Snowling and Taylor, 1994).

B (4) Child is presented with two puppets. The tester says "This puppet says BRISH. This puppet says BRIS. Which puppet said BRIS?". Child has to point to the appropriate puppet (from Vance, 1996a).

K (5) The tester times how long it takes for a child to repeat the syllables [pə tə kə] and compares this time with the norms for chronological age 6–13 years (from the *Time-by-Count Test of Diadochokinetic Syllable Rate*, Fletcher, 1978).

H (6) The child is asked to produce as many words as they can that begin with /k/ (e.g. alliteration fluency subtest from the *Phonological Assessment Battery - PhAB,* - Frederikson, 1995).

KEY TO ACTIVITY 4.6

Locating the last two questions in the framework within the speech processing model

Does the child have language specific representations of word structures?

This question is the missing C. It goes between question letters B and D.

Does the child reject his /her own erroneous forms?

This question is L and goes between letters K and A.

Chapter 5
Profiling Children's Speech Processing Skills

The purpose of collecting assessment information is to arrive at a greater understanding of a child's needs. However, the results of a test are limited in value if viewed in isolation. A bit of assessment information is like one piece of a jigsaw puzzle; it is therefore necessary to collate results from different procedures and tests in a systematic way. The aim of psycholinguistic profiling is to fit together all the pieces to form a picture of the child's strengths and weaknesses in terms of input, representation and output skills. On the basis of this profile a comprehensive individual remediation programme can be designed, which takes into account the nature of the child's processing difficulties. Without this, less obvious factors, such as subtle auditory processing deficits, can easily be overlooked, particularly when there appears to be a very obvious explanation for the child's speech problems. The presence of a structural tongue-tie is a good example of this since, contrary to what is often assumed, this may not be related to speech difficulties at all (Stackhouse, 1980). It is only by profiling the child's phonological processing skills that the true extent of the difficulties can be confirmed.

This chapter illustrates how to draw up a profile of a child's speech processing skills for the purposes of planning a remediation programme. A child's profile is constructed by providing answers to some or, ideally, all of the questions A–L from the assessment framework described in Chapter 4 (see Figure 4. 4). For the purpose of recording a child's speech processing skills, a profiling sheet has been devised based on these questions (see Figure 5.1). This profiling sheet comprises the questions A–L plus space for administrative information about the child (e.g. name, date of birth, age, date of profile and name of profiler) and for general comments.

The focus in this chapter is on two children of contrasting ages and presenting difficulties. Jenny is a 3-year-old girl from London, with obvious speech difficulties which might lead to her being seen by a speech and language therapist in a community clinic setting. Richard

SPEECH PROCESSING PROFILE

Name:

Age: d.o.b:

Date:

Profiler:

Comments:

INPUT

F Is the child aware of the internal structure of phonological representations?

E Are the child's phonological representations accurate?

D Can the child discriminate between real words?

C Does the child have language-specific representations of word structures?

B Can the child discriminate speech sounds without reference to lexical representations?

A Does the child have adequate auditory perception?

OUTPUT

G Can the child access accurate motor programs?

H Can the child manipulate phonological units?

I Can the child articulate real words accurately?

J Can the child articulate speech without reference to lexical representations?

K Does the child have adequate sound production skills?

L Does the child reject his/her own erroneous forms?

Figure 5.1: A Speech Processing Profile Sheet

is an 11-year-old boy from Manchester with specific reading and spelling difficulties (dyslexia), who had not been referred to a speech and language therapist before. These contrasting cases show how profiling can help to identify strengths and weaknesses in speech processing skills in very different kinds of children.

Jenny

Jenny started at a local nursery school when she was 3 years of age. She presented as a quiet and shy little girl. Jenny's mother was aware that people found Jenny difficult to understand but was satisfied that her speech was progressing. However, she had noted that Jenny's 2-year-old sister's speech appeared to be at a similar level. Jenny's hearing had been queried on routine screening at a local clinic. However, at 3;6 Jenny passed a repeat hearing test administered by the health visitor.

Jenny's speech difficulties could not be attributed to any serious abnormality of the oral structure. She had healthy dentition but with an open bite (this allowed her tongue to protrude centrally between the front top and bottom teeth even when her back teeth were closed together; this does not happen in a 'normal' bite) which may have accounted for some of her interdental (lisp) articulation. This in itself is not uncommon and does not normally lead to unintelligible speech. It can be difficult to assess oral function objectively around the age of 3 because of the wide range of normal variability (Williams, 1996). However, it was noted that when Jenny was asked to try and touch her nose with her tongue, she had difficulty elevating her tongue tip, particularly when concentrating on this activity. She also gave a very tense grimace when trying to copy a happy face expression and was not able to copy a sad face expression or blow out her cheeks at all. There were therefore some indications of oral-motor immaturity.

This was reflected in her problems with repeating individual speech sounds, which suggested articulatory immaturity. Although she repeated [p b t d k g m n f s z w] perfectly well, she had difficulty with the following sounds:

Target	*Response*
/v/	Obviously difficult Reluctant to produce this sound Finally produced [z]
th /θ/	[f]
the /ð/	[z]
sh /ʃ/	[ç]
zh /ʒ/	[ʑ]
ch /ʧ/	[ts]

j /ʤ/	[dz]
/r/	[w]
/l/	Obviously difficult Reluctant to produce this sound Finally produced [l] with exaggerated tongue protrusion
y /j/	[j] but very hesitant

Jenny appeared to have appropriate understanding and expressive vocabulary. Her intelligibility noticeably decreased in connected speech, which sounded jerky with wide pitch changes, giving an impression of immaturity. Jenny did not attempt to correct her speech errors at any time during this assessment.

Routine speech and language screening (CA 3;8)

Standardized assessments were used to screen Jenny's speech and language development at the age of 3;8. Table 5.1 summarizes these assessment results.

Jenny co-operated well with these routine test procedures. The results confirmed the observation that she had age-appropriate language comprehension skills and vocabulary development. She responded well to specific questions about pictures in the *Renfrew Action Picture Test* (Renfrew, 1989) for example (T: Tester, J: Jenny):

Picture: Girl hugging a golly

T What's this girl doing?
J hugging that black thing,

Picture: Girl fallen down stairs and broken her glasses

T What's happened to the girl?
J fell over
broken her glasses

Picture: Boy climbing up a ladder which is leaning against a house roof. On top of the roof is a cat

T Tell me what the boy is doing?
J going on a ladder
and catching a cat

In contrast, she had tremendous difficulty retelling the *Bus Story* (Renfrew, 1991) about the naughty bus who runs away from his driver. She was told the story with the picture book in front of her and then

Table 5.1: Results of Jenny's initial speech and language screening tests at CA 3;8

Test	AE	Score	Ranking
Input			
Verbal comprehension			
Reynell Developmental Language Scales	3;11	s.s. 0.2	—
Receptive vocabulary			
British Picture vocabulary Scales	3;8	s.s. 101	%ile 52
Auditory discrimination			
Auditory Discrimination and Attention Test*	<3;0	s.s. -1.7	—
Output			
Expressive language			
Renfrew Action Picture Test			
Information	4;0	—	—
Grammar	3;6	—	—
Renfrew Bus Story*			
Information	<3;0	Raw score: 3, off scale (Range for CA: 3;0 = 11-19, mean=15)	
Mean length of utterance	<3;0	Raw score: 3, off scale (Range for CA: 3;0 = 5-7, mean=6)	
Expressive vocabulary			
Renfrew Word Finding Vocabulary Scale	4;00	—	—
Speech			
Edinburgh Articulation Test*	<3;0	s.s. 87	—

AE = Age equivalent; s.s. = standard score; %ile = percentile rank.
* Tests where Jenny performed below age appropriate.

was asked to tell it back to the tester with the help of the pictures. She responded as follows:

> (Began story where the bus runs away with a gasp and facial expression of 'oh, no' but there was no vocalization)

"train
bus
bus
jump over there
policeman (J demonstrated blowing the whistle)
bus
over there
and jump over fence
push in the mud"

Jenny's mother was not surprised at this restricted version of this story. She had observed that Jenny did not seem to be able to remember stories from even quite familiar books.

Jenny performed at the lower end of normal limits on the *Edinburgh Articulation Test* (Anthony, Bogle, Ingram, et al., 1971), which is a test of articulatory maturity (standard score 87; normal range: 85–115). As this test uses single word naming (from pictures of e.g. MONKEY, ELEPHANT, CHIMNEY, TOOTHBRUSH) it did not capture her difficulties with connected speech.

Similarly, her performance on discriminating minimal pair words with pictures (e.g. FAN/VAN, TEA/KEY, GRASS/GLASS) on the *Auditory Discrimination and Attention Test* (MorganBarry, 1989) was of some concern (standard score: -1.7). As she was performing at the lower end of average on both auditory discrimination and speech and clearly had associated expressive language difficulties, further investigation was indicated.

Before we examine these further investigations, we can summarize what we know about Jenny so far.

ACTIVITY 5.1

Aim: To profile Jenny's speech processing skills on the basis of routine assessment results.

First, decide which questions on Figure 5.1 have been addressed by the procedures and tests already reported. Now answer each question with reference to Jenny's performance on these tasks. Put a tick under each question where the answer is 'yes' and a cross under each question where the answer is 'no'. Use a red pen for crosses and a blue pen for ticks. The use of colour highlights the child's strengths and weaknesses at a glance.

Where possible, answer the questions on the basis of standard scores or age equivalent measures. Sometimes, however, your answers will be based on observation only. Put a question mark (?) if you have a specific query about how to answer a particular question or where her performance is borderline. You can add any notes you wish under the questions that will help you to remember key points about Jenny's performance and jot down any general points under 'Comments' at the top of the sheet.

Check your response with Key to Activity 5.1 at the end of this chapter, then read the following.

We can put a tick under question A because Jenny has recently passed a routine hearing test, though you may want to monitor this, given her history. No tests have been administered as yet to answer questions B, C, D, or F on the input side. Jenny's performance of standard score -1.7, however, on the *Auditory Discrimination and Attention Test* (MorganBarry, 1989) should lead you to putting a cross under question E (see the discussion of Activity 2.1 in Chapter 2, about tests of auditory discrimination with and without pictures, for a reminder of why this test answers question E and not question D).

On the output side, Jenny was administered two naming tests on which she performed differently. You should therefore have both a tick and a question mark (or maybe you put a tick and a cross) under question G. On the *Word-Finding Vocabulary Scale* (Renfrew, 1972) Jenny performed slightly above age appropriate (AE of 4;0 at CA 3;8). She therefore gets a tick when she is compared with her chronological age group on *supplying* the names of pictures and does not appear to have any word-finding difficulties at this point in her development. In contrast, on the *Edinburgh Articulation Test* (Anthony, Bogle, Ingram, et al., 1971) where she is being compared to her chronological age group on her *accuracy of pronouncing* the names of the pictures, she does less well. On this articulation test she performs below age appropriate (< CA 3) and therefore you may have been tempted to put a cross. Strictly speaking, as she is at the lower end of the 'within normal limits' range for her age in terms of her standard score (standard score. 87, range: 85–115), she should not be given a cross for this performance. However, given her unintelligibility in conversation it would be unwise to put a tick here on the basis of one test of single word production. We have therefore put a question mark at G to remind us that her speech needs further investigation.

No tests have yet been administered to help us to answer questions H–J on the output side, but we can put a cross under question K because of her difficulties with copying nonverbal movements (such as facial expressions) and individual speech sounds. Finally, because we have noted that Jenny does not attempt to correct her speech errors on the naming tests or in conversation, we can also put a cross under question L.

Preliminary psycholinguistic information about Jenny's speech and language development has been gathered at CA 3;8 from this routine battery of assessments. She has age-appropriate: vocabulary development (see *British Picture Vocabulary Scales* and *Renfrew Word-Finding Vocabulary Scales*); verbal comprehension (*Reynell Developmental Language Scales*); and grammatical expression in a structured context (see *Renfrew Action Picture Test)*. However, her expressive language problems are more apparent when sequencing a story (see *Bus Story*) and her memory for verbal information may be reduced.

On the input side of the speech processing profile, there is no hearing impairment to explain her difficulties but auditory discrimination problems which may be affecting her lexical representations (E) are present. On the output side, Jenny's speech difficulties are not related to word-finding difficulties but do increase in connected speech (G). In part her speech difficulties can be accounted for by lower level articulatory difficulties (K) and an additional problem is her lack of self-monitoring of her speech output (L).

Activity 5.1 has shown that any test designed to investigate a child's speech and language development can give psycholinguistic information if the results are interpreted within the framework suggested. Although the framework focuses on children's *speech* processing skills, findings from tests specifically addressing *language* abilities are crucial when considering the overall picture of the child's strengths and weaknesses.

Investigations of Jenny's speech processing skills at CA 4;0

In order to follow up the preliminary findings, further tests were administered to Jenny around her fourth birthday. These were drawn from a series of test procedures designed to investigate the psycholinguistic processing skills that underlie speech and literacy development. Control data had been collected from normally-developing children in the age range of 3–7 years for comparison with children with speech and language difficulties (Vance, Stackhouse and Wells 1994, 1995; Vance, Donlan and Stackhouse, 1996).

Auditory discrimination

Jenny was asked to listen to pairs of real words (e.g. KIT/KIT, MISS/MIT, MITTS/MISSED) and nonwords (e.g. BIS/BIS, DIT/DIS, BLEIST/BLEITS) to judge if each pair was the same or different (after Bridgeman and Snowling, 1988). The mean score for 4-year-olds on this test was 18.33/24. Jenny's score of 13/24 (8/12 real word items correct, 5/12 nonword items correct) was significantly below this.

Baa Baa Black Sheep perfectly well (apart from speech production errors) when asked which rhyme she liked best. Jenny was also able to fill in missing gaps when the tester recited: *Twinkle Twinkle Little Star* (e.g. How I wonder what you ——); *Jack and Jill*; *Humpty Dumpty*; and *Incey Wincey Spider* showing that she had receptive knowledge of these rhymes. However, she would not attempt to recite them herself.

Rhyme judgement

Jenny was administered two rhyme judgement tasks comprising six practice items and 12 test items on each: one task was presented auditorily for her to say if two words rhymed or not (e.g. COT ~ KNOT; PLANE ~ FOOT) and the other was presented visually for her to say if two pictures rhymed or not (e.g. MOUSE ~ HOUSE; CHAIR ~ DUCK). It was clear from administering the practice items that there was little point in administering the test items. Jenny scored zero on both rhyme judgement tasks. In contrast, the mean performance of a group of 20 4-year-olds on these tasks was 8.6 correct out of 12 items with a standard deviation on both tests of 2.2 (Vance, Stackhouse and Wells, 1994).

Rhyme production

A similar situation arose on the rhyme production task where Jenny was asked to say as many rhyming words as she could in 20 seconds.with a given target, e.g. BOY. The 20 normally developing 4-year-olds who had also performed the rhyme judgement tasks above produced on average 6.7 (out of a total of 15 items) first responses correct to each target and had a mean total of rhyme responses of 13.5. Jenny again scored zero and was only given the practice items. When asked what rhymed with CHAIR, she replied "house"; with SPOT she replied "spot is pot is potty"; and with SPOON, she replied "eat with, boo".

ACTIVITY 5.3

Aim: To complete Jenny's speech processing profile.

On the profiling sheet presented in Figure 5.1, slot in the results of the above rhyme tests by answering the appropriate questions in the same way as you did for Activities 5.1 and 5.2.

Check your answer against Key to Activity 5.3 at the end of this chapter, then read the following.

We can now answer questions D and F on the input side of the profile and H on the output side. As Jenny scored zero on both of the rhyme judgement tests, we can conclude that she does not yet understand that a simple CVC word can be divided into onset and rhyme. As she was at 'floor' on this test, i.e. she could not do them, we have marked her performance as xxx on the profile (converting her zero score to a z-score will result in a $z = 0$ score which would be misleading). The three crosses at question D mark her poor performance on the auditorily presented rhyme judgement. We can compare this to her performance on the auditory discrimination of real words (after Bridgeman and Snowling, 1988) where she performed better than on the rhyme task but still had some problems (one cross). This result indicates that she understands the task of same/different judgement but is better at detecting differences between onsets than between rhymes which is a more difficult concept to understand.

Jenny's rhyme performance on the rhyme string production test answers question H. Clearly, she has a lot of difficulty producing rhyme. This may be because either she does not yet understand *what* to do or that she does not know *how* to do it. As most 4 year-olds are able to produce some rhyming words her performance of zero has been marked on the profile with three crosses. Her restricted nursery rhyme knowledge may be the most important indicator of a delay in rhyme skills since Jenny has been exposed to rhymes and songs both at home and at school.

We have now answered each question on the profile apart from C. We do not test legal and illegal word knowledge routinely in children like Jenny who are monolingual and who do not have serious auditory processing difficulties (see Chapter 4). For three of the questions (D, E and G) we adminstered two tests which allowed a comparison of tests to be made *within* the same level. For example, the comparison of real word auditory discrimination and real word rhyme judgement above (D); the comparison of the auditory lexical decision task and the *Auditory Discrimination and Attention Test* (MorganBarry) and the comparison of the naming tasks involved under question G (i.e. the *Renfrew Word-Finding Vocabulary Scales* and the *Edinburgh Articulation Test* – see Activity 5.1).

The completed profile is presented in Figure 5.2. It summarizes at a glance the findings of this initial assessment of Jenny's speech processing skills. We can see that her speech output difficulties are more severe than might be predicted from a routine articulation screening test (the *Edinburgh Articulation Test*). Although she can access stored motor programs and therefore does not have a word finding difficulty (see *Renfrew Word-Finding Vocabulary Scales*), her pronunciation of words on both naming and repetition tasks are below age appropriate. These pronunciation problems are not derived from one locus of difficulty. Jenny has auditory discrimination problems (B and D) even when words are familiar (D). Such problems on the input side are likely to interfere with the laying down of precise

SPEECH PROCESSING PROFILE

Name: Jenny

Age: 3;8–4;1 d.o.b:

Date:

Profiler:

Comments:

Receptive vocabulary and verbal comprehension within normal limits. Check expressive language, sequencing skills and connected speech.

INPUT

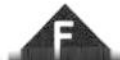

Is the child aware of the internal structure of phonological representations?

✗✗✗ (rhyme/pictures)

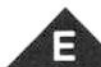

Are the child's phonological representations accurate?

✗ (ADAT) ✓ (aud. lex. dec)

Can the child discriminate between real words?

✗✗✗ (rhyme) ✗ (aud. disc)

Does the child have language-specific representations of word structures?

not tested

Can the child discriminate speech sounds without reference to lexical representations?

✗ (nonword aud. disc)

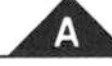

Does the child have adequate auditory perception?

✓ (hearing)

OUTPUT

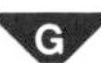

Can the child access accurate motor programs?

✓ (word finding)

✗✗✗ (naming – pronunciation) ? ✓ (EAT)

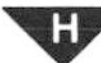

Can the child manipulate phonological units?

✗✗✗ (rhyme production)

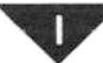

Can the child articulate real words accurately?

✗✗✗ (real word repetition)

Can the child articulate speech without reference to lexical representations?

✗✗✗ (nonword repetition)

Does the child have adequate sound production skills?

✗ (sound repetition)

L

Does the child reject his/her own erroneous forms?

✗ (No attempts to correct errors)

Figure 5.2: Jenny's completed profile.

phonological representations and indeed there is a query about her performance at E. Given that the phonological representations are the foundation for the assembly of stored motor programs it is not surprising that she had difficulties compared to her peer group on naming accuracy (at G) and real word repetition (at I). In addition to these T-D processing problems, there are also B-U difficulties. Her poor perform- ance on nonword repetition (at J) suggests difficulties with assembling new motor programs and her immature oral motor skills (at K) suggest lower level articulatory problems. In addition, the profile reveals that Jenny is not yet able to perform phonological awareness tasks involving reflecting on the structure of utterances as in the rhyme tests at D, F and H. A further lack of awareness is evident in her self-monitoring skills at L; she does not attempt to correct her own speech errors.

This initial psycholinguistic assessment of Jenny's speech difficult- ies comprised a number of familiar test procedures. It did not take long to administer yet yielded important information about the severity and pervasiveness of her speech difficulties. The indications are that Jenny is also at risk for literacy problems and that she would benefit from speech and language therapy not only to improve her intelligibility but also to help her prepare for starting school and literacy instruction.

Implications for Jenny's therapy

It is beyond the scope of this book to go into the detail of carrying out therapy within a psycholinguistic framework. However, it is clear from Jenny's profile that a number of areas need to be targeted in therapy. The following activities were suggested for her initial therapy programme and were discussed with Jenny's mother.

(1) Verbal memory and expressive language

Activities might include sequencing of pictures to make a story. Initially this would be a silent task to build up Jenny's confidence in sequencing her ideas. Jenny would listen to the therapist telling the story from the pictures and would then be asked questions about the story. To begin with, these questions would involve 'yes' or 'no' answers only, but gradually more expressive language demands would be made. Eventually Jenny would be asked to tell back the story from the pictures and specific grammatical structures would be targeted.

(2) Speech input

Listening to similarities and differences between familiar and unfamiliar words.

Activities would include some items on which she makes speech errors to link with her production work in (3). Initially pictures of the items would be included in the activities so that she can be supported by T-D processing skills. Two puppets would then be introduced, one of whom makes speech errors. Jenny has responded well to puppets in the past and would be encouraged to identify when one puppet said a target differently from the other. This provides a visual focus for an auditory discrimination game which once the picture stimuli are removed provides B-U auditory discrimination training. However, as many cues as necessary would be introduced to enhance her listening ability, e.g. symbols of different kinds (see (3)).

(3) Speech output

Sound production would be targeted through accompanying gestures from *Cued Articulation* (Passy, 1990a) and letter shapes (e.g. from *Letterland* which she will be using at school), and linked with (2) above. Help would be given with the sounds that she could not produce in isolation following traditional speech and language therapy techniques. Motor programming of sound sequences to produce new names for nonsense characters would only include sounds that she could produce with ease.

(4) Phonological awareness

Audio and video tapes of nursery rhymes would be introduced for increasing awareness of popular rhymes. Selected rhymes would be used to work on rhythm and gap filling tasks. Once Jenny was proficient at gap filling, identifying rhyming words through picture games would be introduced. Gradually *Letterland* characters (or plastic letters) plus *Cued Articulation* would be introduced with the pictures to demonstrate how to divide a word into its onset and rhyme. Rhyme production games would not be introduced until Jenny clearly demonstrated that she had understood the concept behind rhyming words.

We cannot be more specific about Jenny's therapy programme at this point because we have not included in this chapter on psycholinguistic profiling the full phonological analysis of her speech errors (see Grunwell, 1987; and Ingram, 1989 for guidelines on this). Without this phonological analysis of her speech errors we cannot list the precise stimuli for each of the above therapy areas. This highlights the complementary roles of the psycholinguistic and linguistic perspectives when planning therapy. The psycholinguistic profile will indicate the areas which should be targeted in therapy and how a child's strengths and weaknesses can be balanced in a therapy programme. However, it is the linguistic analysis which describes the child's speech and/or language problems which will determine which grammatical structures or lexical items or sounds will be used as targets in the therapy areas (cf. Chapter 9). For further therapy ideas see Hodson and Paden (1991), Stackhouse (1992c), Connery (1992), Howell and Dean (1994), Dodd (1995), and Layton and Deeney (1996).

Profiling

You have now worked through a speech processing profile with reference to a preschool child. If this was your first attempt at profiling, it may have taken you some time. However, do not be put off. It is the process of completing the sheets that is important and with a little practice inserting ticks and crosses on profiling sheets can be done very quickly.

Comparing Jenny's performance by standardized scores (an inter-child comparison) emphasizes the developmental perspective of the profile since the degree of her difficulty was relative to her peer group. This developmental perspective is essential for identifying children's strengths and weaknesses, but can only be gained if tests that have normal control data are used. Results from tests without such control data are difficult to interpret since you will not know whether a given score of for example, 18/25, is better than age appropriate, within the normal range or a significant deficit.

Some of the tests used to investigate Jenny's speech processing skills had been specifically designed for such a purpose. However, it would be wrong to give the impression that this is the only way that you can gather psycholinguistic information about a child. The initial screening of Jenny's speech and language development was through traditional standardized tests. When these results were interpreted within the psycholinguistic assessment framework they made an important contribution to our understanding of Jenny's difficulties (see Activity 5.1).

Psycholinguistic investigation is more than administering a few tests. Specifically designed tests, though helpful, are not essential. Rather, it is the ability to *interpret* the results from a range of different tests within a common framework that is the key to uncovering the nature of a child's difficulties. This is illustrated in our next case, Richard an 11-year-old boy with dyslexia, who was referred for an assessment of his spoken language skills. A number of tests were used, none of which was specifically designed for the purpose of completing the profiling sheet. However, in Activity 5.4, which follows the presentation of Richard's assessment results, you will have an opportunity to practise profiling on the basis of quite disparate material.

Richard

Richard was referred by his parents for a speech and language assessment at the age of 11;8. They had been concerned about his poor progress at school and had requested an independent assessment of his literacy skills prior to his speech and language assessment. The results of this assessment confirmed that Richard was a boy of above average intelligence but who had specific reading and spelling difficulties (dyslexia). At the age of 11 years he had a reading age of 8;9 and a spelling age of 7;2.

Richard's parents queried whether his dyslexia might be related to spoken language difficulties. Although they had not considered Richard to have had any specific speech difficulties they did think that he 'mumbled' and was sometimes difficult to understand. However, this was the first time he had been referred for a speech and language therapy assessment.

At the assessment reported here, Richard presented as a friendly but quiet boy who was indeed sometimes difficult to understand. He was very co-operative and completed all of the assessments He was most communicative when talking about his hobby – marine life. In a recorded conversation of him talking about sharks he used a wide range of grammatical structures and showed an ability to describe quite complicated structures.

Grammar

Richard's comprehension of grammatical structures was investigated using the *Test for Reception of Grammar* (Bishop, 1989), on which the tester reads a sentence aloud and the child has to choose the matching picture out of four. Richard passed 19/20 blocks on this test giving him, an age equivalent score of over CA 11;0 with a percentile rank of 95.

Richard was given two subtests investigating grammatical knowledge from the *Fullerton Language Test for Adolescents* (Thorum, 1986). The first, *Morphology Competency*, involves the child making up a sentence using a spoken word by the tester. For example, when asked to make a sentence using the word DISHONEST, Richard said "He was dishonest about money". He scored 18/20 on this test which is appropriate for his age.

In the second subtest, *Grammatic Competency*, the child has to listen to a sentence, decide if it contains grammatical errors and if so to correct it. For example, Richard recognized that the sentence "JOHN TOLD ME WHY WAS HE MAD" was wrong and corrected it to: "John told me why he was mad". On this subtest, Richard score 19/20 which was well above the expected 15/20 for his age.

In summary, Richard's understanding and use of grammar when listening and speaking was at least appropriate for his age and certainly superior to his written language. In fact, there was a marked discrepancy in content and fluency between Richard's spoken and written performance. He had been working hard on improving his handwriting skills but in general his written language was limited and laboured. Difficulties in the form of sentence structure, organization and spelling were apparent (see Figure 5.3).

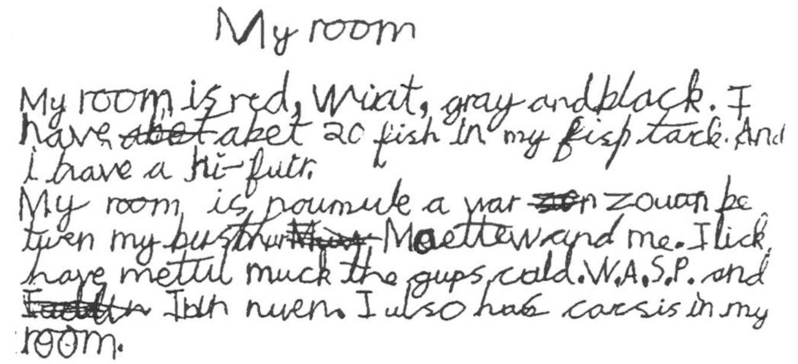

My room

My room is red, wiat, gray and black. I have abet 20 fish in my fisp tarck. And I have a hi-futr.
My room is poumule a war zouan be twen my busthur Maettew and me. I lick have mettl muck the gups cald. W.A.S.P. and Irdh nuen. I also has carsis in my room.

Read back as: My room is red, white, grey and black. I have about 20 fish in my fish tank. And I have a hi-fi in my room.

My room is normally a war zone between my brother Mathew and me. I like heavy metal music the groups called W.A.S.P. and Iron Maiden. I also have cactus in my room.

Figure 5.3: Richard's free writing.

Letter-name knowledge

These written language difficulties could not be explained by poor letter-name knowledge. Richard had no problems on the *Aston Index* (Newton and Thomson, 1982) subtest of producing letter names and sounds from their printed form. He had learned his alphabet by rote but described himself as being "out of practice" with this - he only omitted one letter 'S' but this threw him. He was able to recite the days of the week fluently and knew the four seasons. Months of the year were more difficult and he omitted MAY and OCTOBER.

Reading

In order to investigate if Richard could apply speech processing skills to reading, a series of nonwords of increasing complexity were presented. Richard read 5/12 one-syllable nonwords correctly, e.g. <tib>, <zog>, and 2/12 two-syllable nonwords: <agwop>, <lumseg>. In one-syllable words, his errors included intrusive sounds , e.g. <shup> → "shump" [ʃʌmp], <fid> → "flid" [flɪd], and vowel substitutions, e.g. <pab> → "pib" [pɪb]. In addition to these error types, in the two-syllable nonwords syllabic and sequencing errors became evident: ‹stipnoc› → "sliˈponic, sliˈtonic" [slɪˈpɒnɪk] [slɪˈtɒnɪk] ; <ildpos>→ "idliˈops" [ɪdlɪˈɒps] (see Snowling, Stothard and McLean, 1996 for a standardized nonword reading test.)

Spelling

In order to investigate Richard's segmentation skills when spelling, he was asked to spell words of increasing syllable length (after Snowling, 1985; see Goulandris, 1996, p.98 for complete list of test items). He produced the correct spelling for seven of the 10 one-syllable words (e.g. PET, LIP) but only spelt one of the 10 two-syllable words correctly (TULIP), and could spell none of the three-syllable words presented (e.g. MEMBERSHIP). Richard performed below the level expected for his reading age on this test. However, all of his errors bore some relationship to the sound pattern of the target. Most of his errors on the two-syllable words were phonetic in nature, for example:

APPLE → ‹appul›
PUPPY → ‹pupe›
KITTEN → ‹kitun›.

The three-syllable spellings were semiphonetic in nature, being only partially related to the target. In each case, however, syllable structure was preserved, for example:

CONTENTED → ‹curtnted›
REFRESHMENT → ‹refashmnt›
UMBRELLA → ‹umbualar›.

In summary, preliminary investigation of Richard's literacy skills suggested that he was having problems applying speech processing skills to reading and spelling. We therefore investigated his speech input and output processing and in particular his phonological awareness and lexical skills. The following summarizes our findings.

Auditory skills

Recent hearing tests had revealed no difficulties with auditory acuity. Three tests were administered to investigate Richard's auditory discrimination abilities.

Real and nonword auditory discrimination (Bridgeman and Snowling test, 1988)

Richard was asked to detect if real and nonword pairs were the same or different (e.g. LOST~LOTS, VOST~VOTS). He had no difficulties with this and scored 30/30 correct.

Complex nonword auditory discrimination (from Stackhouse, 1989)

He was also able to discriminate betwen same and different complex nonword pairs (e.g. IKIBUS~IBIKUS, KIRIVIN~KIVIRIN) and scored 27/28 correct on this test. The only error (MITIBOKE/MIKIBOTE) occurred at the end of the test and may have been due to a lapse in concentration. Richard requested repetition of two of the test items but then responded correctly.

Auditory lexical decision (from Stackhouse, 1989)

Single words were spoken (without pictures) by the tester for Richard to decide which were real words (SPIDER, SNOWMAN) and which were nonwords (SPODER, SNEEMON). Again, he had no difficulties with this and scored 30/30 correct.

Vocabulary

Receptive vocabulary

Richard's comprehension of vocabulary was tested using *The British Picture Vocabulary Scales* (Dunn, Dunn, Whetton, et al., 1982). On this test the tester reads out a word and the child has to select the appropriate picture out of a choice of four. Richard performed within the average range (age equivalent 11.4, percentile rank 42).

Expressive vocabulary

On *The Boston Naming Test* (Goodglass, Kaplan and Weintraub, 1983), a graded picture-naming test, Richard scored 45/60 correct. However, he was able to recall 10 further items when given the first sound of the target word as a cue, e.g. for ESCALATOR he responded "lift, stairs"; and for HAMMOCK he produced "bunk"; but he produced the correct name for both of these targets following a phonemic cue. Unfortunately, reliable inform- ation about how children of Richard's age could be expected to perform is not available for this test. However, the indications were that Richard's performance was low average for his age.

Therefore, although Richard's vocabulary development is within normal limits when compared to normal controls (a between-child comparison), there was clearly a mismatch between his low average vocabulary skills and his above average grammatical skills (a within-child comparison).

Rhyming skills

Three rhyme tasks were administered.

Silent rhyme detection (from Stackhouse, 1989)

Richard was asked to select the two pictures out of three that rhymed (e.g. BALL/WALL/BELL). He got all 16 items correct on this test.

Rhyme production (from Stackhouse, 1989)

Richard was asked to say as many rhyming words as he could with a given target. This was difficult for him. Although he could produce one rhyming word for each of 10 targets, he could not go on to produce a fluent rhyme string. He produced two responses correctly on eight of the items, and on one item (BEAR) was able to produce three correct responses. His best response was to the target LOG when he produced a rhyme string of four. However, when he did produce more than one rhyming word he repeated the target word before each new response, e.g. LOG: "log dog, log fwog, log mog, log nog". These rhyme sequences also contained occasional errors, e.g. MAP: "map ap, map flap, map mat". This strategy of repeating the target and the inclusion of similar sounding errors was very like the young normal control children (age range 3–7 years) reported in Vance, Stackhouse and Wells, (1994).

Another distinct strategy in Richard's rhyme string production was that his initial response to the first six items was to produce a rhyming word beginning with [m], e.g. HAT: "mat"; KEY: "me"; COMB: "moan"; BIN: "min"; DRAWER: "more". This meant that even though his first responses were accurate in terms of being an acceptable rhyme response, he had restricted rhyme production skills and limited rhyming fluency. This use of a restricted number of onsets when generating rhyme strings was also typical of younger normally-developing children. In fact the onset [m] was one favoured by preschool children (Wells, Stackhouse and Vance 1996).

Rhyme subtest (Bradley, 1984)

This involves the presentation of four spoken words (without pictures), three of which rhyme. The task is to say which is the odd one out (e.g. FUN, <u>PIN</u>, BUN, GUN). Richard was not able to perform this task. However, when the number of items presented was reduced to three (e.g. FUN, <u>PIN</u>, BUN), he was able to identify the odd one out correctly. His score of zero placed his performance below the 5-year level (mean correct for CA 5 = 3)

Sound segmentation

Three tests of sound segmentation skills were administered.

Initial consonant subtest (Bradley, 1984)

As above, this involved producing the odd one out in four items. However, this time the decision was based on the onsets of the word rather than the rhyme (e.g. PIP, PIN, <u>HILL</u>, PIG). Even when only three items were presented, Richard only performed at chance level on this task (4/8 correct). This put him below the 5-year level (mean correct for CA 5 = 4).

Final consonant subtest (Bradley, 1984)

Again Richard had to produce the odd one out of four words but here the words differed in their codas (e.g. COT, HOT, FOX, POT). He found this easier than the other subtests from the *Bradley Test of Sound Categorisation* and scored 7/8 correct even when four items were presented. However, he could not explain on what basis he was making his decision. On this subtest his performance was equivalent to the normally-developing 6-year-old controls.

Spoonerisms (Perin, 1983)

This procedure was used to see how Richard tackled more advanced sound segmentation tasks. He enjoyed the process of spoonerizing on his own name but was unable to transpose the onsets of the test items. Only four of the more simple items were attempted:

CHUCK BERRY	→	"Bruck Kerry"
JOHN LENNON	→	"Glon Glennon"
BOB DYLAN	→	No response
BOB MARLEY	→	"Barley for his last name Marley Barley Bob Marey".

Spoonerisms are difficult and deliberately chosen to tap segmentation problems in older children. However, as Richard scored zero on this test, he performed below the level expected for his age.

Syllable segmentation

Counting the beats in words is an important skill when it comes to spelling. Richard was able to say how many beats were in his name and in some common words. However, on the syllabification subtest of *The Fullerton Language Test for Adolescents* (Thorum, 1986) which involves identifying the number of syllables in words (e.g. BRANCH; CONSECUTIVELY; HUMANITARIANISM) and sentences (e.g. COME HERE; WE WON THE FOOTBALL GAME LAST NIGHT) he scored 10/20 (5/10 for both the word and sentence condition) which is significantly below the 17/20 correct expected for his age. Richard was able to identify the number of syllables in three-syllable words, but made an error on TABLE saying that it only had one beat. He could not identify how many syllables were in four-syllable words and on the words longer than four-syllables he knew there were a lot of beats but could not count the precise number. Similarly, on the sentences he was accurate only on sentences containing up to five syllables, with one exception: WOULD YOU BELIEVE IT IF I TOLD YOU?, which he identified correctly as having nine beats.

Sound blending

Two sound blending tasks were adminstered.

Silent sound blending

Richard was able to identify simple words (by pointing to pictures) from their segmented sounds spoken by the tester, e.g. P-IE [p aɪ] (picture choice: PIE or TIE), SH-I-P [ʃ ɪ p] (picture choice: SHIP or SHOP).

Production of sound blending

The sound blending subtest from the *Aston Index* (Newton and Thomson, 1982) was administered. Richard was 100 per cent correct on this and was able to blend long words such as DELICATE as well as the nonwords. However, it is possible that these tests were too easy for Richard who may have difficulties with sound blending if longer words were presented. It was noted that when asked to present the tester with segmented words for her to blend, he initially found this difficult. For example, although he produced "ti-ge-sh-ark" [taɪ gə ʃ ɑk] for TIGER SHARK, he segmented MERMAID'S PURSE as "me-a-te-pe-se" [mə æ tə pə sə].

Speech

Richard's connected speech can be difficult to understand even though he can imitate the full range of English speech sounds. He has a quiet voice and longer words are indistinct. However, his hearing was within normal limits and there were no obvious problems with oral structure and function. Two speech repetition tests were administered and an analysis of his connected speech was carried out.

Simple nonword repetition (from Stackhouse and Snowling, 1992b)

This test comprises simple words (e.g. DAKS, BIKUT) and assesses the child's ability to assemble new motor speech programs since the material is unfamiliar. Richard had no difficulties with this (30/30 correct).

Multisyllabic real and nonword repetition (from Snowling, Stackhouse and Rack, 1986)

More complex words (e.g. INSTRUCTED) and matched nonwords (e.g. INSPRUCTID) were used. This test is more challenging than the simple nonword repetition test above, because it involves longer words. Richard made two errors on both the real word and nonword conditions as follows:

HAZARDOUS	→	"hadardous"	['haedədəs]
SWIBBERY	→	"swigery"	['swɪgəri]
STATISTICS	→	"sas-sasis-sasistiks"	[s əs s ə'sɪs s ə'sɪsˌtɪks]
SPAPISTICS	→	"spapiskits"	[spə'pɪskɪts].

These four errors illustrate the main features of Richard's 'hidden' speech difficulty. There are no problems with individual sounds, which is perhaps the main reason for his speech difficulties having been overlooked at school. His errors are typical of the older child with persisting subtle speech difficulties (see Stackhouse, 1996) and include the following characteristics:

(a) difficulty changing place and manner of articulation quickly - hence the two [d] sounds in HAZARDOUS;
(b) sound errors as a result of the phonetic context within the word (in SWIBBERY this triggered the backing of [b] → [g]);
(c) problems programming longer words that contain clusters (e.g. SP, ST, SK, SPL, SKR). In STATISTICS, the problem is compounded by the stress being on the second rather than the first syllable which is less common;
(d) sequencing problems such as in the transposition of sounds known as 'metathesis' (in SPAPISTICS [t] and [k] are reversed).

Although he did not make many errors on this test, it is only a test of single words. Further difficulties arose in spontaneous connected speech where Richard wanted to use complex words in complex sentences. For example, he had to practise the pronunciation of new vocabulary before he could use it in his speech. This was particularly the case when discussing hobbies. Names of fish and sharks are complex. He had had to rehearse these. For example THE GREATER SPOTTED DOG FISH had caused him particular difficulty and he reported consciously practising the production of this until he got it right.

Analysis of Richard's connected speech

The following short extract illustrates why Richard's connected speech was sometimes difficult to follow. The sounds in brackets were omitted from his speech which resulted in the words 'running together' and sounding 'mumbled'.

(1) Whe(n) I we(nt) dow(n) f(or) my hol(i)day in Poole
[wɛ aɪ wɛ daʊ fmaɪ hɒʊdeɪ ˌn pul].

(2) they('ve) got a(n a)quarium
[ðɛɪ gɒʔ: əkwɛəjəm].
(3) they('ve)got (to) turn over on th(eir) stoma(ch)
[ðɛɪ gɒt:ɜn əʊvə ɒn ðstʌməʔ].

The following features were also noted in Richard's connected speech:

(i) /t/ was often pronounced at the middle and end of words as a glottal stop, i.e. without contact of the tongue tip/blade against the teeth ridge. This is more common in Richard's speech than is usual for his regional accent, and made it hard for the listener to identify the word.
(ii) /n/ was frequently pronounced without tongue contact at the end of words, even though some nasality on the preceding vowel was generally audible. This made it hard for the listener to identify the word boundary, as in "whe(n) I" in (1) and in "a(n a) quarium" in (2).
(iii) Some other consonants were pronounced weakly on occasions, e.g. /v/ in the phrases "most vulnerable" and "a bit vicious" (produced in his conversation about sharks) which was pronounced without contact betwen the lower lip and upper teeth. This may be when such consonants are preceded by another consonant in connected speech, as in these examples. There are also occasional consonant omissions, especially in final position, as in "stoma(ch)" in (3).
(iv) Richard also omitted vowels, or even whole syllables sometimes, in longer phrases, which caused problems for the listener. Vowel omissions are evident in the three examples above, e.g. the vowel of "for" and the middle vowel of "holiday" in (1); the first vowel of "aquarium" in (2); and in (3) the whole of "to" and the vowel of "their".

ACTIVITY 5.4

Aim: To complete Richard's speech processing profile on the basis of the information gathered from a range of tests.

Summarize the results of Richard's test results on the speech processing profile sheet (see Figure 5.4). Start from the section Auditory Skills (on Page 127) and work through to the end of the section on Connected Speech above. Any additional background information from the previous sections that you consider to be relevant can be added under Comments.

Check your answers with Key to Activity 5.4 at the end of this chapter, then read the following.

SPEECH PROCESSING PROFILE

Name: Richard

Age: 11;8 d.o.b:

Date:

Profiler:

Comments:

INPUT

F Is the child aware of the internal structure of phonological representations?

E Are the child's phonological representations accurate?

D Can the child discriminate between real words?

C Does the child have language-specific representations of word structures?

B Can the child discriminate speech sounds without reference to lexical representations?

A Does the child have adequate auditory perception?

OUTPUT

G Can the child access accurate motor programs?

H Can the child manipulate phonological units?

I Can the child articulate real words accurately?

J Can the child articulate speech without reference to lexical representations?

K Does the child have adequate sound production skills?

L Does the child reject his/her own erroneous forms?

Figure 5.4: Blank Profile Sheet for Activity 5.4

Working through the profile from A–L, you should have a tick under question A because no hearing acuity problems have been identified. You should also have a tick at B because Richard successfully completed both simple and complex nonword auditory discrimination tasks. There were no data for question C as this was not considered appropriate to test in an initial routine assessment for the same reasons as given in Jenny's case earlier in this chapter.

We put a tick at level D because Richard was able to discriminate between real words on the Bridgeman and Snowling Test (1988) perfectly well. However, our cross with a question mark at the same level needs further explanation. This cross was for his poor performance on the syllable number identification task (Thorum, 1986) which involved listening to the test item, holding it temporarily while the number of syllables were segmented and counted. You may have been tempted to put this test higher up on the input side — perhaps under level F — because it involves awareness of the syllable structure of the word. However, all the other tests grouped at level F (see Appendix 2), require the child to access their own representations from pictures and no stimuli words are spoken by the tester. The syllabification test is more like the tests at level D because, although real words are involved, the child does not *have* to know the word to count the number of syllables and therefore could perform the task without accessing his/her lexical representations.

When performing this test, however, it is worth noting that children often produce the word in order to rehearse their syllable segmentation. What therefore appears to be an input task may in practice be another form of a word repetition task. The corollary of this is that a child may fail on this task because of speech *output* difficulties. In this sense, we could put our cross for Richard's performance on this task on the output side at level I. Our compromise was therefore to put a cross with a question mark at level D to mark that he may not have an *input* problem here and a cross at level I because he had difficulties repeating the longer words on the syllabification test. Further, Richard's performance on all of the other input tasks suggests that this may be justified. He was able to complete the silent blending task and make auditory lexical decisions (E) and could perform the silent rhyme task (F). Questions E and F are therefore also ticked.

Looking down the output side of the profile we can see that there are many more crosses than appeared on the input side of the profile. When answering question G we need to keep in mind the two components of the question (see Chapter 4). First, let us consider Richard's ability to access lexical items, i.e. can he get the correct label regardless of the pronunciation? The answer here is 'yes' as on the *Boston Naming Test* (Goodglass, Kaplan and Weintraub, 1983) he performed within the low average range (between-child comparison). However, we need to note here that this is a poor performance for him (a within-child comparison) given his other abilities e.g. with grammar. We have therefore added a question mark (?) by the side of the tick to remind us that further investigation of his namimg skills would be advisable (e.g. see tests by German, 1989, 1990, 1991 and the procedures adopted by Constable, Stackhouse and Wells, in press). Second, we need to address the question of whether he is accessing accurate motor programmes, i.e. not just getting the label but producing it with acceptable pronunciation. Here the answer is 'no' as he has a number of speech errors in his spontaneous conversation which require further investigation through tests at subsequent levels on the profile.

Richard's most severe problem compared to normal controls was on the output phonological awareness tasks. We gave him three crosses at H for his rhyme production performance, which was like much younger normally-developing children. Similarly, he performed around the 5–6 year level on the tests of sound categorization (Bradley, 1984). We have classified these as output tests because the child is required to produce the word that is the odd one out in the series. It is clearly a complex task which involves remembering and comparing the words with each other in order to make a decision about which is the odd one out. There are therefore a number of levels at which the child may fail this task. One way of checking if a child has output rather than input problems on this test would be to administer the same task but with a silent response, e.g. by presenting four characters, each one 'says' a word in the series and the child points to the one that said the odd one out. Thus, the answer does not have to be spoken and performance can be compared on the silent response vs spoken response task.

Clearly, Richard understood what he had to do on the odd one out task but had difficulties remembering the four items. This again may be because of speech output problems interfering with his rehearsal of the test items. Remembering and manipulating the test items was also problematic for him on the spoonerism task. However, he gets only one cross for this as it is a more challenging task and, in contrast to the other tasks at H, he is not so far behind his peer group.

We gave him one cross under question I to note that although he made only two errors on real word repetition, repeating more complex real words (e.g. STATISTICS) caused him some problems, and longer words were described in the assessment as being 'indistinct'. This also confirmed our suspicion on the syllabification test that Richard had problems repeating real words. However, we gave him a tick under I for his performance on the *Aston Index* sound blending subtest, but noted that we should follow this up by asking him to blend longer words.

Our decision to put two crosses under question J was based on information gathered outside a formal test situation. As Richard made only two errors on the nonword repetition tasks you would be justified in putting just one cross as we had done under I for real word repetition. However, Richard revealed an important piece of information when he told us that he had to practise new words (i.e. in effect nonwords) over and over again as in the GREATER SPOTTED DOG FISH example. New word learning therefore requires some attention, hence the two crosses under J. More positively, we can also use this information to give him a tick under question L since his awareness of his need to rehearse new material shows that he is monitoring his output and attempting to correct his erroneous forms.

We have put a tick under question K because there was no obvious abnormality of oral structure or function and he was able to produce the full range of English speech sounds in isolation. However, no further testing of level K was done at this initial assessment. For completeness, the *Time-by-Count Test* (Fletcher, 1978) could be used to check diadochokinetic rates.

Under Comments we have noted additional information that we need to take into account when summarising Richard's strengths and weaknesses as a basis for planning his therapy/teaching programme. It is here that any significant diagnoses or conditions can be recorded. In this case we have written 'dyslexia'. In addition, we note that Richard has good spoken expressive language skills and that he knows the names and sounds of letters. When planning therapy/teaching activities for Richard, we will need to take into account the effect of his output difficulties on his 'short-term' verbal memory, and we have also put down 'handwriting' to remind us that he will need some help with this (see Taylor, 1996).

Perhaps the most important contribution of this psycholinguistic assessment to Richard's case was that it *uncovered* the specific speech output processing difficulties which were underpinning his dyslexia. Hitherto, these difficulties had gone unnoticed, mainly because of his good spoken expressive language skills and generally intelligible (though 'mumbley') speech. The speech processing profile therefore provided evidence, in a systematic way, that Richard did indeed have spoken as well as written language difficulties. The result of these difficulties was that Richard had been underachieving at school. Thus, although Richard's problems had not appeared severe or obvious to his teachers, they were none the less serious and needed extra attention.

The recommendations for Richard's therapy programme targeted output phonological awareness tasks (see Hatcher, 1994), lexical fluency, new word learning, motor programming exercises, and articulation and phrasing in connected speech. Its aim was to improve intelligibility and strengthen the speech processing skills necessary for reading and spelling. Clearly, this work needed to be linked with the curriculum at school and be carried out in collaboration with the teaching staff involved with Richard on a regular basis.

You have now completed two speech processing profiles, one on Jenny, a preschool child with speech and language problems and one on Richard, a school-age child with dyslexia. If you compare their profiles you will see that Jenny has quite pervasive speech processing problems affecting both input and output sides of the profile, while Richard's speech processing problems are on the output side of the profile. You can now profile other children in the same way and examine what other possibilities exist.

ACTIVITY 5.5

AIM: To profile one of your own cases.

Select a child known to you. Collect together recent reports and assessment results and fill in a speech processing profile summary sheet. A blank master is included at the end of this book as Appendix 3 for you to copy. If there are gaps on the profile, i.e. unanswered questions, think of at least one assessment that would address the question(s) needed to help you plan your intervention. If possible, administer the test (or tests) to the child. If you cannot think of a suitable test and would like to construct your own, you are advised to read Chapter 11 of this volume before doing so!

Compare the profile of your case with Jenny and Richard above.
Try profiling other children with whom you are working.
Discuss children's profiles with colleagues, or present a profiled case to a special interest group.

Summary

The following points have been raised in this chapter.

- The profiling sheet is a means of systematically organizing assessment results within a common framework in order to provide an overall picture of a child's speech processing skills.
- The profiling sheet is designed to provide an easy visual record of a child's strengths and weaknesses. Colour coding and/or graded numbers of ticks and crosses are helpful.
- You do not need results from specifically designed psycholinguistic tests to complete the profile sheet. Data collected from a variety of sources, including your observations, can form the basis for psycholinguistic profiling.

- A test designed to investigate input skills may involve output skills if the child rehearses the test items via speech.
- Completing the profile sheet requires interpretation of data collected and not just the entering of test results.
- Where possible, comparisons should be made with normally-developing children, in order to give the child's profile a developmental perspective (between-child comparison).
- Sometimes it is helpful to make within-child comparisons to show relative strengths and weaknesses which may or may not be within the normal range.
- Not all questions on the profile sheet will be, or need to be, completed on every child at each assessment point.
- Profiling sheets can be used with any age group as long as the assessments used are appropriate for that age group.
- Psycholinguistic assessment identifies the areas to be targeted in therapy/teaching and how weaknesses can be balanced with strengths.
- Linguistic analysis is necessary to identify precisely what stimuli should be incorporated into a child's teaching/therapy programme.

KEY TO ACTIVITY 5.1

Jenny at CA 3;8 — profile from routine tests

SPEECH PROCESSING PROFILE

Name: Jenny

Age: 3;8 d.o.b:

Date:

Profiler:

Comments:

Receptive vocabulary and verbal comprehension within normal limits. Check expressive language skills, connected speech and verbal memory

INPUT

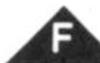

Is the child aware of the internal structure of phonological representations?

Are the child's phonological representations accurate?
✗ (ADAT)

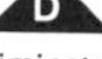

Can the child discriminate between real words?

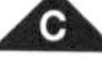

Does the child have language-specific representations of word structures?

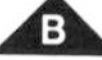

Can the child discriminate speech sounds without reference to lexical representations?

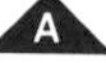

Does the child have adequate auditory perception?
✓ (hearing)

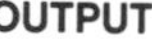

Can the child access accurate motor programs?
✓ (word finding) ? (pronunciation)

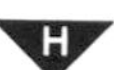

Can the child manipulate phonological units?

I

Can the child articulate real words accurately?

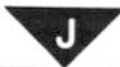

Can the child articulate speech without reference to lexical representations?

Does the child have adequate sound production skills?
✗ (sound repetition/oral examination)

Does the child reject his/her own erroneous forms?
✗ (No attempts to correct errors)

KEY TO ACTIVITY 5.2

Jenny at CA 4;0 — profile of auditory discrimination and speech skills

SPEECH PROCESSING PROFILE

Name: Jenny

Age: 4;0 d.o.b:

Date:

Profiler:

Comments:

INPUT

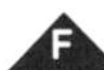

Is the child aware of the internal structure of phonological representations?

Are the child's phonological representations accurate?
✓ (aud. lex. decision – lower range of within normal limits)

Can the child discriminate between real words?
✗ (Bridgeman and Snowling test – real words)

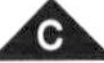

Does the child have language-specific representations of word structures?

Can the child discriminate speech sounds without reference to lexical representations?
✗ (Bridgeman and Snowling test – nonwords)

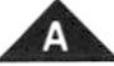

Does the child have adequate auditory perception?

OUTPUT

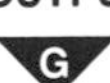

Can the child access accurate motor programs?
✗✗✗ (naming – pronunciation)

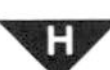

Can the child manipulate phonological units?

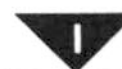

Can the child articulate real words accurately?
✗✗✗ (real word repetition)

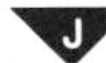

Can the child articulate speech without reference to lexical representations?
✗✗✗ (nonword repetition)

Does the child have adequate sound production skills?

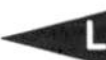

Does the child reject his/her own erroneous forms?

KEY TO ACTIVITY 5.3
Jenny at CA 4;1 — profile of rhyme skills

SPEECH PROCESSING PROFILE

Name: Jenny

Age: 4;1 d.o.b:

Date:

Profiler:

Comments:

INPUT

F

Is the child aware of the internal structure of phonological representations?
✗✗✗ (picture rhyme judgement)

E

Are the child's phonological representations accurate?

D

Can the child discriminate between real words?
✗✗✗ (auditory rhyme judgement)

C

Does the child have language-specific representations of word structures?

B

Can the child discriminate speech sounds without reference to lexical representations?

A

Does the child have adequate auditory perception?

OUTPUT

G

Can the child access accurate motor programs?

H

Can the child manipulate phonological units?
✗✗✗ (rhyme production)

I

Can the child articulate real words accurately?

J

Can the child articulate speech without reference to lexical representations?

K

Does the child have adequate sound production skills?

L

Does the child reject his/her own erroneous forms?

KEY TO ACTIVITY 5.4
Richard's speech processing profile at CA 11;8

SPEECH PROCESSING PROFILE

Name: Richard

Age: 11;8 d.o.b:

Date:

Profiler:

Comments:

Dyslexia. Above average spoken language skills/poor written language skills. n.b. handwriting. Speech output problems affecting rehearsal and intelligibility in connected speech. Knows letter names/sounds.

INPUT

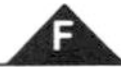

Is the child aware of the internal structure of phonological representations?

✓ (picture rhyme)

Are the child's phonological representations accurate?

✓ (silent blending)
✓ (aud. lex. dec)

Can the child discriminate between real words?

✓ (Bridgeman and Snowling real words)
✗ ? (syllabification)

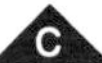

Does the child have language-specific representations of word structures?

(not tested)

Can the child discriminate speech sounds without reference to lexical representations?

✓ (nonword aud. disc)

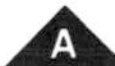

Does the child have adequate auditory perception?

✓ (hearing)

OUTPUT

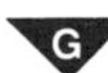

Can the child access accurate motor programs?

✗ (spontaneous speech)
✓ ? (naming but n.b. low average)

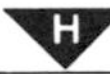

Can the child manipulate phonological units?

✗✗✗ (Bradley test and rhyme prod)
✗ (spoonerisms)

Can the child articulate real words accurately?

✗ (complex word repetition) ✓ (blending)

Can the child articulate speech without reference to lexical representations?

✗✗ (n.b. needs to practise new words)

Does the child have adequate sound production skills?

✓

Does the child reject his/her own erroneous forms?

✓ (aware of problems with new words)

Chapter 6
Building a Model

In the preceding chapters, we have seen how various kinds of assessments can be located on the simple speech processing model introduced in Chapter 1 (Figure 1.2). From this it is clear that these assessments make different demands in terms of input processing, output processing and access to stored representations. For many practical purposes of assessment and remediation, there is no need to be more specific than that about the processing mechanisms involved. This was illustrated in Chapter 5 where case studies were presented in terms of the assessment framework. However, in order to have a greater understanding of children's speech and literacy difficulties from a psycholinguistic perspective, for research purposes, or to communicate with other professionals using a psycholinguistic approach, it is helpful to be more explicit about the levels of processing and processing routes that are being assumed by the framework.

The conventional way of representing levels of processing and routes between them is an information processing model in the form of a diagram consisting of boxes (levels of processing) and arrows (processing routes). In this chapter, we will build up such a model by drawing on the arguments that have been used in previous chapters to justify different types of psycholinguistic test. The aim of the chapter is primarily to demonstrate what lies behind model construction. A minimum requirement for any model, and that includes the one presented here, is that it should be compatible with the data under consideration; beyond that, we do not intend to suggest that our model is in any sense definitive. It is, for us, merely a useful way of conceptualizing what might be happening when children are being tested according to the psycholinguistic framework. Interested users are encouraged to pull the model apart and reconstruct it in the light of further data, practical experience and theoretical insights derived from other studies. The model presented here has already been through numerous versions and it is expected that boxes and arrows will be added or deleted in the light of future work. We have drawn freely on work by other researchers, and have been influenced in particular by the models presented in Waterson (1987) and Hewlett (1990). We have not incorporated more recent theoretical developments that use a connectionist approach, where theoretical claims about children's linguistic development are tested by computational modelling of behaviour (cf. Plunkett, 1995), since very few studies of normal phonological development, let alone developmental speech disorders, have been undertaken using this approach (Vihman, 1996).

Everybody already has a model of some kind to conceptualize what happens when we speak, and when speaking goes wrong. Lay people, as well as those with a specialist interest in speech and language, have notions about input and output. Most obviously, everyone knows about deafness. We are all aware that if speech cannot be heard, then it cannot be understood and if a child has been profoundly deaf from birth, then speech production difficulties will ensue. There are some less accurate conceptions around too. For example, children with unclear or unintelligible speech may be called 'lazy' – suggesting that they are failing to put enough effort into speech production. Another account offered for speech difficulties is that the child is 'tongue-tied', suggesting that the child has a specific physical problem with the tongue which is restricting articulatory ability. The implication of this statement is that a child's speech difficulties are occurring at the 'bottom right' of the assessment framework presented in Chapter 4, i.e. in the mouth. However, 'tongue-tie', an anatomical anomaly where the tongue is anchored to the floor of the mouth resulting in restricted movement of the tongue tip in particular, does not necessarily impair speech development (Stackhouse, 1980).

Other children with problematic speech may be called 'slow' or described as having learning difficulties, suggesting that the speech problems arise from more general delay in cognitive development. In terms of the framework, such a cognitive delay would be likely to have an impact on the development of processing strategies and hence on the lexical representations at the top of the model. While it is true that many children with learning difficulties do have delayed speech and language development, there is a popular misconception that the converse is also the case: that children with speech and language difficulties have a more general cognitive delay. Clearly, this is not always so. For reasons such as this, it is important to move beyond 'lay' models of speech disorders.

Professionals working with speech and language disordered children have more sophisticated models of what is happening when processing spoken and written language, and of what might be happening when speech and literacy do not develop along normal lines. However, there are two aspects in particular which many practitioners still find problematic when trying to conceptualize developmental speech and literacy difficulties in 'model' terms. The first is the desire to have a *comprehensive* model, i.e. to conceptualize within a single model all the different factors that they wish to include, for example:

- How does input processing relate to output processing?
- How can we incorporate visual information (e.g. lip reading) in a speech processing model?
- How can we relate phonological representations to semantic representations?
- How can the model capture the relationship between orthographic representations (for spelling) and phonological representations (for speech)?
- Where does grammar fit in?
- How can we incorporate the effect of pragmatics and context on speech processing?

It would be difficult to include all these factors within a single model, and harder still to represent them on a sheet of paper. Some psycholinguists have made the attempt (e.g. Levelt, 1989). However, much of the model building in the psycholinguistics and cognitive neuropsychology literature is found in papers which are concerned with a relatively small part of the processing system: typically a model is devised to explain the findings of a series of experiments designed to investigate a particular aspect of processing.

The model that will be developed here does not attempt to address all the questions that might be posed in relation to children's speech and literacy difficulties. Most obviously, although it attempts to handle the processing of connected speech and the influence of phonetic context, it does not deal in any detail with sentence processing and grammatical development. Within this limitation, it attempts to be reasonably comprehensive in respect of the assessment framework outlined in Chapter 4, so that users can use it to interpret a speech processing profile of the kind described in Chapter 5.

The second difficulty in constructing a model for children's speech disorders is in incorporating the *developmental* perspective. The issue of comprehensiveness, described above, applies equally to models of normal adult processing, and also to models which aim to capture what happens to speech and language processing in cases of acquired speech and language disorders such as aphasia, apraxia of speech, or acquired dyslexia (cf. Ellis and Young, 1988). These models are concerned with what happens within a relatively stable system (that of normal adults), and what happens when that previously intact system breaks down. In the case of children a further, dynamic, dimension has to be added, because the processing system is changing and developing as the child matures. Consider how children change year by year; there is a huge difference between 1-, 3-, 5-, 7- and 9-year-olds in terms of speech, language and literacy skills. A developmental model needs to be able to show how children can acquire knowledge (e.g. new words with semantic and phonological representations) and skills (e.g. the ability to rhyme, segment, blend or to pronounce complex sequences of consonants). In order to understand and remediate children's disorders of speech and literacy, we need not only to be able to identify *where* the processing is breaking down, but also *when* that ability normally develops and, in model terms, *how* it develops, i.e. what processes are involved. In building a model, we therefore need to draw on psycholinguistic research into the normal development of speech and literacy skills.

In this chapter, the model is presented in information processing terms. It is built up box by box, in order to help the reader to become familiar with the box and arrow approach and the terminology used. In Chapter 7, we will discuss speech processing from a developmental perspective to try to capture how the model needs to change over time to reflect how the child develops and tackles new tasks.

Input Processing

In Chapter 1 (Figure 1.2), we presented a basic model of speech processing in the form of an ear, mouth and lexical representations. This model was used in subsequent chapters to build up our assessment framework. We can now express this model in information processing terms using a box and arrow format (Figure 6.1). Plain boxes represent levels of processing, while those enclosed in bold represent stored knowledge. Arrows represent flow of information.

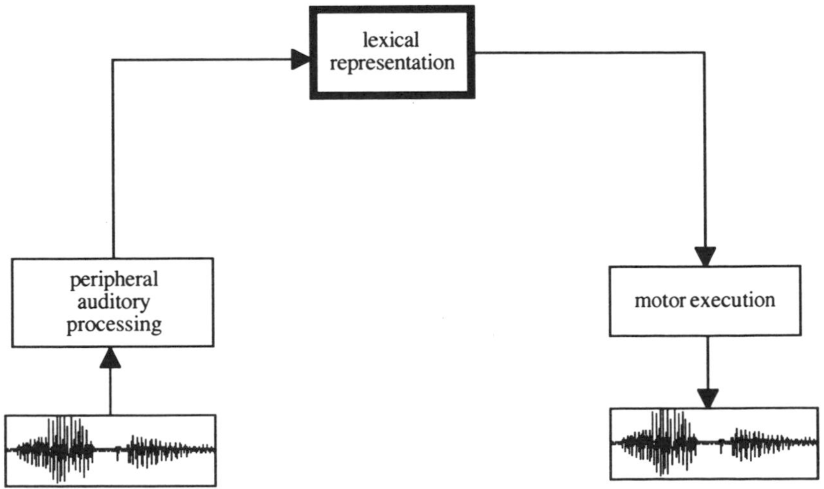

Figure 6.1: A simple information processing model based on Figure 1.2

Peripheral auditory processing

The most peripheral point on the input side, on the left here, was represented by the ear in Figure 1.2 and represents general auditory ability, not related to speech in particular. In the model presented in Figure 6.1, the ear is represented by the peripheral auditory processing box. As yet, there are no intermediate levels of processing between the level of peripheral auditory processing and the lexical representation. However, we need to fill in this gap since we know that there are children with normal peripheral hearing who have difficulties with higher level auditory processing.

Speech / nonspeech discrimination

The precise nature of auditory processing difficulties varies across children. Some children with acquired language problems, for example following convulsions or a road traffic accident, may retain their hearing acuity but be unable to distinguish between speech and environmental noises (Vance, 1991; Lees, 1993). This indicates a prelinguistic level of processing in normal children in which speech is discriminated from other sounds, before being sent on for further decoding. We therefore need to add a box for speech / nonspeech discrimination, to account for this ability present in normally-developing children but not in children with severe language difficulties involving auditory agnosia (Figure 6.2).

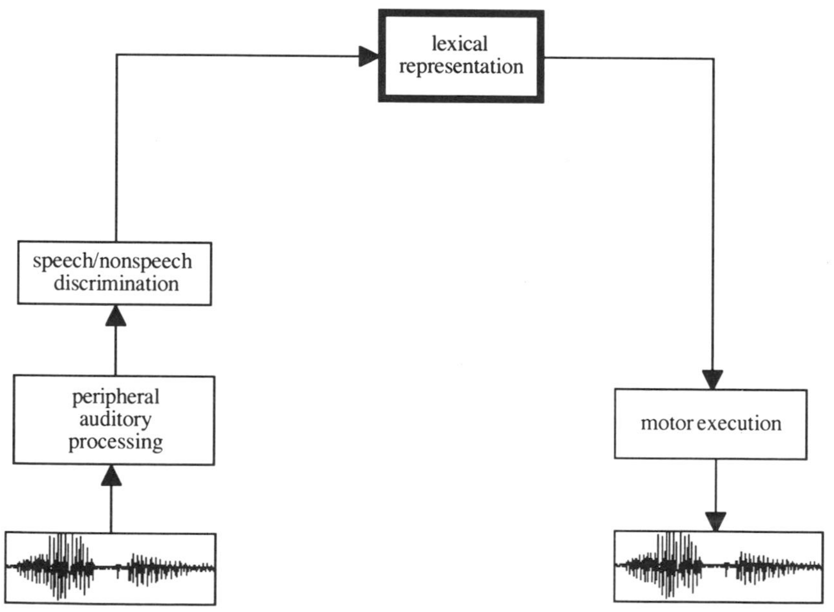

Figure 6.2: Model Building – Speech/nonspeech discrimination added

Phonological recognition

Now that the child is attending to speech as distinct from other noises, the next step for the child is to determine whether the speech belongs to a language that is familiar. Leaving aside for the moment the case of bilingual children, and assuming a child with English as a first and only language, we can posit a level of processing at which speech input is recognized as English, and sent on for further decoding, while unfamiliar (in this case, non-English) speech is not processed further. Compare the experience of a monolingual English speaker tuning in a radio, who recognizes and passes over broadcasts in foreign languages until an English broadcast is found. Tests were described in Chapter 4 that investigate the child's ability to discriminate legal nonwords, which conform to English phonological patterns but happen not to be words of English e.g. BLIK, from illegal nonwords, which contain English sound types but in non-English sequences, e.g. BNIK; and from exotic nonwords, which contain sound types not found in English, e.g. [βɲix] (see also Chapter 11). It is hypothesized that the child distinguishes between these by matching the input against an inventory of familiar (English) phonetic patterns, enabling exotic phonetic sequences and sound types to be filtered out. The level of processing at which this occurs will be referred to as phonological recognition.

Phonetic discrimination

Although, for the purposes of processing familiar language material, exotic phonetic sequences and sound types can be filtered out and disregarded, children and adults have the ability to recognize phonetic distinctions found in unfamiliar languages, such as the distinctions between stop consonants made with different types of airstream mechanisms – the clicks, implosive and ejective sounds found in some African languages, for example. Such sounds are often used paralinguistically, in languages where they do not function as part of the sound system. Thus, one kind of click is used in English to encourage horses, while another is used to express disapproval ("tut tut"). English speakers clearly have the ability both to recognize and produce such sounds. When the situation arises where the individual has to learn a second language, these general phonetic abilities are essential for recognizing and learning unfamiliar sound patterns and distinctions — for example the front rounded vowels found in French words such as LUNE, PEU, FLEUR, which do not occur in English. Even within English itself, English speakers gain the ability to recognize and identify a much wider range of phonetic items than they use in their own speech. This ability is needed to make sense of unfamiliar regional accents, which are likely to contain sound types quite as exotic as those found in other languages. Thus, ejective consonants (made with glottalic airstream) are used by speakers of some Northern British English accents at the end of words like BET and BOOK, whereas in the accent of Liverpool, the final /k/ in BOOK can be produced as a voiceless velar fricative [x], as in German BUCH. The range of different vowels found in accents of English around the world is even greater than for consonants. In order to understand speakers of different accents, the English speaker needs to draw on phonetic discrimination abilities much broader than those required by his or her own accent. For this reason, an off-line level of processing called phonetic discrimination is included in the model, to indicate that this type of phonetic processing can be called upon as circumstances demand. How this level of processing might be affected in children with speech disorders has not yet been investigated in any detail, but clearly it has implications for the child's ability to tackle new languages, as well as for the ability to comprehend the child's own first language in all its variety (Nathan, Wells and Donlan, 1996). On our model, off-line processing units such as Phonetic Discrimination appear as shaded boxes. Broad arrows indicate that information flows between boxes as part of a learning process, rather than in the on-line processing of familiar input.

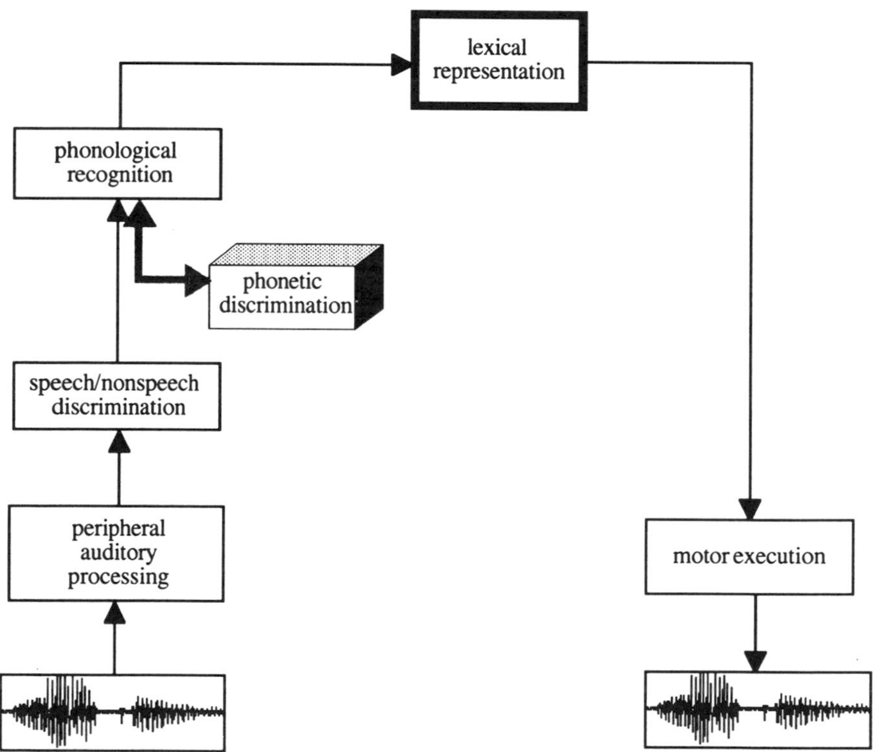

Figure 6.3: Model building – Phonological recognition and phonetic discrimination

There is a close relationship between the general phonetic abilities that permit phonetic discrimination of the kind just described, and the ability to identify a phonological unit of one's own language and accent correctly – the ability to identify that the word spoken was PIN rather than BIN or TIN, for instance. Because this latter ability is needed to process material spoken in one's own language, it can be seen as an aspect of phonological recognition: once the language material has been accepted as familiar, it can be processed further in order to identify the sound patterns it contains.

This process can be thought of as consisting of two parts: the input material has to be segmented, or parsed, into its constituent units, and those units have to be identified. Where the input is connected speech, as is normally the case, an initial level of parsing will have to identify where word boundaries occur. In English, bottom-up phonetic cues to word boundaries include the phonetic prominence associated with the stressed syllable. This is not a very precise cue, but there is usually one stress per multisyllabic word, and the majority of bisyllabic words in English have a 'trochaic' pattern, whereby the stress is located on the first syllable (e.g. 'RABBIT, rather than GI'RAFFE). Research suggests that English-learning infants are sensitive to this pattern (Jusczyk, Cutler and Redanz, 1993). Consonant sequences that are illegal within a syllable but which can occur at syllable and word boundaries (e.g. [kʃ] as in BLACK SHOES) provide a further cue for segmenting the speech stream. However, children will also use their prior linguistic knowledge (i.e. top-down processing) to try to make sense of what they hear. For example, the phrase 'my son John' from a popular nursery rhyme was interpreted as 'mice and John' by a normally-developing 4-year-old. Similarly, a 3-year-old singing '*Row Row Row the Boat*' ended with "Life is butter cream" instead of "Life is but a dream" — perhaps being confused by the unusual syntax of the target phrase. Adults too make such 'errors' when there are insufficient linguistic or contextual cues to guide interpretation. For example, an (English) student in a linguistics lecture, on hearing for the first time Chomsky's famous example of a semantically ill-formed but syntactically well-formed sentence, "Colourless green ideas sleep furiously", transcribed it in her notes as "Colourless green-eyed ears sleep furiously".

Once the spoken input has been parsed into constituents such as word and syllable, the individual phonological units have to be identified. In earlier chapters, mention was made of children who are able to discriminate real English word pairs, but not some pairs of nonwords, even though the nonwords are perfectly possible, though accidentally non-existent, words of English (e.g. VOST vs VOTS). Such tests tap a level of phonological recognition that does not involve access to the lexical phonological representations, but draws solely upon knowledge of the phonological units (consonants, vowels) and sequences (clusters, syllable types etc.) found in English. In order to discriminate pairs of words, both real and non, it is suggested, following Waterson (1987), that the listener latches on to the salient phonetic features perceived for each word, which form an auditory pattern; then on this basis synthesizes a phonetic pattern for each word and compares them. If, as seems likely, the synthesis process draws on articulatory rehearsal, this account offers some insight into why some children with speech *output* difficulties can have problems with input processing, and in particular in processing nonwords, i.e. those for which the child cannot refer to a previously stored lexical phonological representation (Bridgeman and Snowling, 1988; Raaymakers and Crul, 1988).

Figure 6.3 summarizes the levels of input processing discussed so far. The child has to be able to hear the full range of sounds involved in speech (peripheral auditory processing), and to identify the input as speech (speech / nonspeech discrimination). The child then has to be able to recognize the phonological 'landmarks' specific to English – those that facilitate the segmentation of the input into words, syllables and smaller units – and to identify each of these units accurately (phonological recognition). When the input contains novel phonetic material, e.g. from an unfamiliar accent of English, or from an unfamiliar language, the child needs to be able to sort out the unfamiliar material in phonetic terms, for example by mapping the percept onto new articulatory routines in an attempt to reproduce the unfamiliar sound (phonetic discrimination).

Lexical Representations

None of the levels of input processing described so far requires the child to have access to the lexicon. However, as we saw in Chapters 2–4, some input tasks do make this demand, for example when the child is presented with two pictures (e.g. CROWN and CLOWN), the tester pronounces one or the other, and the child has to decide which word has been spoken (MorganBarry, 1988). To succeed on this, the child has to recognize the pictures via the visual system, accessing the semantic representations of each word, and thereby activating prior knowledge about the phonological structure and content of each of the two words. This phonological information, referred to as the phonological representation, can be thought of as part of the child's knowledge of each word form stored in memory. The phonological representation does not exist in isolation, since the child's knowledge of a word also includes its meaning: without knowing that the person who makes a fool of himself at the circus and has a red nose and funny costume is referred to by the label CLOWN, the child will be unable to access the phonological representation on seeing the picture, since it is not possible to go directly from a visual stimulus to a phonological representation without accessing the semantic representation first. The phonological representation and semantic representation are linked to a third aspect of the lexical representation, which specifies the gestures required for the accurate pronunciation of the word: the motor program. These components of the lexical representation, first introduced in Chapter 1 (see Activity 1.2), will be explained in more detail later. In Figure 6.4, the semantic representation, phonological representation and the motor program are presented as separate but connected components of the lexical representation. All are enclosed in bold, as they represent stored knowledge. The broad black arrows indicate that not only is there an on-line flow of information between these components (for example, from the semantic representation to the motor program, in a naming task), but there are also links between these different aspects of the word that are a permanent part of the child's lexical entry for that word: it is assumed that phonological information and semantic information about a word are linked together. Thus, the child's stored knowledge of a word consists not only of the phonological representation, the semantic representation and the motor program, but also of the links between them.

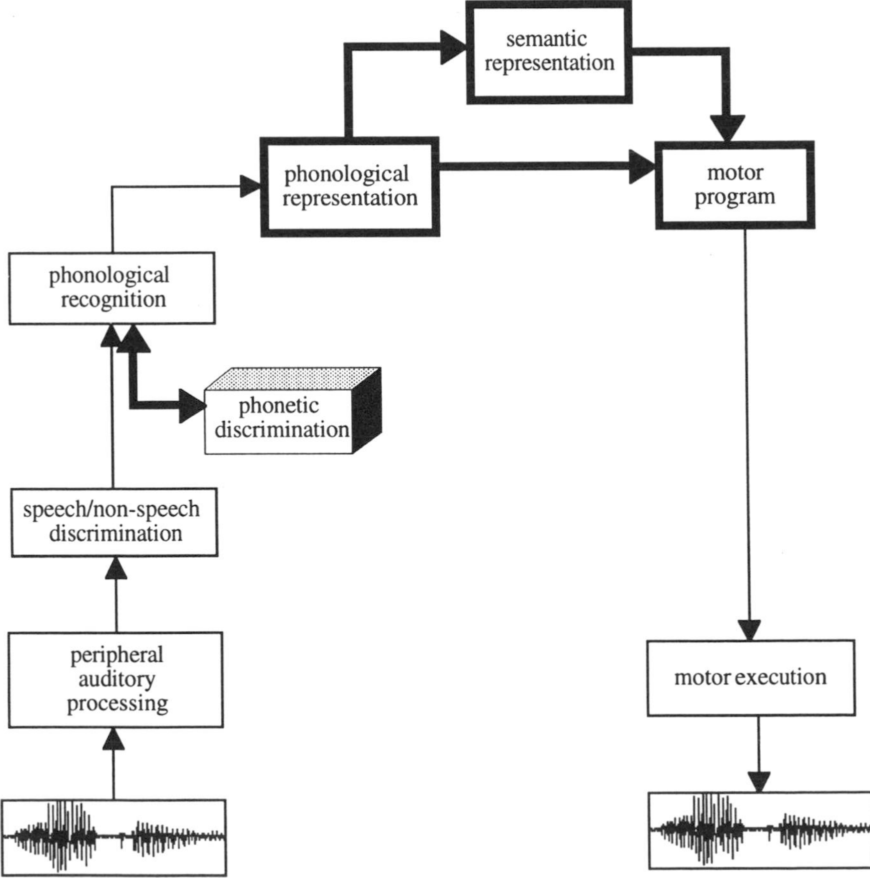

Figure 6.4: Model building — components of the lexical representation added

Now that we have completed the input side of the model, we can trace the processing routes involved in some of the input tasks that are incorporated in the assessment framework. This allows us to see the demands a task makes on a child's processing skills.

ACTIVITY 6.1

Aim: To understand the psycholinguistic properties of popular auditory tasks by drawing their routes through the input side of the model presented in Figure 6.4.

For this activity, you will need transparencies (ideally – but tracing paper will suffice if transparencies are not available), coloured pens and the diagram in Figure 6.5. This diagram depicts the boxes from the model in Figure 6.4, without the arrows.

Tracking a processing route involves drawing lines to connect each box you believe to be involved for the successful completion of the task, with arrows to indicate the direction of flow of information. All routes begin at the peripheral auditory processing box. None of the routes will involve the right-hand side of the model since none of the tasks in this activity requires any spoken output from the child. Draw each route on a separate transparency in a different colour (this is necessary to complete Activity 6.2, when you will overlay transparencies to compare and contrast the processing routes involved in different tasks).

On the diagram in Figure 6.5 draw the processing routes involved in the following auditory tasks. The letters in brackets refer to the speech processing profile presented in Figure 5.1 (see Chapter 5).

(a) Real word discrimination, e.g. "Are these two words the same or different: BIN, PIN ?" (D)

(b) Nonword discrimination, e.g. "Are these two words the same or different: 'IKIBUS, 'IBIKUS ?" (B)

(c) Auditory lexical decision, e.g. Child looks at a picture of a CAR. Tester asks: "Is this a [tɑ]" (i.e. tar)? (E)

(d) Nonspeech discrimination, e.g. Child listens to electronically generated pairs of tones presented with different time intervals between them: Tester asks "Did you hear one sound or two?" (A)

Check the routes you have drawn against Key to Activity 6.1 (i) – (iv) at the end of this chapter, then read the following.

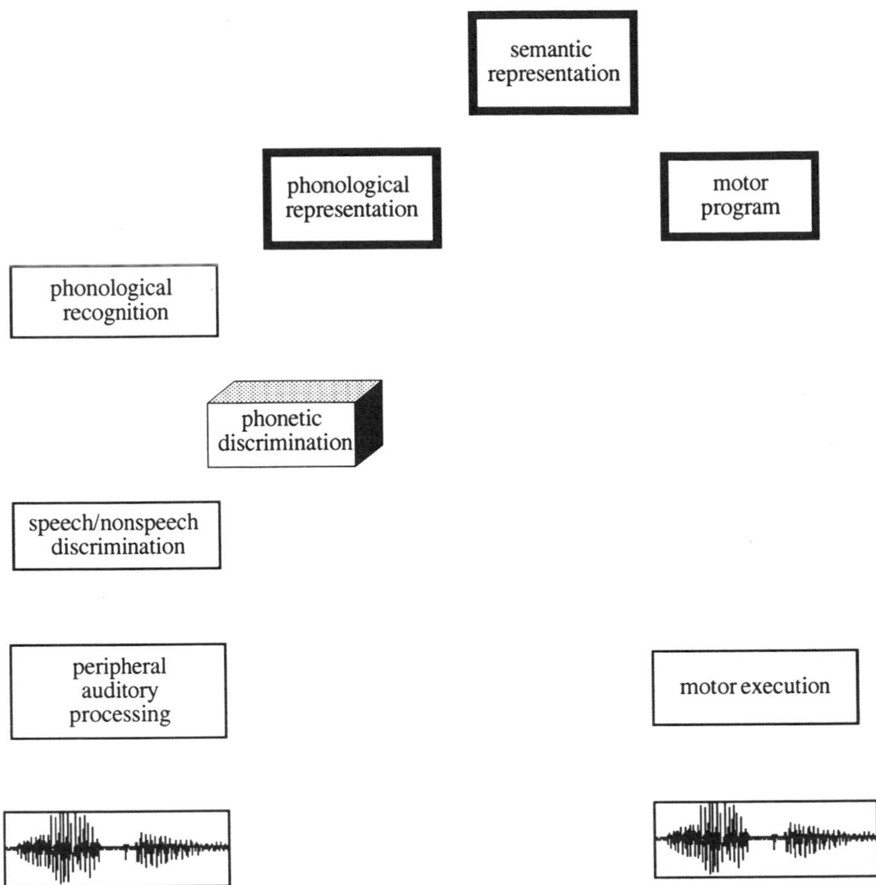

Figure 6.5: Input side of the model, minus arrows

In order to respond successfully in task (a), real word discrimination, the child has to have hearing good enough to perceive the two words and detect the phonetic differences between them, so adequate peripheral auditory processing is essential. The stimulus consists of speech, and is identified as such (speech/nonspeech discrimination). Phonological recognition is the essence of this task. Having identified BIN and PIN as conforming to English phonological patterns, the child has to discriminate between two possible syllable onsets of English, phonetically [p] and [b]. A successful response can therefore be achieved without further processing: see Route 1 in Key to Activity 6.1(i).

In addition, the child *may* access his/her phonological representations of the two words PIN and BIN, to support the process of discrimination: discovery that these are indeed two distinct words already in the child's vocabulary may help to confirm the decision that the two stimulus words are different, i.e. that the relatively small phonetic difference between them is not just accidental or 'free variation', but does in fact have a contrastive function. This then extends the processing route to the phonological representation: see Route 2 in Key to Activity 6.1(ii).

In task (b), nonword discrimination, the same steps are needed as for task (a), since the stimuli are possible English words. The route is therefore the same: Route 1 in Key to Activity 6.1 (i). The difference between tasks (a) and (b) is that Route 2 is not an option in task (b): the child cannot make use of phonological representations to support or confirm a decision, since these nonwords have no previously established phonological representations.

In task (c), auditory lexical decision, the stimulus is a possible English word, and so passes through the first three boxes, as in (a) and (b). This time, however, the comparison is with a form that has not been spoken, but which the child has to summon up on the basis of the picture. The picture provides access to the semantic aspect of the lexical representation, which in turn gives access to the phonological representation of CAR. This can now be compared to the form that has been processed auditorily:[tɑ]. The processing route thus extends to the semantic representation and the phonological representation within the lexicon: see Route 3 in Key to Activity 6.1 (iii).

In task (d), nonspeech discrimination, the stimulus is not speech, and so processing is completed at the level of peripheral auditory processing: see Route 4 in Key to Activity 6.1 (iv).

We have now drawn four routes, to illustrate the processing demands in a selection of popular input assessment tasks. Next, we can compare and contrast the processing routes involved for the different tasks and spot the commonalities and differences between them.

ACTIVITY 6.2

Aim: To compare and contrast the processing routes involved in the input tasks included in Activity 6.1.

Take your transparencies of the four routes drawn in Activity 6.1. Overlay them on the diagram in Figure 6.5 as follows, looking for the commonalities and differences between pairs of routes:

(i) Routes 1 and 2. Check against Key to Activity 6.2 (i);
(ii) Routes 2 and 3. Check against Key to Activity 6.2 (ii).

Then read the following.

(i) Comparison of Route 1 and Route 2. This demonstrates the extra support available by accessing the lexicon on a same / different task when the words are familiar (Route 2), as opposed to nonwords (Route 1).

(ii) Comparison of Route 2 and Route 3. This demonstrates the role of semantic knowledge in performing an auditory lexical decision task (Route 3), as opposed to a same / different auditory discrimination task (Route 2).

Components of the Lexical Representation

Having explored the input side of the model in some detail, we now consider the components of lexical representations in greater depth. In addition to the three components already mentioned (semantic representation, phonological representation, motor program), the lexical representation also contains *grammatical* information – for example, whether the word is a noun or verb etc., and whether it has irregular forms (e.g. BRING ~ BROUGHT, MOUSE ~ MICE). Once the child starts learning to read and spell, *orthographic* information is added to the lexical representation. These pieces of information about the word are not discrete. The semantic and grammatical representations are linked, since the grammatical class of a word is closely bound up with its meaning ('things' having the grammatical category of noun rather than verb, for example). Similarly, in English, the phonological and orthographic aspects are linked, since for regular words there are many predictable relationships between phonological units and graphemes. The lexical representation of a word therefore has a number of components – what the word means (semantic representation), what grammatical function(s) it has (grammatical representation), what it sounds like (phonological representation), how it is produced in speech (motor program), how it appears in writing (orthographic representation) and how it is produced in writing (orthographic program). Figure 6.6 depicts the distinct but interconnected parts of a lexical representation.

Thus, an adult's lexical representation of the word MOUSE might contain:

- a semantic representation: a small rodent, with long tail, fond of cheese, dwelling in skirting board etc.;
- a grammatical representation: animate count noun, with irregular plural form (MICE);
- an orthographic representation of letters in the appropriate sequence that enables the word to be recognized in various typefaces, sizes, handwriting styles etc.;
- an orthographic program for writing the letters ‹m o u s e› in that sequence, with appropriate links; or for typing the letters in the correct sequence;
- a phonological representation, e.g. /maʊs/ (but see next section);

- a motor program for speech: closure of lips accompanied by vibration of vocal folds and nasal escape of airstream; followed by open vocalic articulation with raising of velum (soft palate), lips opening to unrounded position, tongue low in mouth, followed by progressive raising of tongue body toward soft palate and rounding of lips, close approximation of tongue blade to alveolar ridge creating turbulence, accompanied by opening of vocal folds.

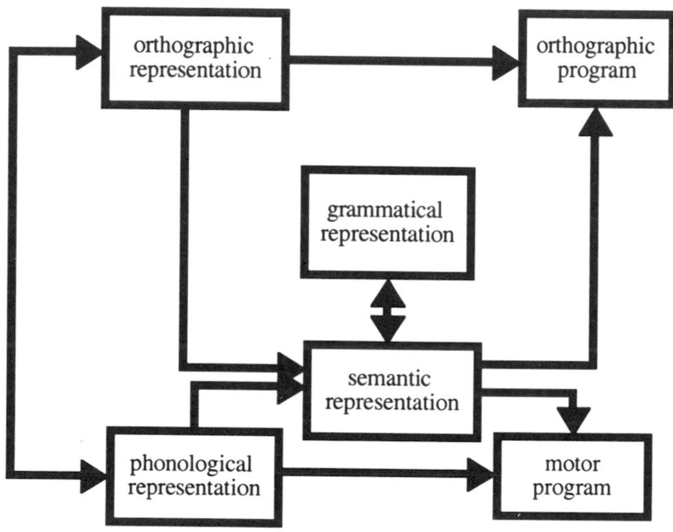

Figure 6.6: Components of the lexical representation

The information given here for each component of the lexical representation of MOUSE is very limited. A great deal more semantic and grammatical detail could be added, but is not central to the topic of this book. The phonological representation is discussed at greater length in the next section. The information given for the motor program in the traditional terms of articulatory phonetics serves to give some indication of the complexity of gestures involved in a simple monosyllabic word. The orthographic representation and program are discussed further in Chapter 8.

Phonological representations

For a word to be correctly identified from spoken input, the phonological representation must be accessed. For this to happen, the phonological representation has to contain enough phonological information to identify the word uniquely (e.g. as CROWN as opposed to CLOWN). However, it is unlikely that the phonological representation contains much more than the minimum amount of information required for recognition purposes since, as already mentioned, the word has to be recognized using input from a wide variety of sources such as speakers of different ages, genders and regional accents. Having too detailed phonetic information about the word could result in failure to identify variant pronunciations that did not conform to the stored form. Instead, it can be assumed that phonological representations only contain sufficient information to make the word distinctive from other words, i.e. information that is abstract enough to be shared by variant pronunciations of the word.

The internal structure of the phonological representation

In the past, it was generally assumed that phonological representations took the form of strings of phonemes (contrastive sound segments, i.e. vowels and consonants), of the kind given for MOUSE: /maus/. However, evidence from studies of different languages, as well as from psycholinguistic investigations of adults and children, has shown that this is not a tenable hypothesis about the way in which human language is organized. Instead, phonological representations are considered to have an internal hierarchical structure, in which units 'higher up' are at least as important as units lower down (Hogg and McCully, 1987), and may also be mastered earlier developmentally (Treiman and Zukowski, 1996). In simple monosyllabic words such as MAT, MAD and MAN the highest level segmentation of the syllable is into its onset and its rhyme, as has been described in earlier chapters. The rhyme is everything from the vowel nucleus to the end of the syllable, i.e. [at] in MAT. The onset is everything that precedes the vowel nucleus, i.e. [m]. Figures 6.7 and 6.8 shows how this structure can be represented.

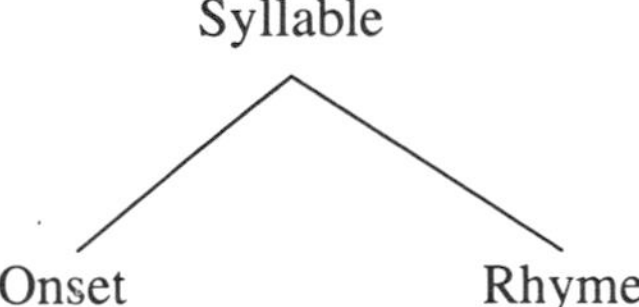

Figure 6.7: Onset/rhyme segmentation

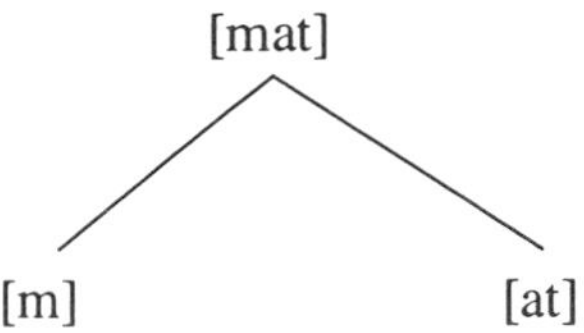

Figure 6.8: Syllable structure of MAT

The rhyme can then be further subdivided into the nucleus (i.e. the vowel) and the coda (the consonant or consonants following the vowel) as in Figures 6.9 and 6.10.

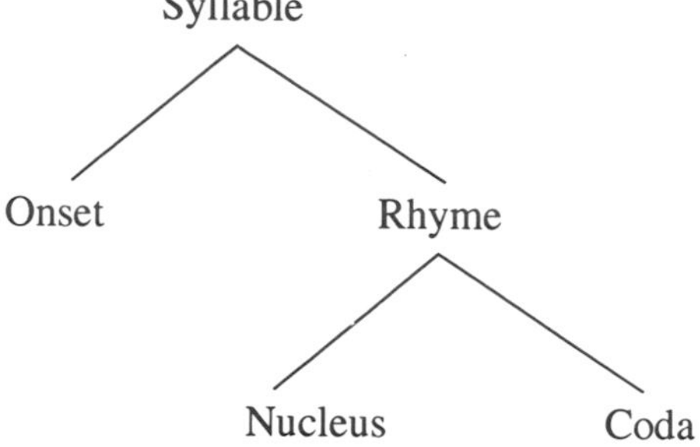

Figure 6.9: Nucleus / coda segmentation

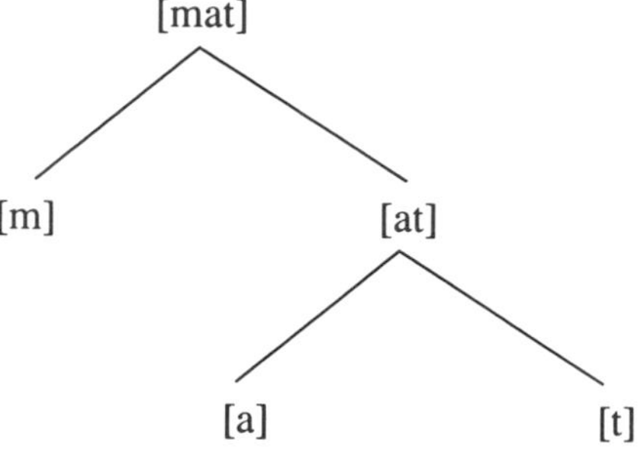

Figure 6.10: Nucleus / coda segmentation of MAT

The term 'rhyme' (sometimes spelt 'rime') has a technical sense here, to describe a major constituent of the syllable; but it can be readily seen how, at least for monosyllabic words, this sense of rhyme closely matches our lay use of the term when we ask children to think of words that rhyme with, for example, MAT. We expect them to produce words that share the same vowel and final consonant(s), i.e. have the same rhyme, but differ in the initial consonant(s), i.e. have a different onset, e.g. HAT CAT RAT. Because of this correspondence, we can see that when we ask a child to detect two words that rhyme in a picture presentation task rather than from spoken input, we require the child to summon up his/her phonological representation of each of the words depicted, and then to segment the phonological representations into their major constituents of onset and rhyme in order to decide which two words have the same rhyme. This is why in the assessment framework presented in Chapter 4, such tests were described as tapping the child's awareness of the internal structure of phonological representations.

Before investigating the nature of phonological representations further, let us briefly consider words of more than one syllable. These necessarily have a more complex representation, in which each syllable has its own internal hierarchical structure. One complexity involves the assignment of consonants to abutting syllables. For example the word RABBIT, though it has ‹bb› in the orthography, has only a single consonant between the two vowels in pronunciation. Which syllable should this be assigned to? Should we segment as [rɑ] [bɪt] or [rɑb] [ɪt]? In fact, there is no theoretical objection to permitting the single consonant to be ambisyllabic, i.e. to belong to both syllables, functioning as the coda of the first syllable and the onset of the second. This can be represented as in Figure 6.11.

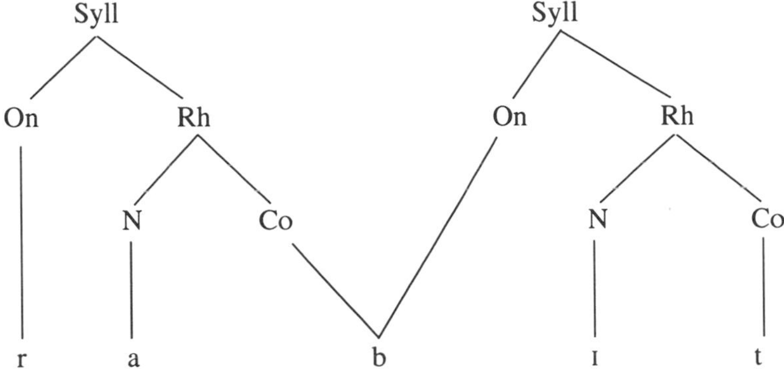

Figure 6.11: Syllable structure of RABBIT.

Figures 6.10 and 6.11 have illustrated the hierarchical structure of phonological representations, but are misleading with regard to the actual content of the phonological constituents. The terminal constituents in Figure 6.10 were represented by phonetic symbols [m], [a], [t]; but in fact it is generally held that the content of phonological representations is quite abstract: they only contain the information necessary to distinguish the unit in question (e.g. the onset [m]), from other units that can occur in the same place in English monosyllables, e.g. [n], [t], [k] etc. For instance, although [m] is pronounced with voicing, this voicing is not specified in the phonological representation, since any unit in English that is nasal, like [m] and [n], is automatically voiced. It is therefore unnecessary to refer to the phonetically important but phonologically redundant voicing of [m] in order to identify it as [m]. By contrast, it is essential to refer to the nasal feature, since this is what distinguishes [m] from [b] in pairs such as MAKE and BAKE. One consequence of this underspecification is that the way in which phonological representations are presented is quite technical, using distinctive phonological features (Spencer, 1988). For practical purposes, however, it is rarely necessary to present phonological representations in formal terms. The important point is that the phonological representation does not contain all the phonetic information needed to pronounce the word correctly, but only the information needed to distinguish that word from other words.

This information relates primarily to acoustic / auditory properties of the word, such as voicing, nasality, friction, vowel quality. However, important visual information is available too, for example the lip closure that is visible at the onset of both MAKE and BAKE, and of the second syllable of RABBIT, the lip-rounding visible throughout words such as HOOP and RUDE, or at the onset of the first syllable of RABBIT; and the lip spreading evident throughout words such as LEAN or SITTING, in many accents of English. Such distinctive visual information, like auditory phonetic information, is incorporated into the phonological representation, thereby contributing to recognition of the word. Listeners with hearing impairments are particularly dependent on such visual cues.

Motor programs

If, as has been suggested, the information in the phonological representation is abstract and rather sparse, then the phonological representation cannot of itself serve as a sufficient basis for speech output, which requires detailed specification of articulatory gestures if it is to result in accurate pronunciation of the word. For pronunciation, the child has access to another aspect of the lexical representation, referred to in Figure 6.6 as the motor program.

The motor program for a word consists of a series of gestural targets for the articulators (tongue, lips, soft palate, vocal folds), stored in the lexical representation, that are designed to achieve an acceptable pronunciation of the word, i.e. a pronunciation compatible with the phonological representation. One of the questions in the assessment framework of Chapter 4, question G, asks whether the child can realize motor programs accurately. If the child has an accurate phonological representation (E) and has adequate sound production skills (K), yet is unable to pronounce a word in such a way as to distinguish it clearly from other (phonologically similar) words, this suggests that the motor program is deficient. As will be discussed in Chapter 7, this is evident in many young children, who fail to signal contrasts such as KEY ~ TEA in their speech, even though they can perceive the difference.

For some speech production activities, notably spontaneous speech and picture naming, no input processing of auditory information is required: the spoken output is generated from the semantic representation. Since the word to be uttered is by definition already known, and the phonological representation is not required for recognition purposes, the motor program can be accessed directly from the semantic representation, leading to a more automatic production than would be the case if the semantic representation first accessed the phonological representation, which in turn accessed the motor program.

Output Processing

Motor programming

The semantic representation, phonological representation and the motor program are presented as separate components of the lexical representation, linked by arrows (see Figure 6.6). This helps us see what is involved in activities such as spoonerisms and rhyme production, listed under question H in the assessment framework: *Can the child manipulate phonological units?* In the case of spoonerism tasks (using monosyllabic words, for simplicity), the child initially has to segment the phonological representations into onset and rhyme, e.g. SHARP KNIFE, pronounced [ʃɑp naɪf], into [ʃ] + [ɑp]; [n] + [aɪf]; then to reassemble the onset of one word on to the rhyme of the other: [n] + [ɑp]; [ʃ] + [aɪf], in order to create motor programs for the new words: [nɑp ʃaɪf].

Similarly, in a rhyme string production task where the child has to produce as many words as possible that rhyme with a given target, e.g. FAT, the child has to segment the phonological representation into [f] + [at], select a new onset, add it to the rhyme, and create a new motor program. Normally-developing children routinely produce nonwords, e.g. [lat], [gat], as well as real words (e.g. "cat", "mat") in responding on this task (Vance, Stackhouse and Wells, 1994), which indicates that they create new motor programs, rather than relying on pre-existing ones. This points to the need for a component in our model where new motor programs are created: motor programming. Because it is not used in all cases of speech production, but only when the speaker is having to produce previously unfamiliar words, motor programming is located to one side of the main processing route. This is shown in Figure 6.12, where it can be seen that motor programming on the output side parallels phonetic discrimination on the input side. The test most commonly used to assess the child's ability to construct new motor programs, and thus to assess the functioning of motor programming, is nonword repetition, although this test also taps other processes of discrimination and segmentation.

Constructing a new motor program

Motor programming can be thought of as comprising a store from which phonological units are selected, and a process of assembling these units in new combinations. An analogy would be a child's box of letters, from which you can make a selection, then sequence them in new combinations to create new words. However, in the case of speech, the phonological units are unlikely to be segment-sized, particularly for the younger child. Following our earlier discussion of the nature of phonological representations, the store can be thought of as containing the set of the possible onsets and of the possible rhymes of English. For each onset or rhyme, information is stored about the gestural targets that, if achieved, will result in an acceptable production. For each onset or rhyme, alternative gestures are included, to cover the different combinatorial possibilities; for example, the gesture for the onset /k/ in KEY is different from the onset /k/ in CAR or COOL because of the influence of the following vowel. In a rhyme production test, the child, having segmented the stimulus word into onset and rhyme, has to activate motor programming to select new onsets, then attach the new onset to the rhyme. A similar process is involved when the child is asked to produce strings of words beginning with the same onset.

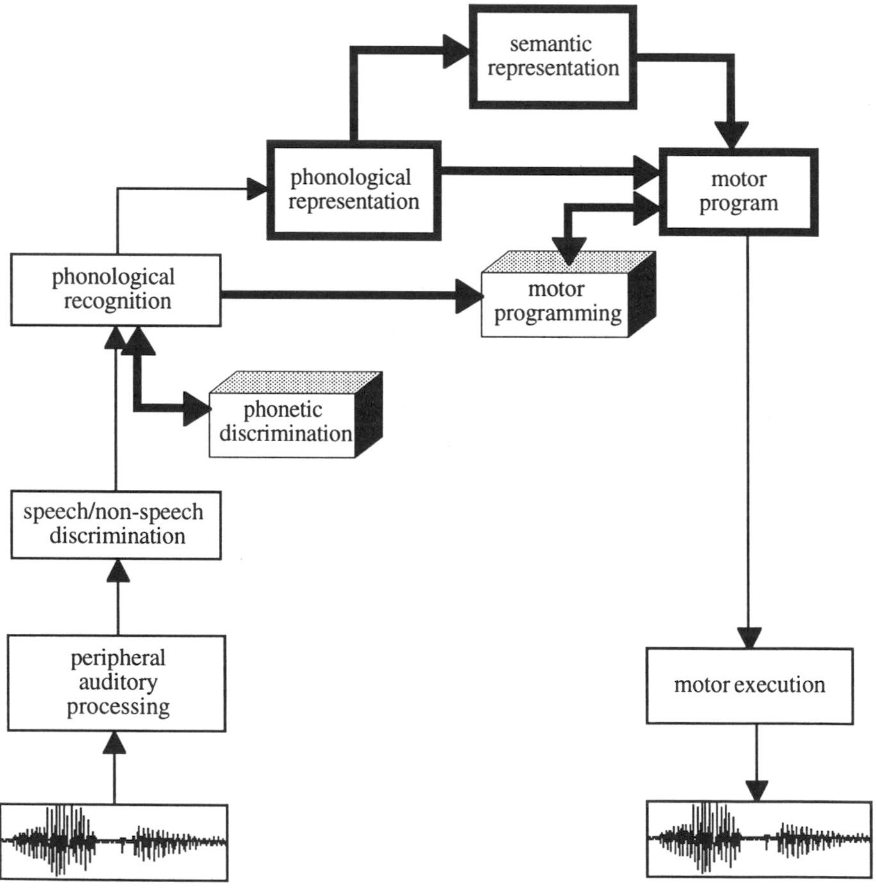

Figure 6.12: Model Building — Motor programming added

Motor planning

Any of the tasks in the assessment framework that require a spoken output require the child either to access a pre-existing motor program which is part of a lexical representation, or else to create a new motor program. Once the motor program has been retrieved or created for each word to be uttered, the various gestural targets have to be assembled in the correct sequence in real time, taking account of the contextual requirements that will influence the eventual production. These include the rhythmic and intonational patterns selected, and the grammatical structure. This stage of processing is easier to illustrate for utterances greater than a single word, since these have a richer grammatical, intonational and rhythmic structure. But even in the case of single words, we can see that the pronunciation will be influenced by factors such as: how quickly the word is to be spoken; whether it is to be spoken with an expressive intonation, with wide pitch movement, or in a whisper; whether it is to function as a question, in which case it may have a rising intonation; or a statement, in which case the intonation is more likely to be falling. The pronunciation of an individual word will also be affected by the context in which it finds itself. Thus the gesture for the rhyme of CAT, which we can symbolize /at/, is quite different when (in casual speech) the word is followed by a word beginning with a [p] as in THE CAT PURRED, as opposed to when it is followed by a vowel, as in THE CAT ATE. These aspects of the utterance have to be achieved through neuromuscular activity, which has to be planned in advance. This level of processing, where the motor programs of the individual words are assembled into a single utterance plan, is referred to as motor planning. It is the level of processing at which occasional 'slips of the tongue' can occur in the speech of otherwise unimpaired speakers, both adult and child, when a segment from one word of a planned utterance may replace, or be exchanged for, a segment from another word in the planned utterance. The following examples of spontaneous slips of the tongue are taken from a diary study of two children under the age of 6 (Stemberger, 1989):

> "I found the fin – pin"
> "Prekend – pretend you hold your breath and fall down"
> "I got my secks – socks wet"
> "We could have a fillow fight".

In terms of our model, units of production (in these examples, onset or nucleus) are transposed or replaced following access and sequencing of the stored motor programs for the individual words. While it would be of interest to collect comparable data of spontaneous slips of the tongue as part of clinical assessment, it is impractical to do so on a regular basis. For the purposes of clinical assessment, motor planning skills can be tapped by eliciting connected speech, for example through picture description or sentence repetition tasks.

Motor execution

Finally, we reach the mouth, or more accurately the vocal tract – all the physical organs that are involved in producing speech, including the lungs and the larynx as well as the oral and nasal cavities. If there are anatomical problems with any part of the vocal tract – lips, teeth, tongue, palate, vocal folds, lungs – then the production of speech may be affected. This is also the case if the innervation of these organs is affected, as in dysarthria. At this processing level, the motor plan is actually executed and so gives rise to an acoustic signal. This completes the model (see Figure 6.13).

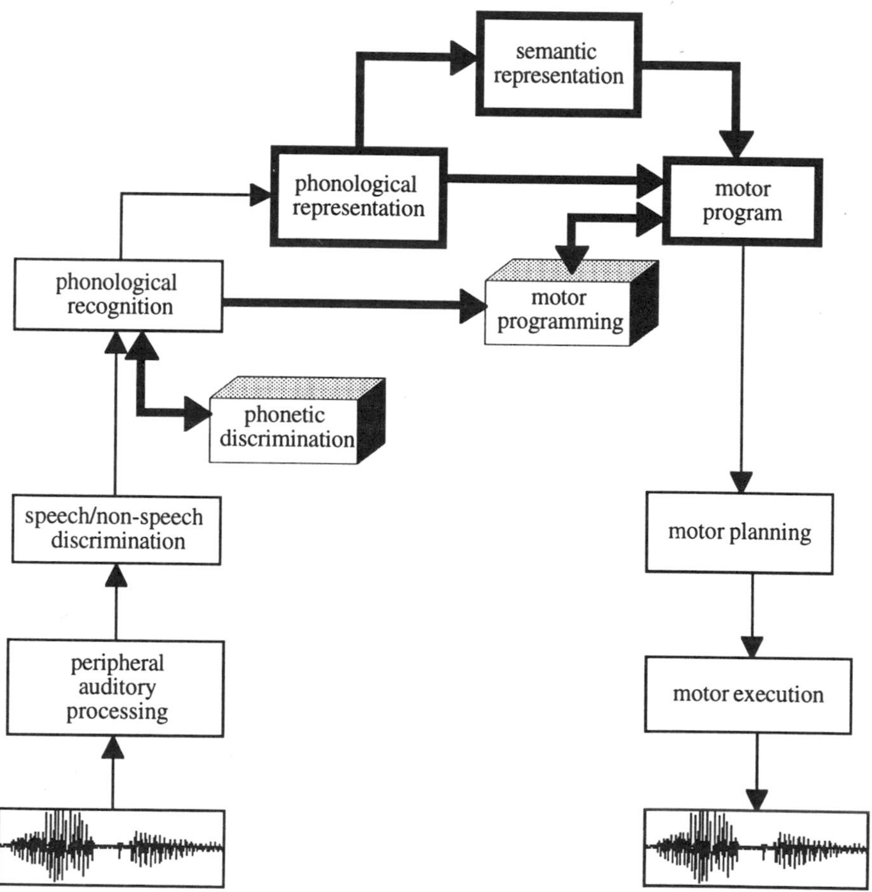

Figure 6.13: The complete model

Now that we have the complete model, we can try to trace the processing routes involved in some of the tasks incorporated in the assessment framework that involve output as well as input.

ACTIVITY 6.3

Aim: To understand the psycholinguistic nature of popular speech output and phonological awareness tasks by drawing their routes through the speech processing model presented in Figure 6.13.

In the tests considered here, some spoken output is required from the child, so the right-hand side of the model comes into play. For this activity, you will require transparencies, coloured pens and the diagram presented in Figure 6.14. This diagram depicts the boxes from the model in Figure 6.13, without the arrows.

As in Activity 6.1, tracking a route involves drawing a line to connect each box you believe to be involved for the successful completion of the task. Again, each route should be drawn in a different colour on a separate transparency.

On the diagram in Figure 6.14, draw the processing routes involved in speech tasks (e) – (g). [Tasks (a) – (d) were tracked as part of Activity 6.1]. The letters in parentheses refer to the speech processing profile presented in Figure 5.1.

(e) Naming, e.g. the child is shown a picture of STAMPS, and is asked: "What's this?" (G).

(f) Nonword repetition, e.g. the child is asked to repeat the following word: PER'PLISTERONK /pə'plɪstəɹɒŋk/ (J) (from Gathercole and Baddeley, 1996).

(g) Rhyme production, e.g. the child is asked to say as many words as possible that rhyme with BOAT (H).

Check your drawings against Key to Activity 6.3 (i) – (iv) at the end of this chapter, then read the following.

In task (e), naming, there is no spoken input since the stimulus presented is a picture, so the auditory processing route required for tasks (a) – (d) in Activity 6.1 is not involved. Processing starts with the semantic representation, which is activated by the picture (provided the child recognizes the picture and knows the word STAMPS). If the word is already well known to the child, s/he is able to access the motor program associated with it in the lexical representation, which has been built up previously by pronouncing the word on many occasions. The motor program is then forwarded to motor planning, where further phonetic aspects of the utterance are planned (tempo, intonation pattern etc.), and instructions sent to the articulators in motor execution, for the co-ordinated movements of lungs, vocal folds, tongue, lips and soft palate required for accurate pronunciation of STAMPS. [See Route 5 in Key to Activity 6.3 (i).]

In task (f), nonword repetition, peripheral auditory processing and speech/nonspeech discrimination are involved, since the stimulus is a spoken word. Although not a word of English, PER'PLISTERONK /pə'plɪstəɹɒŋk/ conforms to English phonological patterns, and thus proceeds to phonological recognition (cf. Route 1 in Activity 6.1). When the child has to repeat a word, s/he is likely to search the lexicon to establish if the word already exists, since, if it does, a pre-existing motor program can be utilized [as for STAMPS in task (e)]. In order to locate the

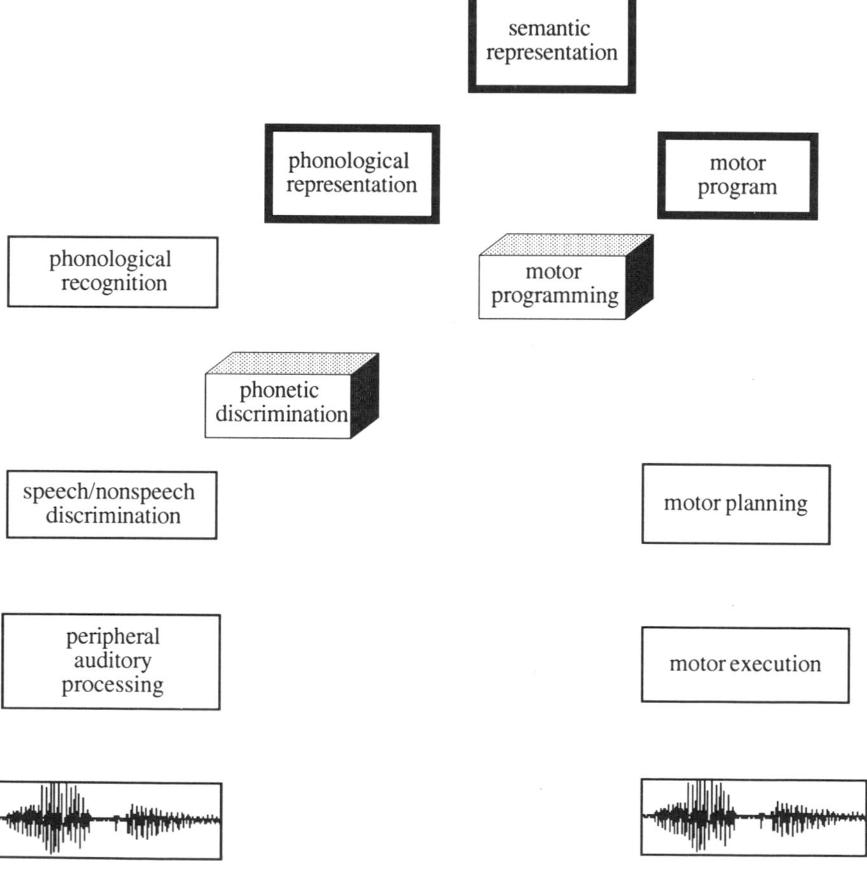

Figure 6.14: Complete model without arrows

word in the lexicon, the child first has to scan the phonological representations stored there (cf. Route 2 in Activity 6.1). On finding no entry for PER'PLISTERONK, the child then has to create a new motor program as the basis for a spoken response. For this to be done accurately, a phonological representation first has to be created, against which subsequent pronunciation can be checked for accuracy. Creation of a phonological representation requires segmentation and parsing of the stored percept into phonological constituents, i.e. syllables, then syllable constituents (onset ~ rhyme), possibly also segmenting the rhymes, e.g. [ɒŋk] into [ɒ] + [ŋk] and even the codas: [ŋk] into [ŋ]+ [k]. This is achieved at the phonological recognition level. Once a phonological representation has been created in this way, it is forwarded to motor programming, where the appropriate phonological units, with gestural targets encoded in them, are located and assembled in the correct sequence. This then forms the new motor program, which is part of a new lexical representation which also contains the new phonological representation (the latter will serve as a basis for recognition if the word is heard again); but there is no semantic representation, as PER'PLISTERONK as yet has not been assigned any meaning. The motor program is then forwarded to the motor planning stage, the remainder of the process being as for STAMPS in task (e). [See Route 6 in Key to Activity 6.3 (ii)].

In task (g), BOAT has to pass through peripheral auditory processing and speech/nonspeech discrimination, and be recognized as conforming to English phonological patterns in phonological recognition, where it then has to be parsed into onset and rhyme: [b] + [əʊt]. The rhyme constituent is then forwarded to motor programming, where a suitable onset is selected, e.g. [l], which is then assembled to the rhyme, to create a new motor program: [ləʊt]. This is forwarded to motor planning, then to motor execution. In order to create more than one rhyming response, the latter part of the route has to be repeated, i.e. from the selection of a new onset through to motor execution. For this to happen successfully, the rhyme has to be held in working memory, which may involve subvocal or audible rehearsal of the rhyme [əʊt] or of the whole target BOAT. This is evident in the strategy adopted by many young children when performing the rhyme production task, of repeating aloud the target word before each attempt, e.g. "boat [ləʊt] boat coat boat dote" (Vance, Stackhouse and Wells, 1994). This rehearsal route involves the motor program, motor planning and motor execution for the word being rehearsed.The child then has to process his or her own speech output, via phonological recognition and motor programming. [See Route 7 in Key to Activity 6.3 (iii)].

There is an alternative, lexical processing route for task (g) which results in real word rhymes only. As for Route 7, BOAT is processed up to phonological recognition. However, instead of being parsed into its constituents, the stimulus directly activates adjacently stored phonological representations that share the same rhyme, e.g. COAT. The phonological representation of the activated lexical item COAT then activates its stored motor program directly, which is in turn forwarded to motor planning and motor execution. [See Route 8, Key to Activity 6.3 (iv)].

As part of Activities 6.1 and 6.3, we have now drawn eight routes, illustrating the processing demands involved in some popular assessment tasks. As in Activity 6.2, we will now compare and contrast the processing routes involved for the different tasks in order to identify the commonalities and differences between them.

ACTIVITY 6.4

Aim: To compare and contrast the processing routes involved in tasks included in Activities 6.1 and 6.3.

Take your transparencies of the routes drawn in Activities 6.1 and 6.3. Overlay them on the diagram in Figure 6.14 as follows, identifying the commonalities and differences between the following pairs of routes:

(i) Routes 3 and 5 Check against Key to Activity 6.4 (i);
(ii) Routes 5 and 6 Check against Key to Activity 6.4 (ii);
(iii) Routes 1 and 6 Check against Key to Activity 6.4 (iii);
(iv) Routes 6 and 7 Check against Key to Activity 6.4 (iv);
(v) Routes 7 and 8 Check against Key to Activity 6.4 (v).

Then read the following.

(i) Comparison of Route 3 (auditory lexical decision) and Route 5 (naming). This demonstrates that the auditory visual lexical decision task and the naming task have one important element in common: both require access to semantic knowledge.

(ii) Comparison of Route 5 (naming) and Route 6 (nonword repetition). This demonstrates that the phonological processing involved in a test of nonword repetition is much more complex than for naming, although the latter (unlike the former) requires semantic knowledge.

(iii) Comparison of Route 1 (nonword auditory discrimination) and Route 6 (nonword repetition). This demonstrates the similarities and differences in processing between two nonword tasks: auditory discrimination and repetition. It shows that one of the difficulties with nonword auditory discrimination is that some steps of processing (e.g. access to semantic and phonological representations) are not available, putting pressure on temporary storage mechanisms. This is equally true of nonword repetition, but here there is the additional burden of carrying out segmentation and assembly tasks, as well as motor execution.

(iv) Comparison of Route 6 (nonword repetition) and Route 7 (rhyme production – nonlexical route). This highlights the similarity, in terms of processing routes, between nonword repetition and rhyme production. Both involve phonological recognition, segmentation, a possible attempt to access the phonological representation and creation of a new motor program. Rhyme production makes a greater demand in terms of temporary storage and the feedback loop, whereas nonword repetition may make greater demands in terms of motor planning and execution, as the stimuli are often longer and more complex than in rhyme production tasks.

(v) Comparison of Route 7 (rhyme production – nonlexical route) and Route 8 (rhyme production – lexical route). This highlights the difference between using a lexical route for rhyme production, through which rhyming responses will all be real words from the child's vocabulary, as opposed to the nonlexical route, which is likely to produce nonwords just as readily as real words.

In Activities 6.1 and 6.3 we traced on the model seven tasks of the kind used when drawing up a speech processing profile, in order to show how the processing demands of different tasks can be compared. You can do the same for any of the other tasks described in Chapter 4 (e.g. rhyme detection, real word repetition) or any other speech processing tasks with which you are familiar. You can also compare the routes involved in any two (or more) such tasks, as we did in Activities 6.2 and 6.4.

As we stated at the outset, the model is intended primarily as a stimulus for thinking about speech processing. It can be used to analyse assessment tasks as we have done here, and to locate children's specific areas of strength and weakness (see Chapters 9 and 10). What it does not do is locate specific disorders in specific boxes. Although one might with some confidence say that the child with a profound hearing loss has a difficulty with peripheral auditory perception or that the child with a cleft lip and palate will have problems with motor execution, this does not disbar them from having deficits at other levels of processing too. For example, although developmental verbal dyspraxia has been described as a motor programming difficulty, it is oversimplistic to isolate the difficulties experienced by such children to one box representing the motor programming function. This would be a limited view to take because, in developmental terms, a problem with motor programming can have far-reaching effects throughout the speech processing system (e.g. on auditory discrimination of complex words and on lexical representations). Further, as discussed in Chapter 1, case study research has emphasized individual speech processing differences between children who have been given the same diagnostic label. The model is therefore best suited to the analysis of individual cases, rather than to the classification of disorders in general terms. Chapters 9 and 10 illustrate how to do this and the model is reproduced in Appendix 4 for you to copy for use with clients.

A final word of caution: the model presented in this chapter is not intended to be in any way definitive, nor does it claim to have neuroanatomical reality. It will inevitably change and develop in the light of research and the experience of practitioners working with children with speech and literacy problems.

Summary

- The model focuses on speech processing and is related to the assessment framework presented in Chapters 4 and 5.
- Building a model helps us to be more explicit about the levels of processing assumed within the assessment framework presented in Chapters 4 and 5.
- Tracking processing routes through the model pinpoints the demands made by different tests in common usage, e.g. how a test can be tapping more than one level.
- Overlaying these routes reveals the commonalities and differences between tests in terms of their processing demands and helps to identify where a child's difficulties might be.
- It is not the case that there is one test for each box, e.g. motor programming will be tapped by both a nonword repetition test and a rhyme production test.
- General diagnostic categories (e.g. dyspraxia, dysarthria, phonological disorder) should not be equated with deficits in particular boxes.
- The model embodies a way of thinking; it is not intended to map on to neuroanatomical 'reality' in a direct way.
- The model is not comprehensive; it is impossible to present all aspects of speech processing in a single two-dimensional model.
- The model is not definitive and will inevitably change.

KEY TO ACTIVITY 6.1

(i) Route 1 – real word discrimination (nonlexical route) and nonword discrimination

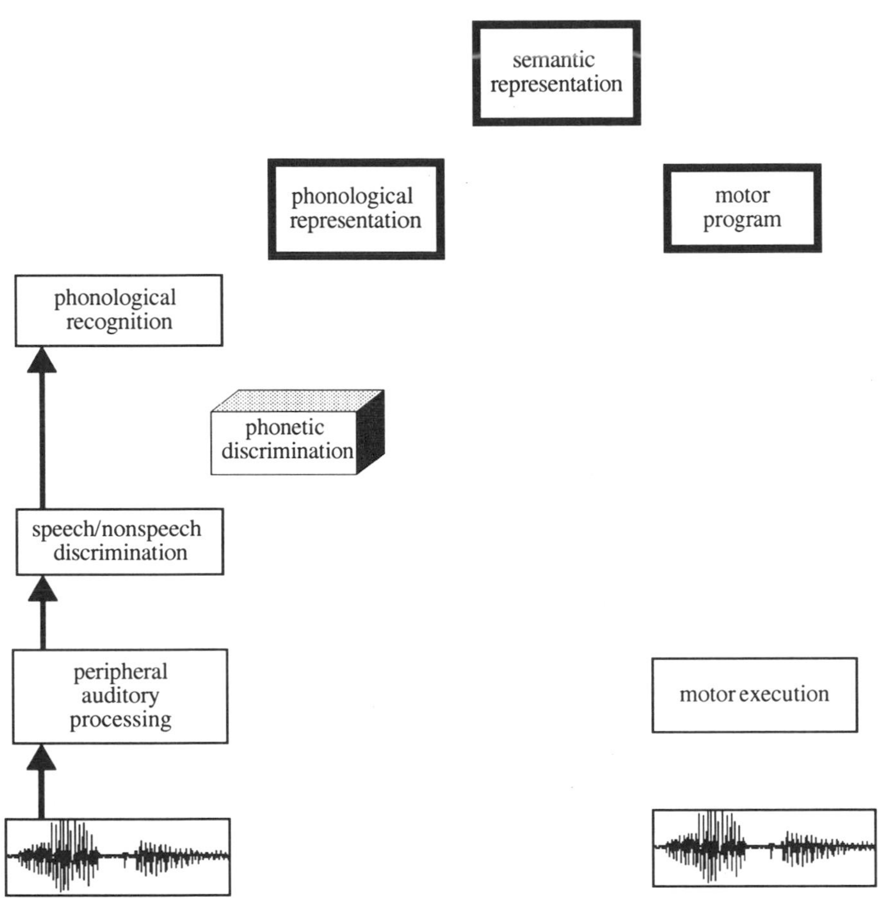

KEY TO ACTIVITY 6.1

(ii) Route 2 – real word discrimination (lexical route)

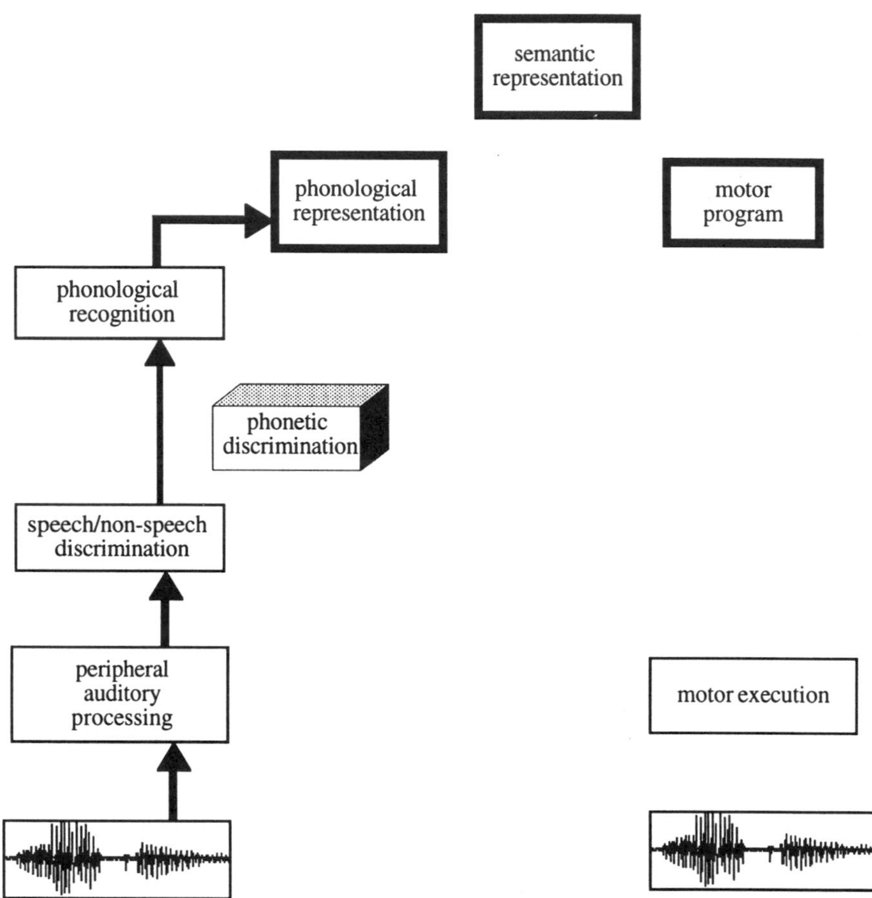

KEY TO ACTIVITY 6.1

(iii) Route 3 – auditory lexical decision

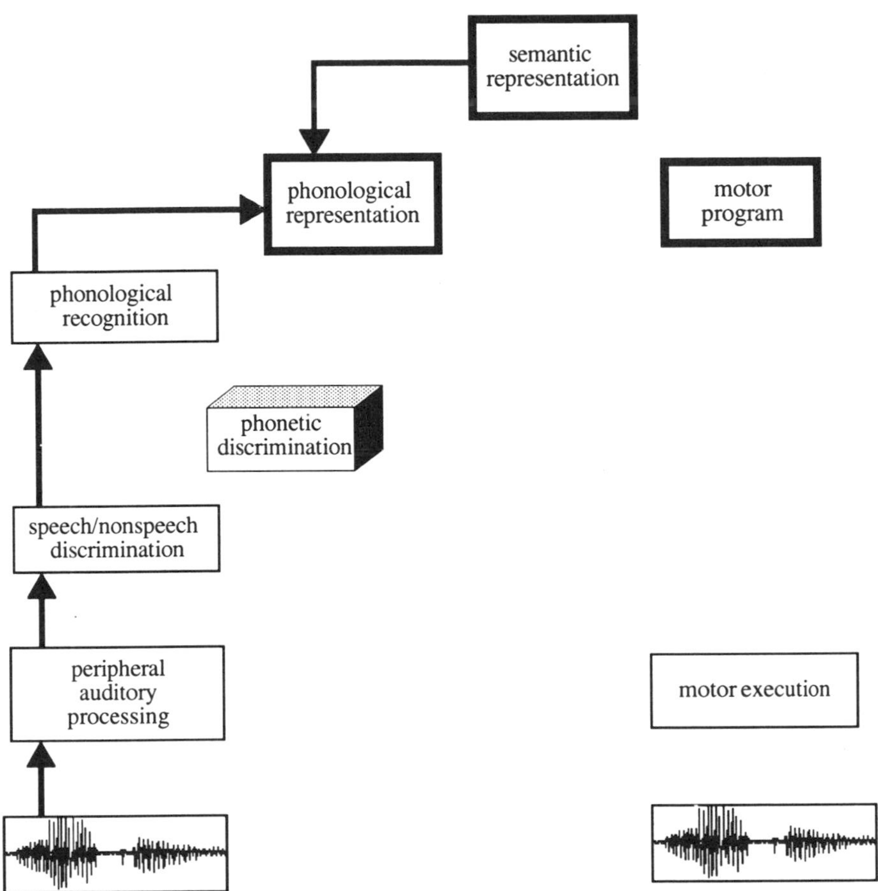

KEY TO ACTIVITY 6.1
(iv) Route 4 – nonspeech discrimination

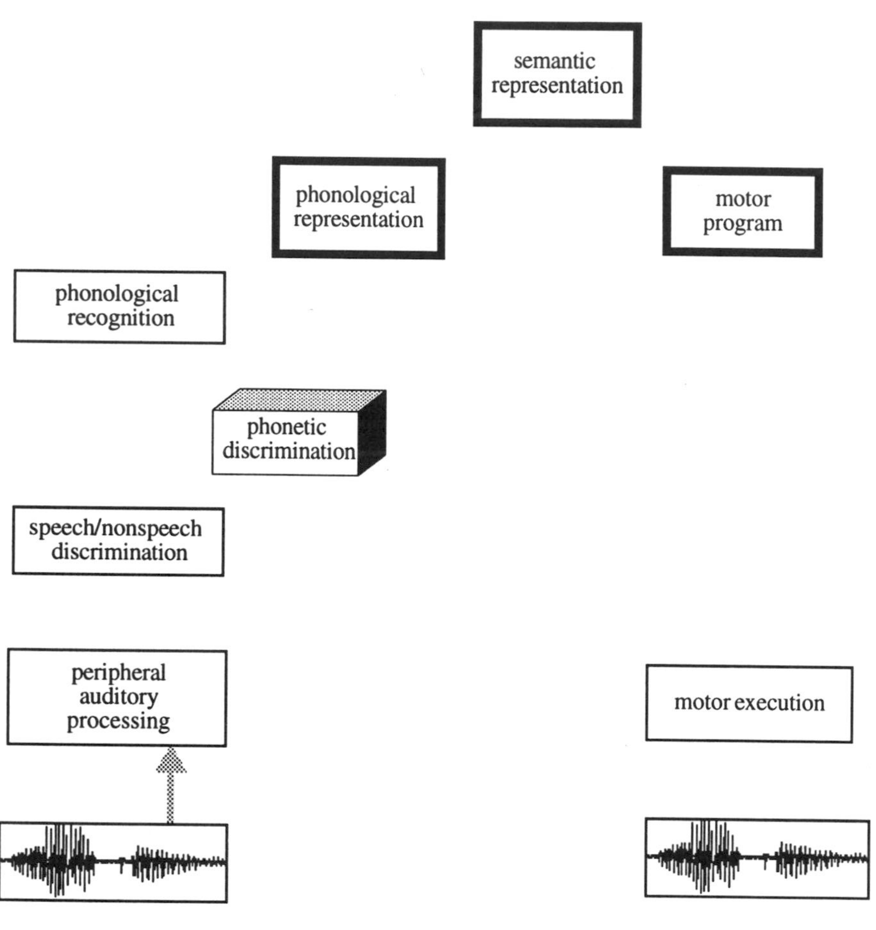

KEY TO ACTIVITY 6.2

(i) Routes 1 and 2 compared

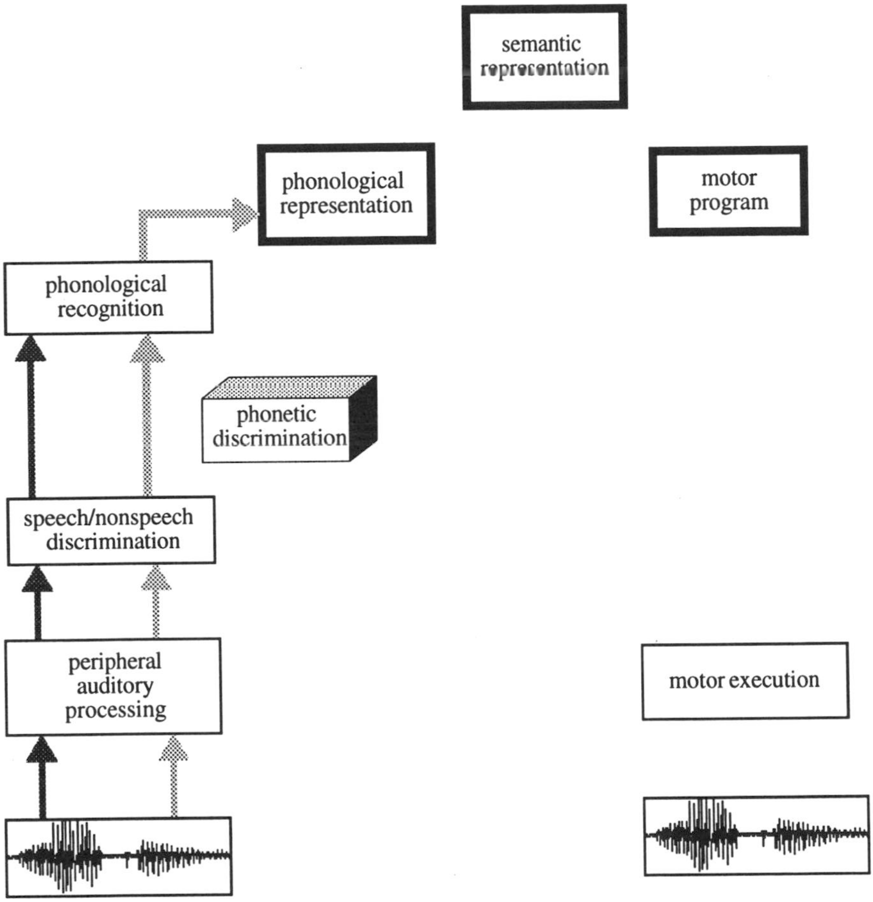

semantic representation

phonological representation

motor program

phonological recognition

phonetic discrimination

speech/nonspeech discrimination

peripheral auditory processing

motor execution

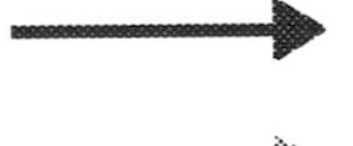

Route 1 – real word discrimination (nonlexical route) and nonword discrimination

Route 2 – real word discrimination (lexical route)

KEY TO ACTIVITY 6.2

(ii) Routes 2 and 3 compared

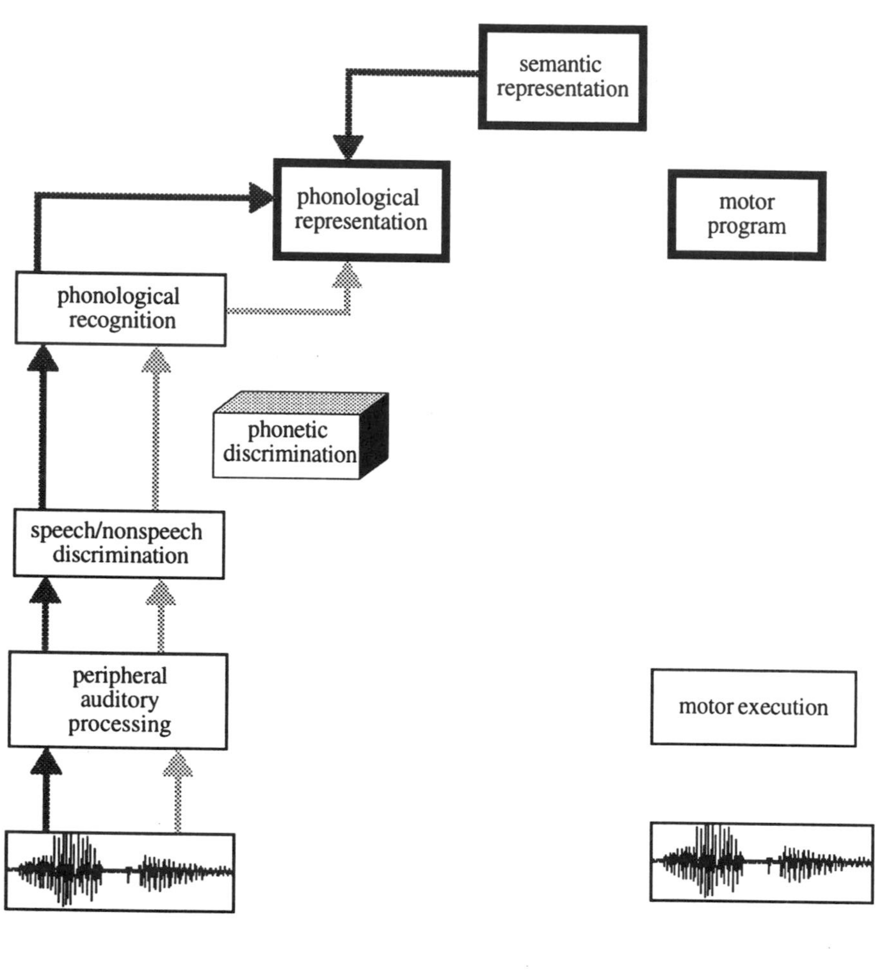

Route 2 – real word discrimination (nonlexical route) and nonword discrimination

Route 3 – auditory lexical decision

KEY TO ACTIVITY 6.3

(i) Route 5 – naming

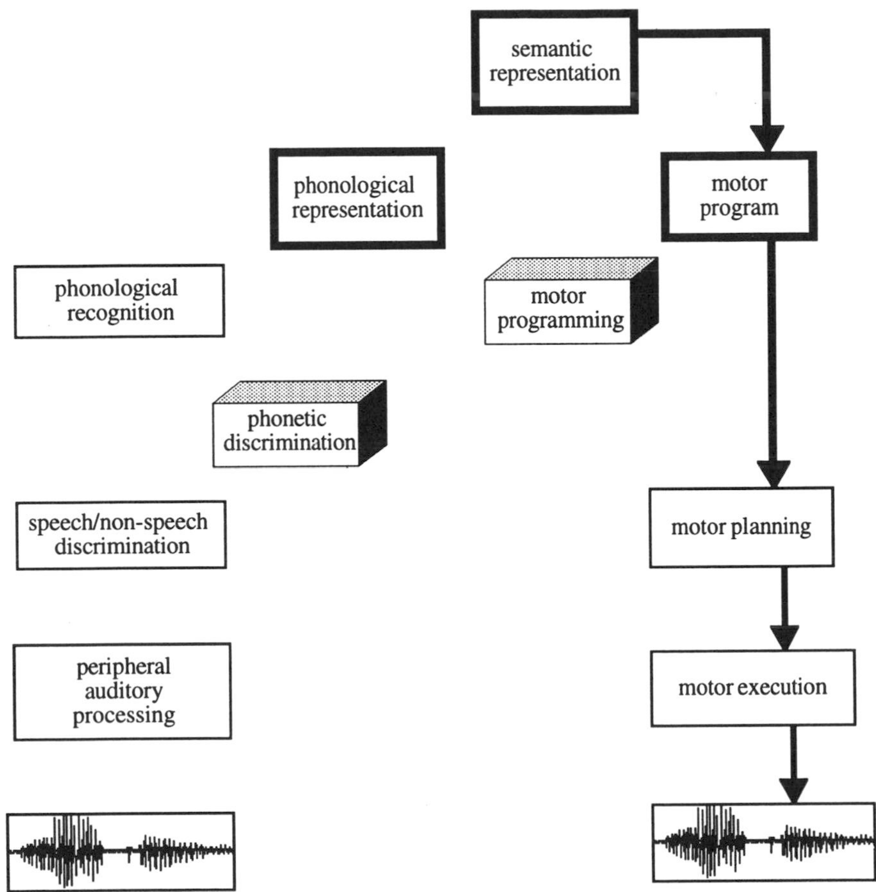

KEY TO ACTIVITY 6.3

(ii) Route 6 – nonword repetition

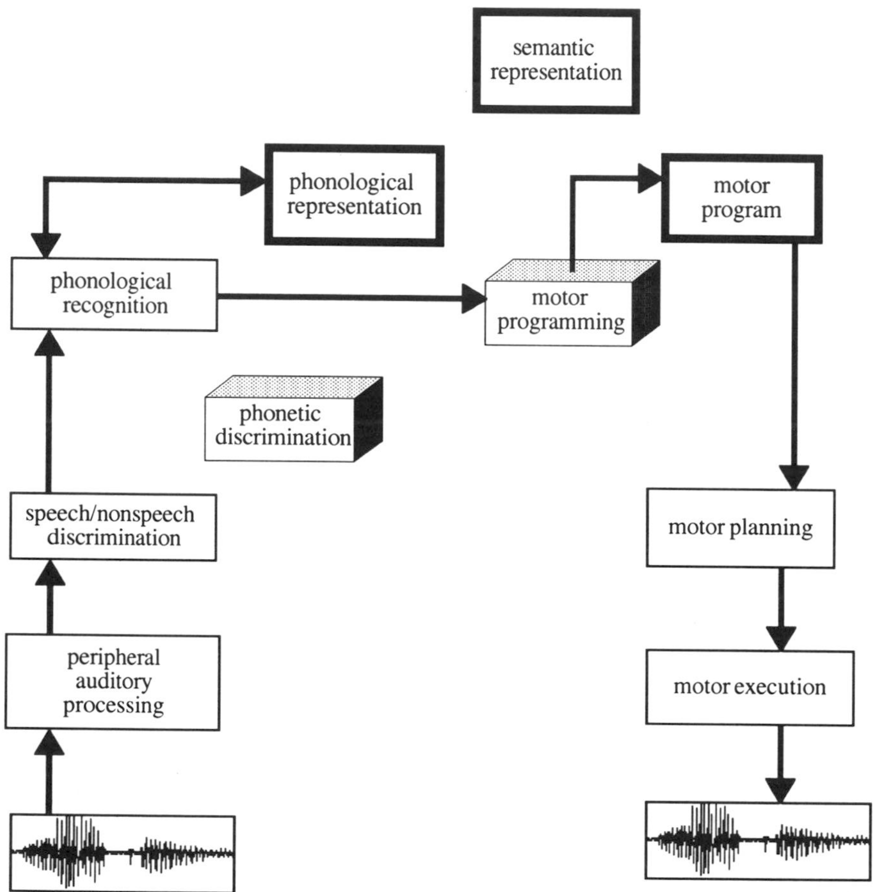

KEY TO ACTIVITY 6.3

(iii) Route 7 – rhyme production (nonlexical route)

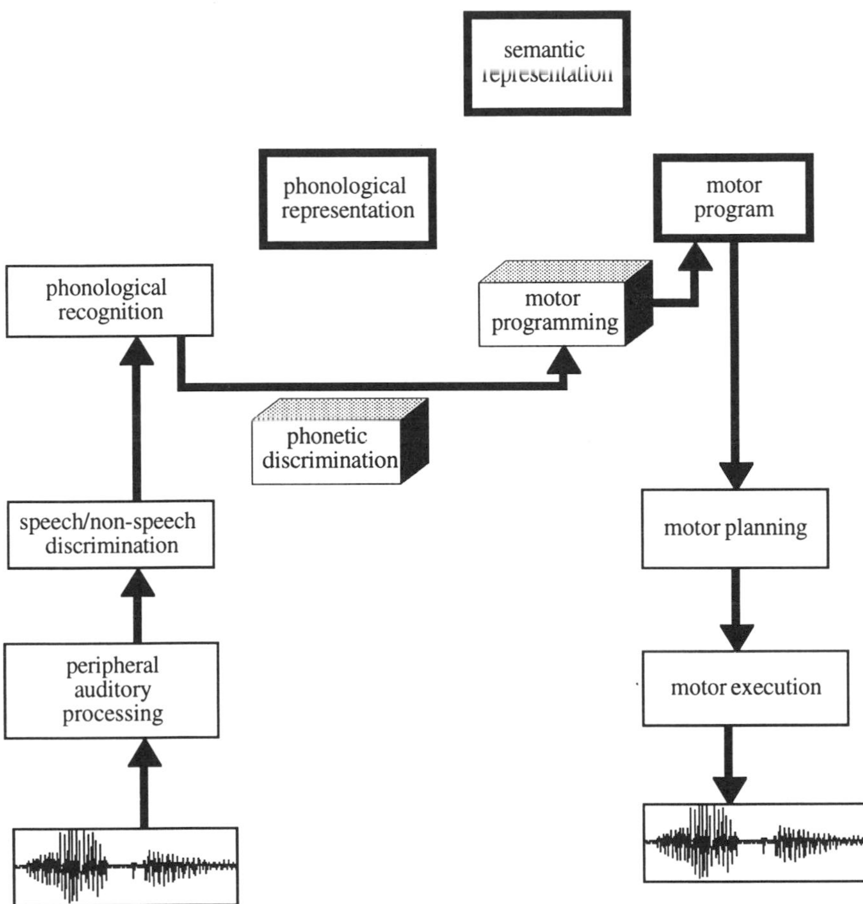

KEY TO ACTIVITY 6.3

(iv) Route 8 – rhyme production (lexical route)

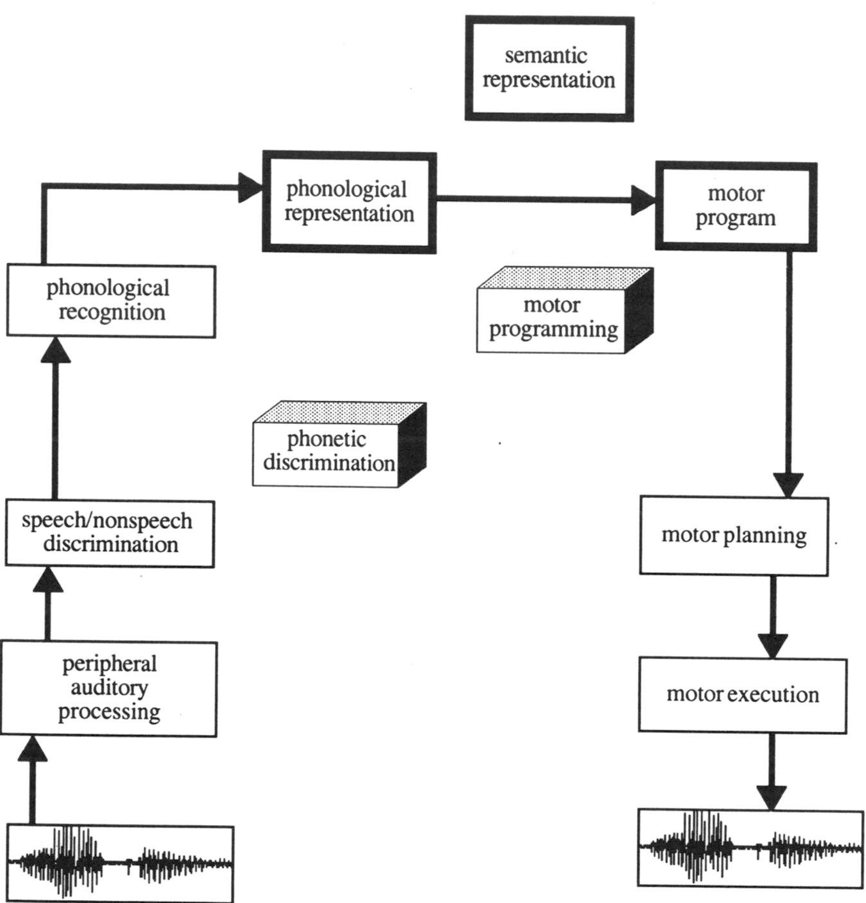

KEY TO ACTIVITY 6.4

(i) Routes 3 and 5 compared

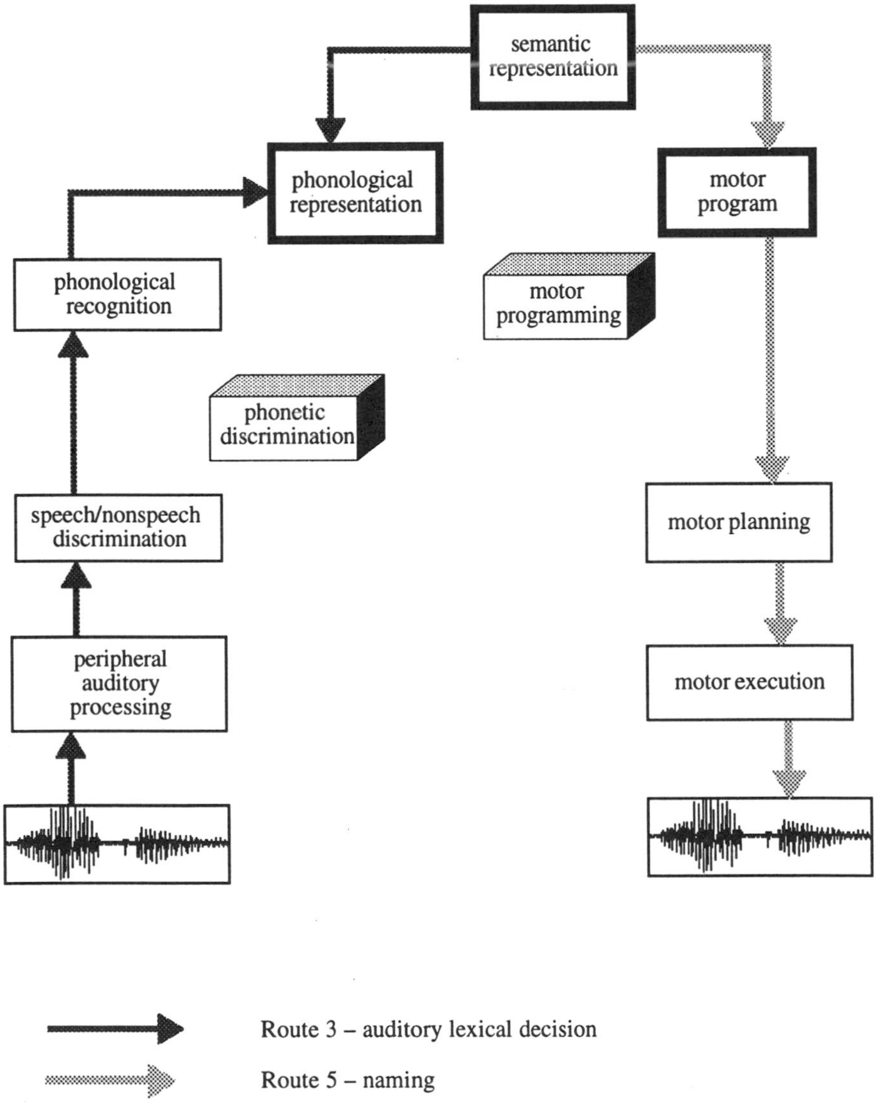

semantic representation
phonological representation
motor program
phonological recognition
motor programming
phonetic discrimination
speech/nonspeech discrimination
motor planning
peripheral auditory processing
motor execution
Route 3 – auditory lexical decision
Route 5 – naming

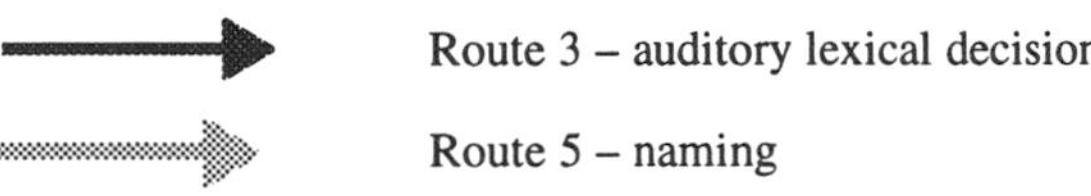

KEY TO ACTIVITY 6.4
(ii) Routes 5 and 6 compared

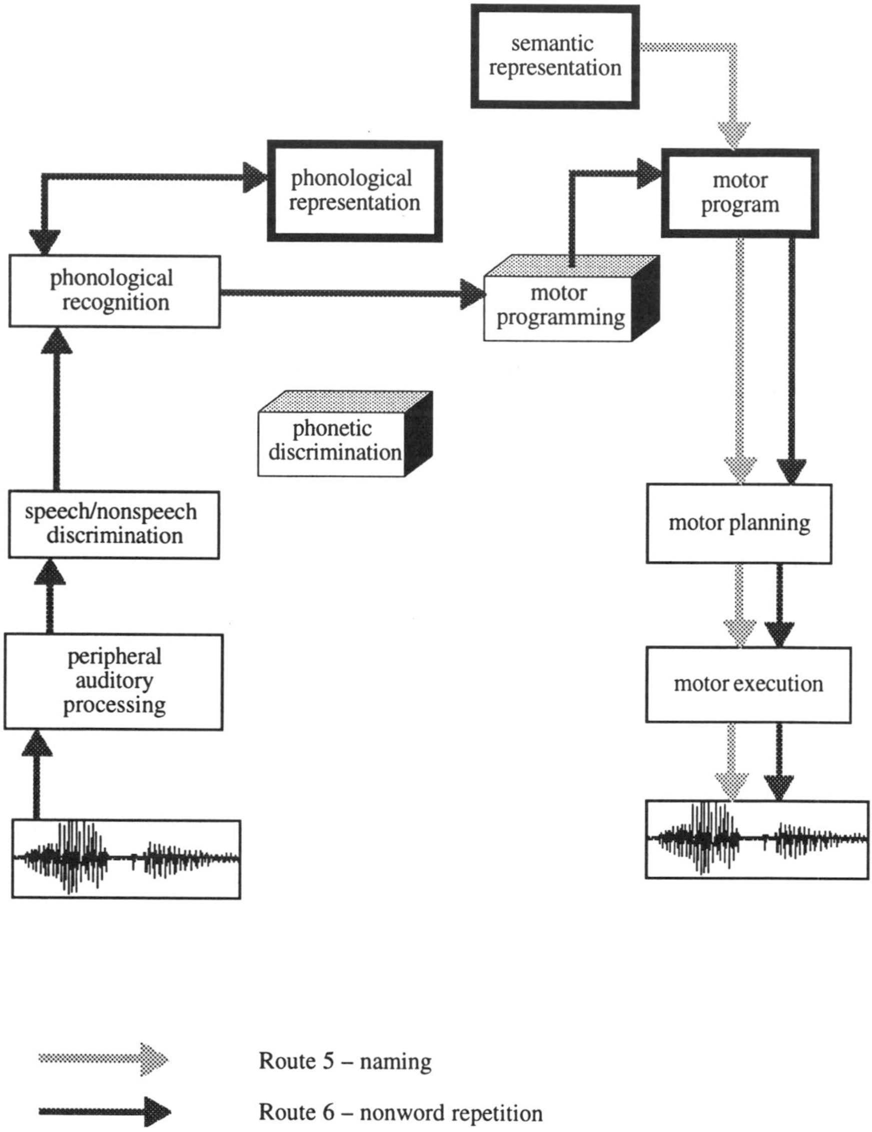

semantic representation
phonological representation
motor program
phonological recognition
motor programming
phonetic discrimination
speech/nonspeech discrimination
motor planning
peripheral auditory processing
motor execution
Route 5 – naming
Route 6 – nonword repetition

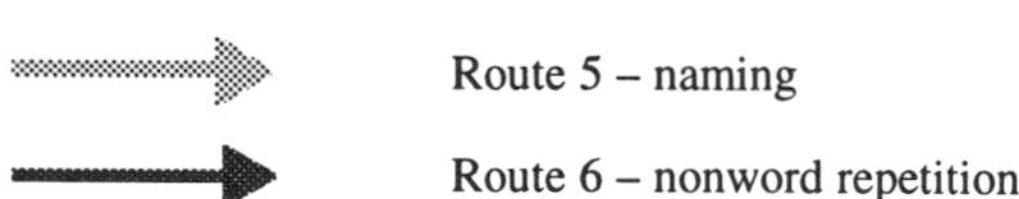

KEY TO ACTIVITY 6.4
(iii) Routes 1 and 6 compared

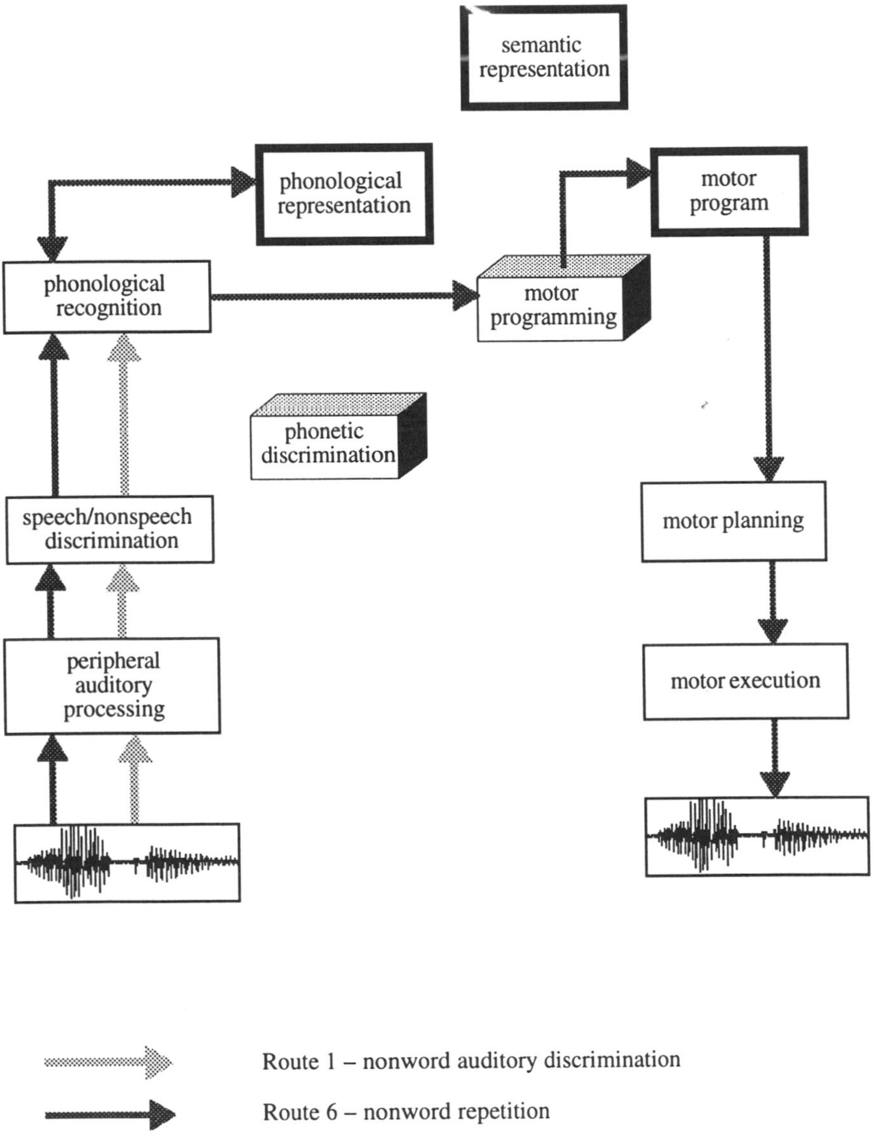

semantic representation
phonological representation
motor program
phonological recognition
motor programming
phonetic discrimination
speech/nonspeech discrimination
motor planning
peripheral auditory processing
motor execution
Route 1 – nonword auditory discrimination
Route 6 – nonword repetition

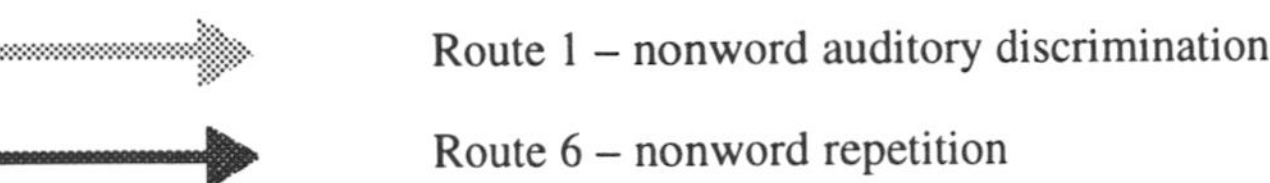

KEY TO ACTIVITY 6.4

(iv) Routes 6 and 7 compared

semantic representation

phonological representation

motor program

phonological recognition

motor programming

phonetic discrimination

speech/nonspeech discrimination

motor planning

peripheral auditory processing

motor execution

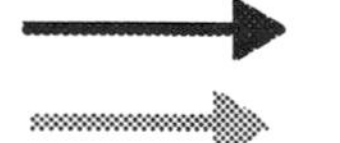

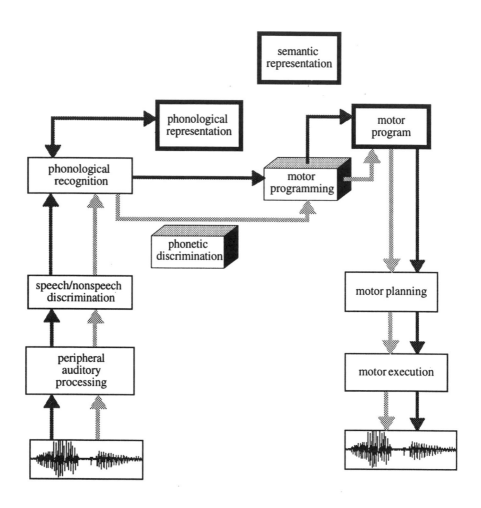

Route 6 – nonword repetition

Route 7 – rhyme production (nonlexical route)

KEY TO ACTIVITY 6.4

(v) Routes 7 and 8 compared

semantic representation

phonological representation

motor program

phonological recognition

motor programming

phonetic discrimination

speech/nonspeech discrimination

motor planning

peripheral auditory processing

motor execution

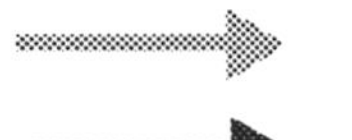

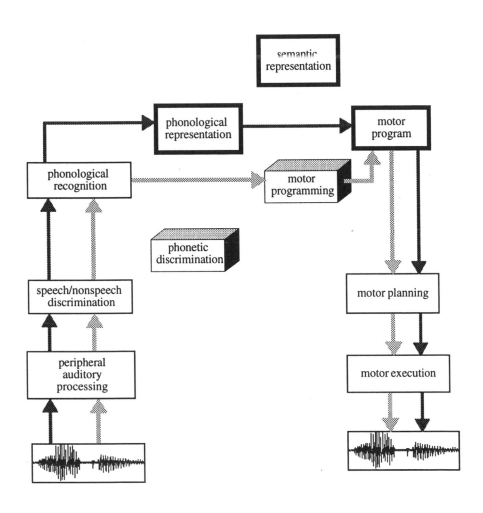

Route 7 – rhyme production (nonlexical route)

Route 8 – rhyme production (lexical route)

Chapter 7
Phases of Development I – From Cries to Words

The information processing model presented in Chapter 6 helps us to understand how children tackle various assessment tasks and at which levels they are having difficulties with speech processing. However, it does not help us to understand whether success or failure at a particular task is to be expected of a child of a particular age. It is one thing to find out that a child cannot do a particular speech processing task and to understand where the processing is breaking down. It is another matter to determine whether failure on the task is only to be expected in a child of that age and phase of development, or whether the failure is indicative of a specific problem. Because we are dealing with children, we need to address the issue of how normally-developing children change over time and how they develop their speech processing skills. With this background knowledge of normal development we can gain a fuller appreciation of the nature of speech processing difficulties in children and how they might best be remediated.

In 1985, Uta Frith discussed the problems of applying processing models that are used to explain acquired dyslexia (as found in some adults following a stroke, for example) to children with developmental dyslexia. Pointing out 'the fallacy that developmental and acquired disorders are one and the same thing', she stressed the importance of moving away from rigid box models when trying to explain the changes that occur in normal and atypical development in children (Frith, 1985). In preference, she adopted a phase model to account for normal development of literacy skills, within which dyslexia is seen as an arrest in development at the logographic phase – an early visual whole word reading phase prior to developing alphabetic skills (see Chapter 1).

Frith's approach helps us to see children with literacy difficulties in a more positive light. They are not 'disordered' or fundamentally different from normally-developing children, but in certain aspects of their development they have not moved on to the next phase in the way that studies of normally-developing children lead us to expect. It is also a useful conceptual framework in which to develop a progressive remediation programme aimed at supporting the child through a phase or phases in which they are having difficulty. In severe cases of arrested development, remediation is aimed at developing compensatory strategies to get round a troublesome phase of development and thus move on to later phases where the child may be able to experience some success. Knowledge of normal developmental progression therefore allows us not only to identify when a child is in difficulties with one or more aspects of their development, but also gives us some insight into how such a difficulty might be remediated.

In this chapter, Frith's general approach is adapted to the study of children's speech development. The aim is to give a developmental dimension to the model of speech processing presented in Chapter 6, by considering how its different components emerge in the normally-developing child. We present an overview of how the maturing speech processing system allows the developing child to undertake more complex and demanding processing tasks. This provides a context for exploring the nature of speech difficulties in children, and the relationship between speech and literacy difficulties.

The phases of speech development outlined in this chapter are descriptive, rather than explanatory stages (cf. Ingram, 1989, Chapter 3). While our aim is to show in broad terms how speech processing behaviour changes over time in the course of normal development, we do not offer detailed arguments for why these phases occur when they do, for example in terms of theories of biological, cognitive or social development. The descriptive framework used is that of the speech processing model presented in Chapter 6. Each phase has a label which derives from the type or types of behaviour which are new at that phase, and thus characterize it. We associate each phase with an approximate chronological age range, as is customary in many developmental linguistic profiles that are designed to have a clinical application (e.g. Grunwell, 1985; Crystal, Fletcher, and Garman, 1989). For example, the Prelexical Phase covers the first year of life up to the emergence of first words. However, the emergence of first words occurs before the first birthday in some children, and well after it in others. The references to age throughout this chapter are thus indicative only and should not be interpreted strictly: the developmental phase approach embodies the notion that one set of behaviours will precede those characteristic of the next phase, irrespective of the precise chronological age at which each phase is reached. A second caveat is that the phases presented are broad in their coverage, and gloss over the detailed development that takes place within each one. Further information about the extensive research into phonological development that underpins this and the next chapter can be found in Ingram (1989), Ferguson, Menn and Stoel-Gammon (1992) and particularly Vihman (1996).

The Prelexical Phase

The neonate

Healthy infants of just a few weeks are feeding, and making the sounds associated with that activity, as well as crying when hungry or uncomfortable, but they do not produce speech-like sounds. They respond to sound, including speech. Using techniques such as measuring change in sucking rate, researchers have shown that normally-developing infants of a few weeks are capable of detecting slight phonetic differences, as between [pa] and [ba]; [ba] and [da] . Furthermore, they are better than adults at discriminating between pairs of speech sounds which are either not present or are not linguistically significant in the language to which they are exposed (e.g. for English infants, the difference between oral and nasalized vowels, which is contrastive in French but not English). For an extensive review of research on the infant's perception and production at this phase, the reader is referred to Chapters 3–5 of Vihman (1996). We will now consider the speech processing capabilities of the neonate, in terms of the model presented in Chapter 6.

ACTIVITY 7.1.

Aim: To establish which components of the psycholinguistic model presented in Chapter 6 are needed to explain the verbal behaviour of a neonate.

Using a transparency (or tracing paper) and a coloured pen, circle the boxes on the speech processing model in Figure 7.1 that are already active in the neonate. (Figure 7.1 reproduces the completed model of speech processing from Figure 6.13.)

Check your answer with Key to Activity 7.1 at the end of this chapter, then read the following.

You have probably circled *peripheral auditory processing*, since the infant's hearing abilities are fully intact. Given the results of the studies mentioned above, we can be confident in also circling the next box up, *speech / nonspeech discrimination* and also include *phonetic discrimination*, since infants show the ability to discriminate between pairs of speech sounds, including sounds not found in the language to which they are being exposed. At this age there is, however, no evidence of a specific bias in auditory responses towards one language rather than another, so we would not circle *phonological recognition*. On the output side, you may have circled *motor execution*, to capture the observation that the child has intact speech organs with the potential to produce speech. However, the kinds of sounds produced, although resembling speech in so far as pitch and loudness vary, have little or no phonetic resemblance to words at this phase. On these grounds, motor execution should perhaps not be circled yet. There is no evidence for any processing higher up on the output side.

The child at 6 months

By 6 months, children are producing more recognizably speech-like sounds: pitch, loudness, friction and trilling can be manipulated, for example. Some are beginning to produce 'canonical' babbling, i.e. consonant–vowel (CV) sequences, starting with a single CV e.g. [ba], which will be reiterated, e.g. [ba ba ba]. The vocalizations of infants at 6 months are not recognizable as coming from one language background rather than another: French adults cannot reliably tell apart the babble

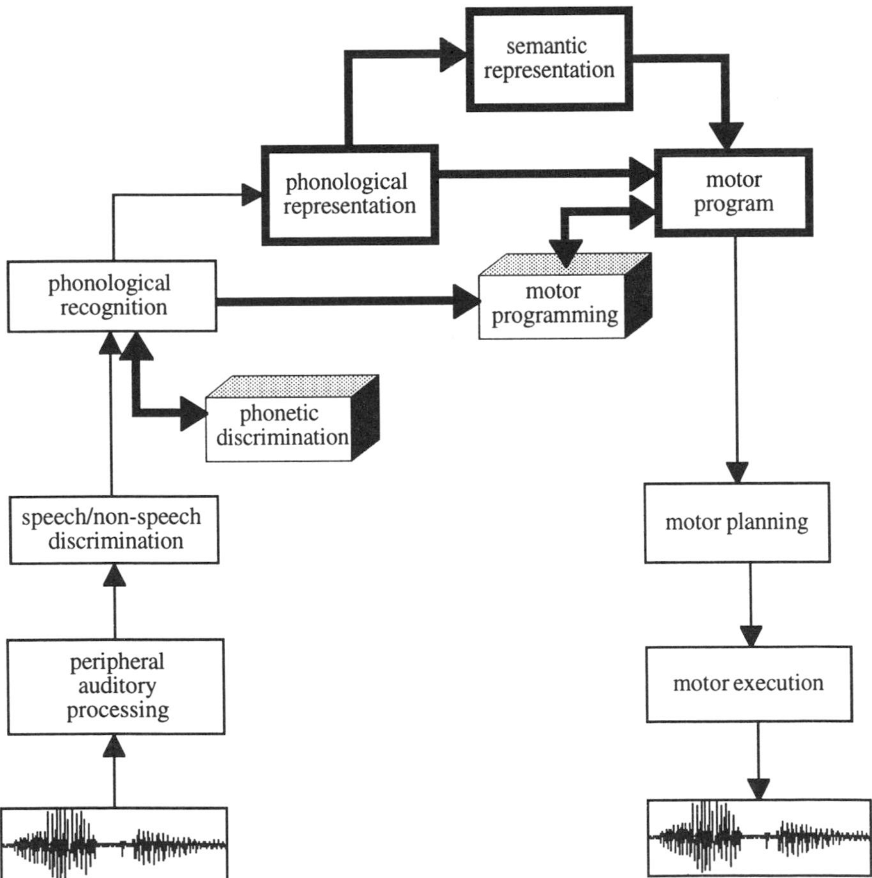

Figure 7.1: The complete model for Activity 7.1

of French infants from the babble of Arabic infants, for example (Boysson-Bardies, Hallé, Sagart, et al., 1989).

From the environmental context within which familiar words are introduced, children begin to recognize some spoken words, e.g. MUMMY, TEDDY. They still do not show a perceptual preference for the phonological contrasts of the ambient language, as opposed to contrasts found in languages to which they are not exposed. This applies to segments, syllables and phonotactic structures (e.g. language-specific sequences of consonants). However, at 6 months there are some first signs of tuning in to the ambient language, on the basis of prosodic features. Thus, a group of 6-month-old American infants demonstrated a preference for a spoken list of English words compared to a matched list of Norwegian words, while the same preference was not evident when English words were presented together with Dutch words. Norwegian words are quite distinct from English words in terms of pitch and other aspects of prosodic patterning, whereas Dutch and English are quite similar in these respects (Juszcyk, Friederici, Wessels, et al., 1993). The psycholinguistic model needs to take these developments into account.

ACTIVITY 7.2.

Aim: To establish what components of the psycholinguistic model presented in Chapter 6 are needed to explain the verbal behaviour of a 6-month-old child.

Using a transparency (or tracing paper) and a coloured pen, circle the boxes on the speech processing model (Figure 7.1) that are already active in the 6-month-old child. Use a different coloured pen to the one you used in Activity 7.1, so that the transparencies, when overlaid, give a picture of normal development.

Check your answer with Key to Activity 7.2 at the end of this chapter, then read the following.

Six-month-old children's ability to recognize some words indicates that they must have laid down lexical representations for those words, and that those lexical representations must include a phonological representation that is adequate for recognition purposes. The *phonological representation* box should therefore be circled. However, there is no evidence that such young children have performed any kind of segmentation or analysis of the perceptual gestalt (e.g. for TEDDY), into constituents such as syllable, onset or rhyme, let alone smaller segments. Indeed, there is only very slight evidence that they are aware that the word is phonetically and phonologically specific to one language, this being prosodic rather than segmental. The *phonological recognition* box does not therefore need to be circled yet.

As well as the phonological representation, there must also be a *semantic representation* for TEDDY within the lexical representation, since the child associates a meaning to TEDDY when s/he hears the word spoken. The semantic representation should therefore be circled, but not linked to the *motor program* within the lexical representation, since the child does not yet attempt to pronounce TEDDY .

Although there are no lexical representations containing motor programs yet, *motor programming* is already active, producing the CV sequences found in the child's babble, and so should be circled. At this phase, the store in the motor programming box is limited, containing perhaps just one or two syllable types (V, CV) and a small set of items that can fill the the V (rhyme) slot and the C (onset) slot, particularly stop consonants and nasals such as [p], [b], [n]. Some more 'exotic' or 'wild' sound types may also occur, i.e. ones which are not found in the ambient language, such as trills in English. Motor programming produces *motor programs*, so that box should be circled too. However, it is important to recognize that a motor program at this phase is not linked to a semantic representation and a phonological representation. To make this clear, the semantic and phonological representations can be included within a single circle, while the motor program is in a separate circle. On the model, this phase of development can be captured by having no arrows to link the semantic and phonological representations to the motor program, as in Key to Activity 7.2.

The observation that deaf children begin to babble in spite of the lack of speech input (Locke, 1983), suggests that at least at this early phase of development, speech output is not necessarily linked to input, i.e. that the ability to babble is not dependent on having heard others talk, or indeed on hearing oneself babble. On the model, this can be captured by having no linking arrows between the left and right sides of the diagram (see Key to Activity 7.2).

On the output side, the motor program (for babble) is given a motor plan, and then is realized through movements of the articulators. As volitional control is very limited at this phase the *motor planning* box should only be circled very faintly! However, *motor execution* is active since, as has been noted, babies at this phase are beginning to produce a restricted range of articulations in babbling.

Implicit in this developmental account is the possibility that one or more components of the speech processing system may not come on stream in the normal way. For example, motor execution will be adversely affected by anatomical or neurological anomalies that affect the vocal tract, such as a cleft lip or palate, or in cases of dysarthria. Depending on the effectiveness of surgical or other medical intervention, such problems will affect the peripheral output processing of speech, giving rise to developmentally unusual speech patterns. A case that illustrates how a child's speech patterns can be attributed to this peripheral level of output processing is presented by Harris and Cottam (1985). Mike, who is from South Yorkshire (England) was seen at CA 4;11. Oral examination revealed no structural abnormalities, but at rest a general laxness of lips and tongue, with lips parted and tongue tip slightly protruding. An element of developmental dysarthria was thought to underlie his speech difficulties. His speech reveals patterns which are in many respects different from those commonly identified in normal development, for example CAKE → [kheːʔs]; CAR → [xɑː], [khɑː]; COTTON → [kxɒsən]; MILK → [mɪʊx]; PAPER → [pheːɸə]; SUGAR → [səsə]. These patterns mainly affect target plosives, and can be summarized as follows:

(a) In all positions, target plosives and affricates may be realized as fricatives at the target place of articulation.
(b) Target plosives may be heavily aspirated, or realized as affricates at the same place of articulation as the target, particularly in word-initial position.

What these patterns have in common is a tendency for consonants that involve a high degree of oral closure – such as plosives [p] [t] [k] [g], where the articulators have to create a complete seal within the mouth so that pressure builds up – to be replaced by consonants that require less closure, such as fricatives [ɸ] [s] [x], where air is permitted to escape in the course of the articulation. Harris and Cottam state that these patterns 'can be attributed to a common underlying problem, one of articulatory weakening. This widespread operation of opening seems to stem from a general difficulty in achieving and maintaining a gesture of total occlusion in the oral cavity, which in all likelihood can be attributed to [Mike's] lack of muscle tone....'. In terms of our model, these patterns in Mike's speech are thus attributable to the level of motor execution, rather than to higher levels of phonological processing and organization. Developmentally, this represents an arrested development at the Prelexical Phase, as such neurological weakness is typically evident before the demands of language are made. However, this does not mean that other aspects of speech processing cannot develop. For instance, children with dysarthria are not particularly at risk for later difficulties with literacy and metaphonological skills such as rhyme (Bishop, 1985; Bishop and Robson, 1989). The same is true for children with cleft palate, another condition that primarily affects motor execution (Stackhouse, 1982).

The child at 9 months

By 9 months, some functional vocalizations are used (e.g. to express delight, anger or needs), often in conjunction with gesture. These typically have no particular resemblance to words of the ambient language, and will disappear later. Babble includes a greater range of CV sequences, and begins to take on characteristics that are peculiar to the ambient language. This is particularly true of features of voice quality, rhythm and pitch, which are markedly different between languages such as French and Arabic. Language-specific trends are also evident in the relative frequency of labial consonants. Vihman (1996, p.120) suggests that the latter development may reflect the great importance of visual information to the infant in acquiring the speech production patterns of the ambient language, since labial consonants like [m, p, b, f, v] are visually very salient. There is evidence that by this age deaf children's babbling is qualitatively different from that of hearing children (Oller, Eilers, Bull, et al., 1985).

On the input side, by 9 months children are showing sensitivity to familiar words as opposed to unfamiliar words from the ambient language (Jusczyk and Aslin, 1995). They begin to show a preference for common phonotactic structures from their own language, such as particular sequences of consonants (Jusczyk, Luce and Charles-Luce, 1994); and also for the most common word-stress pattern of English – the trochaic pattern of 'TIGER, where the stress is on the first syllable, as opposed to the iambic pattern of GI'RAFFE where the stress is on the last syllable (Jusczyk, Cutler and Redanz, 1993).

ACTIVITY 7.3

Aim: To establish which components of the psycholinguistic model presented in Chapter 6 are needed to explain the verbal behaviour of a 9-month-old child.

Using a transparency or tracing paper, circle the boxes on the model diagram in Figure 7.1 that are active in 9-month-old children but which were not active at 6 months. Use a different coloured pen, so that the transparencies, when overlaid, give a picture of development.

Check your diagram with Key to Activity 7.3 at the end of this chapter, then read the following.

On the input and output sides, we can see a drift towards language-specific processing. On the input side, the experimental evidence suggests that language-specific *phonological recognition* is now active, so this should be circled; and that the store of *phonological representations* has increased. On the output side, the store of syllables within *motor programming* is getting larger. Greater use of a wider range of recurrent patterns in babbling suggests that *motor planning* is more developed. The evidence that now babbling takes on features of the ambient language and that deaf children's babbling is qualitatively different from that of hearing children, indicates a link between the input side and motor programming, shown in Key to Activity 7.3 as an 'off-line' link between phonological recognition and motor programming.

As for the children's meaningful vocalizations, these must have a *motor program*, and also a *semantic representation* of some kind. For these vocalizations, then, we need to show the link between semantic representation and motor program, but exclude the phonological representation. This could be shown by drawing a circle that encompasses semantic representation and motor program, while excluding phonological representation. Alternatively, this can be shown by having two different semantic representation boxes, with different links, as in Key to Activity 7.3.

In this account of the Prelexical Phase, several references have been made to prelingually deaf children. In terms of the speech processing model, prelingual deafness can be viewed as a deficit at the peripheral level of auditory processing, which inevitably has consequences for all higher-up levels of input processing and, in turn, for speech output. Even though the deaf child's vocal tract may be fully functional and no different from a hearing child's, the deaf child will be unable to establish accurate phonological representations in the normal way. This is a major obstacle in the way of creating accurate motor programs for words and, for children with profound hearing loss, results in speech patterns which are characterized by 'exotic' vocalic and consonantal articulations, i.e. ones which are not found in the ambient language (Parker and Rose, 1990).

The speech difficulties associated with prelingual deafness can be viewed as the product of arrested development at the Prelexical Phase since, as with cleft palate or dysarthria on the output side, they are manifest before the child is confronted with demands of language. Although prelingual deafness has major knock-on effects for all the other components of the speech processing chain, this does not mean that there are problems with the components themselves – only with the input they are receiving. Thus, the vocal tract of the deaf child may be perfectly normal (motor execution); so too may the motor programming and motor planning components, and the cognitive, if not the auditory, skills required for phonological recognition and phonetic discrimination, as well as the ability to form semantic and grammatical representations. These are strengths that can be built on in teaching and therapy. The condition of prelingual deafness has an important feature in common with cleft palate and dysarthria: these are medical conditions that primarily impact upon the periphery of the speech processing system, and do not necessarily entail higher level deficits in phonological processing. Deaf children, for example, are often able to rhyme and attain good literacy skills (Campbell and Wright, 1988).

The Whole Word Phase

By around 12 months of age children are ready to enter the next phase of speech development, characterized by the emergence of first words. Babbling displays more varied patterns of CV combination, though still with a preponderance of stop and nasal consonants. Simultaneously with this richer, more variegated babbling is the development of meaningful sound sequences which arise independently of the adult language, often referred to as protowords (Stoel-Gammon and Cooper, 1984); and of words that derive from adult forms. With the emergence of these first 'proper' words, the input and output sides of the model come together: children now produce words which they have heard spoken and have understood. This means that the lexical representation for each word now consists of semantic representation, phonological representation and motor program, all linked. The model is therefore complete, in that all the components of the final model presented in Chapter 6 (Figure 6.13) are now in place.

Clearly there is a still a very long way to go before the child's speech is anything like that of an adult. However, subsequent developments in speech processing are not concerned with the basic structure of the processing system so much as with major developments that have to take place within individual components. Most obviously, in motor execution, the child has to develop articulatory skills that are dependent partly on physical maturation as well as on increasingly fine co-ordination of the organs in the vocal tract. Great expansion of the lexicon will occur, as the child learns new words which put huge additional demands on the organization and storage of words in relation to one another. This in turn puts demands on the components involved in phonological analysis and segmentation. In the remainder of this chapter some of these developments will be explored in more detail, by continuing the 'snapshots' of children at important milestones in speech development.

For most children, the first phase of word production, described here as the Whole Word Phase, is characterized at its outset by a range of forms with distinct meanings, which, from a phonological point of view, do not show much evidence of systematicity: it is generally not the case that the child makes use of the minimum of phonetic resources (consonants, vowels) combined in the maximum possible way. The forms clearly have to be within the child's productive capacity (i.e. limited by *motor execution* capacity), and some children, at least, appear to select for their first words adult target words that conform to those limitations. Waterson (1978, 1987) describes Patrick at this early phase (10–14 months) as having a small vocabulary of words which by and large he pronounced in an appropriate way:

BOB	→	[ba]
NO	→	[nəu]
UP	→	[ʌp]
ANNE	→	[æn]
GOOD	→	[gʊd]
BONE	→	[bəun]

Since the vocabulary is very small, and there is no evidence of segmentation or simplification, the lexicon can be thought of at this phase as an unstructured list of lexical representations, consisting of semantic representation, phonological representation and motor program. The *semantic representation* may correspond more or less precisely to the adult meaning: some words may be overextended, others underextended in their meaning, for example. Each *phonological representation* can be taken to be as yet unsegmented, consisting of the most acoustically salient features of the adult form. It does not have the internal structure of onset – rhyme constituents, since there is no need for them, given the small size of the lexicon. In *phonological recognition*, language-specific patterns are found, but again these are best regarded as unsegmented words (or longer stretches), since there is no reason for segmentation to occur, nor any empirical evidence that it does (Juzscyk, 1992). The *motor program* for each word likewise consists of a single, undifferentiated gestalt of gestures, since the motor program does not yet contain segmented constituents such as syllables, onsets, rhymes or smaller segments that could be combined into different motor programs. This phase, where the word is the minimal unit for input, representation and output, is analogous to Frith's logographic phase of literacy development (see Chapter 1), since it is the whole word that is the key structural unit.

As this phase unfolds during the second year, children's vocabulary increases rapidly, and the range of phonetic forms found in output also increases (Waterson, 1978). Another characteristic can be an increased amount of variability in the production of individual words. Ferguson and Farwell (1975) give the example of variant forms of the target PEN, produced within the space of half an hour by an American girl, K, at CA 1;3: [mã]; [ʌ̃] ; [dɛ^{dn}]; [hɪn]; [bõ] [p^{h}ɪn]; [t^{h}n t^{h}n t^{h}n]; [ba^{h}]; [d̪^{h}au^{n}]; [buã]. One notable aspect of the tokens of PEN is that, although in articulatory terms they appear very diverse, each of the different variant forms can be seen to reflect the phonetic content of the target: the child selects some features and reproduces them, though not necessarily in the correct sequence. For instance, in [mã] , there is bilabial closure at the onset, and nasality in the rhyme, as in the target PEN [p^{h}ɛ̃n]. However, the nasality that characterizes both parts of the rhyme (nucleus and coda) in the target, is found over the whole of the child's token, onset as well as rhyme; while the rhyme itself consists of a nucleus without coda. The vowel nucleus has a front, unrounded articulation, like the target, but is more open. Thus, there are many similarities between target and child version. Compare that to another token, [dɛᵈⁿ]. Here, the alveolar place of articulation and the voicing of the target coda of [pʰɛ̃n] are reproduced at onset position, as well as at coda position. The vowel nucleus this time is reproduced accurately.

The development of children's motor skills for speech purposes is central to our understanding of what is happening at this phase. In terms of the model, this means the development of motor programming, motor planning and motor execution. According to recent theories about motor speech development, at the Whole Word Phase the child has stored what we have termed a motor program, for each word as a whole (Kent, 1992, p.81). The variability found in first words (e.g. for PEN in the example just cited) can be attributed to the child's inability to co-ordinate gestures to realize the motor program in a consistent way, i.e. at the level of motor execution.

In the child's versions, it is not simply a misordering of adult segments that is involved. The phonetic ingredients of one particular target segment can be distributed over more than one segment in the child's production, or the ingredients of the target segments can be recombined in the child's forms. The child seems to be latching on to phonetic parameters, rather than individual segments, and paying relatively less attention to linear order. This is illustrated in the following production of MUFFIN (a cat's name) by our daughter at CA 1;6 as [m̩m̥̩ᶠ]. The response has the correct number of syllables and the phonetic features that she has abstracted for production are all found in the target /mʌfɪn/: for the first syllable, nasality, continuance and bilabiality from /m/ and syllabicity from /ʌ/; for the second syllable, voicelessness, labiality and friction from /f/, nasality and continuance from /n/ and syllabicity from /ɪ/. She has not yet established the precise temporal alignment of these features, however (cf. Studdert-Kennedy and Whitney Goodell, 1995).

As the above examples suggest, this phase is parametric in terms of both production and perception. Waterson (1976) in particular argues, mainly on the basis of her son Patrick's production forms, that children attend primarily to the most salient acoustic properties of the words they hear. The evidence for this is that these are the features of the target word that children reproduce in their own speech; and that children's production forms cannot be readily accounted for by one-to-one segmental correspondence 'rules'. Here are some words produced by Patrick at CA 1;5 – 1;6 years:

FETCH	→	[ɪʃ]
FISH	→	[ɪʃ] [ʊʃ]
FINGER	→	[ɲẽːɲẽ] [ɲiɲɪ]
FLY	→	[wæ] [bβæ]
		[βæ] [væ]
FLOWER	→	[væ] [væwæ]

The adult target forms of all five words begin with [f], a voiceless labiodental fricative, but Patrick never uses this. In FISH and FETCH, the initial consonant does not appear at all; in FINGER, the initial consonant is a voiced palatal nasal; and in FLY and FLOWER a range of forms occur, beginning with voiced bilabial or labiodental articulations of different kinds. According to Waterson (1976), there is a systematic relationship between the child's realizations and the adult target form, but it is based on the most salient perceptual features of the target word, rather than on a correspondence between individual segments. Thus in FETCH and FISH, the high frequency aperiodic noise of [ʃ] at the end of the word is much more salient, in terms of both length and intensity, than the fricative [f] in onset position. Waterson argues that this leads the child to attach relatively little importance to the onset consonant by comparison. A similar argument is made with respect to the nasal in FINGER, which is more strongly articulated than the initial [f] and acoustically more salient. The nasal is reduplicated in the child's version, thereby maintaining most of the syllable structure of the target form. In FLY and FLOWER, the [f], as the first part of a cluster, is more forcefully articulated, and also has no competition from consonants elsewhere in the word in terms of perceptual salience. For these words, features of the target initial fricative are maintained: labiality in all realizations; friction in [βæ], [væ], [bβæ]; continuance in [wæ], [βæ], [væ] and labiodentality in [v]. Such data suggest that perceptual factors are as important at this phase as articulatory factors in determining the form that children give to their first words. This supports the view that, at this point, children's words are stored as perceptual gestalts for recognition purposes, i.e. the phonological representations of words are not segmented; and on the output side, the motor program for the word is not yet an invariant linear sequence of gestures, but rather consists of a number of targets, based on perceptual salience, that can be realized in different ways on different occasions.

The speech patterns of young children described in this section are reminiscent of the patterns found in older children with developmental verbal dyspraxia (Stackhouse, 1992b). Such children typically have difficulties with sequencing sounds in words (cf. PEN above); features of the target may be reproduced, but not in the correct sequence, e.g.

TREASURE	→	[ˈstɛɹəz]
CARAVAN	→	[ˈʤælɪbəbæn]
WASP	→	[wɒps]

These examples, taken from Michael, aged 10 and Caroline, aged 11, are qualitatively different from the errors made by normally-developing children aged 3;3–5;6, with whom they had been matched on the *Edinburgh Articulation Test* (Stackhouse and Snowling, 1992b). The younger children almost invariably preserved the linear sequence of the target, making perhaps one or two segmental errors. Michael and Caroline made errors on fewer target words overall, but when they did make an error, sequencing errors as well as segmental errors were found, as in these examples. Such observations suggest that children with developmental verbal dyspraxia may in certain respects be arrested at the Whole Word Phase of speech development (Stackhouse, 1993); this suggestion will be explored further at the end of the chapter.

Another feature of this early phase of speech development is that many children show what has been dubbed 'selection-avoidance' behaviour. That is, the adult target forms of the new words that they acquire in their production tend to conform to their own preferred phonetic patterns. The child avoids adult words that are outside these patterns (Schwartz and Leonard, 1982). In terms of our model, this can be viewed as an interaction between motor programming and lexical representations. At this phase of the child's development, the motor programs that can be generated are quite limited. This can have two consequences. Firstly, the child, cognizant of motor limitations, might devise motor programs only for those words that in the adult form are reasonably compatible with the motor program patterns s/he is currently capable of generating. Experimental studies suggest that children have no problems learning 'unacceptable' words for comprehension purposes, so the processing limitation is on the output side only (Ingram, 1989, p. 212). Secondly, the child could attempt to reproduce many very different adult forms, but pronounce them all in much the same way, i.e. creating a lot of homophony. This does indeed happen. Patrick, at 1;5 years, pronounced all the following words in the same way: TRUCK, JUG, STICK, CRAB, CART, DUCK, CAKE → [gʌk] (Waterson, 1976).

Throughout this phase, children comprehend more words than they produce. This is true of the first 50 or so words, which are acquired relatively slowly, and also of the subsequent period of rapid expansion in vocabulary (Benedict, 1979). One plausible explanation for the discrepancy is the motor limitations on the child at this phase; for production purposes children mainly confine themselves to adult words that can be accommodated within their current motor programming abilities. This hypothesis fits well with the view of phonological representations presented in Chapter 6: the phonological representation is underspecified, containing just enough information to allow it to be distinguished from other words in the child's vocabulary at a particular moment. While the vocabulary is relatively small, the information in the phonological representation will be very sparse, since not much phonological information is needed to distinguish a word from competitors. In this case there will be a large discrepancy between the information contained in the phonological representation and the information needed to pronounce a word, i.e. for a motor program for the word. As a consequence, the child will be able to recognize many more words than s/he can pronounce. As the vocabulary increases, more information will need to be included in each phonological representation, since there will be more words in the lexicon that are phonologically similar and therefore potentially confusable in recognition (cf. Waterson, 1981, 1987). The filling out of the specification of the phonological representation brings it closer in line with the motor program that is required for accurate production (cf. Huttenlocher, 1974; Vihman, 1996, p. 126), predicting that the discrepancy between comprehension and production will progressively reduce.

While this is the case in normal development, some children go on to experience severe 'word-finding' difficulties, i.e. a dissociation whereby they are unable to produce spontaneously many words that they have no problems in understanding. This can lead to behaviour such as the following:

> " key.....oh what do you call them......oh yeah...you put.... you put...with your.....with your..oh.....with your....when you....when someone's stole something.... and...... what do you call them... necklace?.... no......I just don't know the word."

This was the response of Michael, a 7-year-old boy with severe word finding difficulties, to a picture of HANDCUFFS (Constable, Stackhouse and Wells, in press). Michael's performance on matched single word comprehension and confrontation naming tasks revealed that he was unable to retrieve accurately some words that he could understand perfectly well e.g. BINOCULARS → ['nɒkənɜz 'nɒkəmɪlɑz]. On a series of auditory lexical decision tasks Michael accepted matched nonwords as the real words, but only for the items that he had named incorrectly e.g. he accepted [bɪ'nɒkjunəz] and [bɪ'lɒkjunəz] for BINOCULARS. This indicates that Michael had imprecise phonological representations for the items he found hard to name, with the result that minimally different nonwords were accommodated within the representation.

Michael's dissociation between comprehension and retrieval is thus attributable to imprecise phonological representations, which have given rise to inaccurate and / or unstable motor programs. As a consequence, the links between the different components of the lexical representation are faulty, leading to classic word-finding behaviour. This can take the form of phonological trial and error as in CIGARETTE → [sɪʔə sɪɹɪjɛt siːjɛt], which suggests that Michael has accessed a motor program but is unsure about its precise form. Another manifestation of the problem is circumlocution, as in the HANDCUFFS example, which reveals Michael's knowledge of the semantics of the item, coupled with an inability to access a suitable motor program for production purposes. Developmentally, word-finding difficulties of this type can be viewed as a consequence of being unable to progress satisfactorily to the phase where phonological representations are specified fully enough to provide a basis for generating an accurate motor program.

The Systematic Simplification Phase

This is the phase of phonological development that has often been characterized in terms of phonological mapping rules, or simplifying processes, that show the regular ways in which the adult forms appear to be simplified by the child. The patterns of correspondence between child and adult forms become more systematic, with less variability in production. The interpretation of this change in terms of our model will be discussed below. However, it should be emphasized that these phases are not discrete, nor can they be given a precise chronological span. As we will see in the next activity, this is attested by further data from Patrick at CA 1;5. First, however, let us consider the input side.

Phonological perception

Claims have been made for the development of 'phonemic perception' in children of this age, which would support a view that phonological representations are structured phonemically, i.e. in terms of a linear string of segments. However, children at this phase, while able to discriminate between pairs of words already in their vocabulary, can have difficulty when one or both words are unfamiliar, i.e. effectively non-words for the child (Barton, 1976). Thus, less than half the 15 children in Barton's study, aged between CA 2;3 and 2;11, could distinguish FROG from FROCK – a pair of words in which at least one word was previously unknown to all the children. By contrast, the 15 children already knew the words BACK and BAG and all could discriminate between them when tested. Since the phonological contrast being tested is virtually the same, this suggests that the child's perception at this phase is lexically based i.e. that the child accesses lexical phonological representations, rather than more abstract phonological units, when identifying a word. In terms of the model, this suggests that for many children at this phase, the *phonological recognition* box on the input side is not yet developed to the point of containing an inventory of phonological units or segments that can be accessed, for example in a discrimination task where the child has to distinguish between novel words.

A failure to distinguish such pairs also indicates an imprecise phonological representation for the word in the pair that the child does already know. Thus "thish" [θɪʃ] will be heard as FISH, "wabbit" [wabɪt] as RABBIT (Eilers and Oller, 1976). The evidence suggests that during this phase phonological perception is developing gradually (Ingram, 1989). In terms of the model, this entails developments in the specification of existing phonological representations, which will take place as the vocabulary develops when finer distinctions have to be attended to by the child (cf. FROG~FROCK). These refinements involve finer categorization of phonological units (e.g. voiced vs voiceless in this example) and also finer segmentation of the words into phonological constituents, i.e. a growing awareness that phonological contrasts can be found not only across the whole word, or syllable (as at the Whole Word Phase), but also at the onset position only as in COAST ~ GHOST, or the rhyme position only, as in FROCK ~ FROG, MONKEY ~ MUCKY (Eilers and Oller, 1976).

Ingram (1989) emphasizes that another important factor in the development of phonological perception may be the child's own phonological productive capabilities. In this context, it is interesting to note that some older children with severe speech difficulties have specific problems discriminating between nonword pairs. This difficulty is exacerbated when the items to be discriminated contain consonant sequences such as [st] vs [ts]. e.g. VOST vs VOTS (Bridgeman and Snowling, 1988) or where they differ by a transposition of consonants between the onset of different syllables, e.g. IKIBUS ~ IBIKUS (Stackhouse, 1989). There is a parallel with the Systematic Simplification Phase of normal development, where the lexical status of the words being tested affects the child's ability to discriminate. This suggests that the deficit of the older speech-disordered child may derive from a failure to pass satisfactorily through this developmental phase, where the child progressively learns to abstract phonological units from words and store them for phonological recognition purposes, thus permitting accurate discrimination and segmentation of unfamiliar speech material (Vihman, 1996, chapter 7).

Systematic simplification in speech output

The data from perceptual studies of children at this age indicate that there are considerable differences among normally-developing children in terms of the perceptual oppositions that they are aware of. This is matched by a corresponding picture of individual differences in production: some children produce final consonants early, others do not; some produce fricatives from the outset, others do not, and so on. This variability supports the view that the various 'simplifying processes' may have different places of origin within the processing system. This point is discussed in more detail later. First, we will investigate some of the patterns of speech output characteristic of this phase, by considering some more data from Patrick.

ACTIVITY 7.4

Aim: To describe the patterns of correspondence between target forms and child's pronunciations.

In the following words, identify what happens to particular consonants or consonant types in different positions in the syllable. Why is CRAB anomalous?

Target		*Patrick*
PLANE	→	[beɪm]
STAMP	→	[bem]
PRAM	→	[bæ̃], [bæm]
PLUM	→	[bʌm]
DOWN	→	[daun]
CHIN	→	[dɪn]
BIB	→	[bɪp]
PIP	→	[bɪp]
CUP	→	[bæp], [bʌp]
PLATE	→	[beɪp]
GRAPE(S)	→	[beɪp]
TRUCK	→	[gʌk]
JUG	→	[gʌk]
STICK	→	[gʌk]
DUCK	→	[gʌk]
CART	→	[gʌk]
CAKE	→	[gʌk]
CRAB	→	[gʌk]

Compare your answer to Key to Activity 7.4 at the end of this chapter, then read the following.

In studying this data from Patrick at CA 1;5 years, we can see that regular patterns of correspondence between adult and child forms can already be identified. However, it is only when such regular patterns become the dominant feature of children's output that they should be described as having entered the Systematic Simplification Phase. The phases are thus not discrete but are identified by the dominant feature in a child's output. More specifically, the simplification patterns that dominate earliest tend to be ones which have the whole word as their domain, rather than the single segment. These include harmony or assimilatory patterns such as reduplication, consonant harmony and context sensitive voicing and patterns that affect the shape of the entire word, such as syllable deletion or final consonant deletion, most of which are evident in the data in Activity 7.4. Together with the pervasive pattern of cluster reduction, these conspire to create a series of templates, to which the child's word forms have to conform. Thus, the data analysed in Activity 7.4 conform to a simple template: all words have a single voiced stop consonant at onset, followed by a vowel and a final consonant that is either a voiceless stop or a voiced nasal. Furthermore, the two consonants must share the same place of articulation. The specific patterns of correspondence between adult and child form, such as determine the place of articulation of the consonants, the quality of the vowel, and whether the final consonant is oral or nasal, are subject to the more general constraints imposed by the template. One way of viewing the transition from the Whole Word Phase to the Systematic Simplification Phase is as the progressive expansion and loosening of these word templates (Macken, 1980, 1992).

For some children, however, the templates can remain very restricted, thereby impeding intelligibility greatly. Grunwell and Yavas (1988) describe the case of a 9-year-old boy, Graham, who had developed a relatively complete set of vowel contrasts and singleton consonantal contrasts for English, but with a complete absence of consonant clusters. Furthermore, the singleton consonants were restricted almost exclusively to word initial position: in a sample of 170 words sampling the full range of English target syllable and word patterns, Graham produced only seven coda consonants (six of which were [n]), apart from the glottal stop [ʔ] which he used pervasively. In addition to these restrictions on syllable structure, target words of more than one syllable were generally reduced; only 17/65 target two-syllable words were not reduced to a monosyllable, and only 2/9 three-syllable words were not reduced to two or one syllables. As a consequence, many target words were homophonous in Graham's speech, for example:

BLOOD, BROTHER, BRUSH, BUCKET	→	[bʌʔ]
FINGER, FISH, FRIDGE, SWIMMING	→	[fɪʔ]
CRISPS, KITCHEN, SKIPPING	→	[kɪʔ]

Children such as Graham, whose speech output is constrained by a set of word and syllable templates, have not progressed through the transitional phase between the Whole Word Phase and the Systematic Simplification Phase. For Graham, at the age of 9, this is clearly a very serious difficulty, given his age and the pervasiveness of the restrictions on his speech output, with their consequences for his intelligibility.

In other children, template restrictions may be more specific and more easily overcome. Leonard and McGregor (1991) present data from W, an American girl of CA 2;9, whose speech displayed some of the patterns typical of the Systematic Simplification Phase, for example:

Cluster reduction:

DRINK	→	[dɪŋk]
PLAY	→	[pe]
GRAPES	→	[geps]

Stopping of affricates:

CHAIR	→	[tɛə]
JUICE	→	[dus]

However, W also displayed a much more unusual pattern: the target fricatives /f/, /s/, /z/ and /ʃ/, were always omitted in word initial position, but turned up in word final position in W's own speech as [f], [z] or [s], as in the following examples:

FALL, FLY, FOUND	→	[af]
SAW	→	[as]
SCHOOL	→	[kus]
SNAKE	→	[neks]
SHOE	→	[us]
SHIRT	→	[ʌts]

In one respect, these forms are reminiscent of the Whole Word Phase: W assorts the phonetic ingredients in an order that does not correspond to the target. However, there is a difference: W's mis-sequencing is consistent and systematic. The pattern is evidence for a template restriction, whereby the fricatives in question are inadmissible at onset position, but admissible at coda position. W makes use of the greater possibilities at coda to ensure that the onset fricative of the target is signalled in some way, even though its position does not correspond to that of the target. She thereby, incidentally, indicates that the omission of target initial fricatives is not due to perceptual limitations.

W was seen again after 4 months, during which period her mother made efforts to draw attention to initial fricatives by prolonging them when repeating the target form of W's unusual productions back to her. Her pattern was now undergoing change, in the direction of the adult system, e.g. SNAKE was now pronounced correctly. The case of W suggests that some children may have quite specific template restrictions, which can give rise to unusual patterns but which may nevertheless resolve without much trouble, enabling them to progress through the transition to the Systematic Simplification Phase.

As the Systematic Simplification Phase progresses, the patterns that predominate are generally ones that affect individual segments, rather than words or syllables: fronting of velar and postalveolar consonants, stopping of fricatives, /r/ → [w], /θ/ → [f], for example. The exception is cluster reduction, which continues to impose limiting templates on the child's output form (see Grunwell, 1987 for a full account of the chronology of these patterns).

The psycholinguistic origins of simplification patterns

The patterns of simplification characteristic of this phase of speech development can in theory arise at different places in the psycholinguistic model (cf. Aitchison, 1987, chapter 12). It is likely that this is the case in normal development, with different patterns having different origins. Some appear to be perceptual in origin, for example 'weak (pre-tonic) syllable deletion', e.g. BANANA → ['nɑnə]. There is nothing articulatorily complex about the first syllable, but it is unstressed, therefore not acoustically salient, when it precedes the most salient syllable in the word. Even in the adult pronunciation, the first vowel can be virtually absent e.g. [b'nɑnə], while the child at this phase often overlooks the entire syllable. According to this interpetation, such a child would have a phonological representation for BANANA that consists of only two syllables.

Other simplifying patterns are more likely to have a basis in output processing. Reduplication, e.g. PUDDING → ['pʊpʊ], reflects the child's perceptual awareness that the target word has two syllables, in conjunction with inability to achieve phonetic differentiation between two syllables within the same word. In terms of the present model, this can be seen as a developmental limitation on motor programming, which gives rise to an immature motor program for this particular word.

The observation that different common simplifying processes can have different origins in terms of the phonological processing system suggests that it is misleading to lump these patterns together as 'processes' or 'rules' and locate them all at the same place on a psycholinguistic model. If we consider a single simplifying process, such as 'final consonant deletion', one child may fail to signal final consonants because of a failure to perceive or attend to the final consonant, and therefore to store it as part of the phonological representation. For the final consonant deletion pattern to be 'suppressed', it will therefore be necessary for the child's perceptual abilities to develop. Another child may have stored an accurate phonological representation, but be unable to produce the final consonant because motor programming has not yet developed sufficiently to produce templates for motor programs containing a final consonant. What we have termed a motor program is equivalent to what Kent calls a 'gestural score':

> '...the composite of a set of sensorimotor trajectories, where each such trajectory is a neural representation of a movement and its sensory consequences. The production of almost any word requires that several of these sensorimotor trajectories be combined in a gestural score.'
>
> (Kent, 1992, p.81)

According to our developmental model, in the Whole Word Phase the set of sensorimotor trajectories has as its domain the word, but as the child moves into the Systematic Simplification Phase, the domain becomes co-extensive with smaller phonological constituents. Initially these are the syllables: compare reduplicated bisyllabic words, where the same motor gesture is simply repeated, e.g. PUDDING → ['pʊpʊ], with non-reduplicated bisyllabic words, in which two separate sets of gesture are used: PUDDING → ['pʊdɪŋ]. With increasing segmentation of phonological representations into constituents, it can be envisaged that the sets of sensorimotor trajectories will have as their domain parts of the syllable, such as the onset and the rhyme. This allows each rhyme to be combined with each onset, to create many new motor programs from existing motor resources. It is then that children will be ready for rhyme games and songs, and be able to build up phonological awareness skills.

At the same time, the child's planning and control of the gestures themselves, at the levels of motor planning and execution, also have to mature. In his discussion of final consonant deletion, Kent (1992) points out that in some cases the final consonant, though not audible, nevertheless has left traces that can be identified by acoustic analysis. The failure to signal the consonant audibly may be due not so much to any kind of 'simplification process', as to an imperfect attempt to realize the final consonant, which fails because the child does not yet have the motor skills to co-ordinate all the aspects of the gesture precisely, e.g. to ensure frication noise in the case of a final fricative consonant.

Relationship between input and output

So far, in this description of the Systematic Simplification Phase, we have considered the input (perceptual) and output (motor) sides. We now consider how the two are related. In our model, the lexical representation of each word includes a phonological representation and a motor program. The phonological representation contains just sufficient information about the sound structure and content of the word to distinguish it from the other words in the individual's lexicon. Developmentally, this implies that at the outset, this information will be generally sparse, since the number of words in the child's lexicon is small, therefore little information is needed to make a word unique. As the vocabulary develops, more information will need to be encoded. The phonological representation is taken to be the basis for recognition, i.e. for input processing. At the same time it is intimately involved in speech output, inasmuch as the motor program depends on the phonological representation for its own specification. The motor program for each word encodes the articulatory exponents of the word's phonological representation, i.e. it encodes the gestures that are required to produce the word in such a way as to make it distinctive from the other words in the child's vocabulary, along with other gestures that are not phonologically distinctive in this way but are nevertheless part of the pronunciation of the word. As the child's vocabulary increases, this means not only that the phonological representation has to be refined, but so also, as a consequence, does the motor program. For instance, if the child has the word KEY in his/her lexicon, with an associated motor program, and then adds TEA the phonological representation of KEY has to be adapted so that the initial consonant is more precisely specified. Correspondingly, the motor program has to be made precise enough so that the tongue contact for KEY is henceforth distinct (i.e consistently further back) from that for TEA. In the case of a child who hitherto had been pronouncing KEY with a more [t]-like gesture, as is quite common, this means that the motor program has to be revised, i.e. sent back to motor programming for updating of the program, which can then be incorporated into the lexical representation. If this process works smoothly, the child's output will develop progressively in accordance with the expansion in vocabulary.

However, successful revision and updating of the motor program is dependent on a number of factors, any or all of which may be absent. On the input side, the child has to be aware that the new word TEA does indeed sound different from KEY and therefore requires a distinct phonological representation. The child may perceive the two words TEA and KEY as homophonous, just as we have homophones in the adult language, such as WRITE, RIGHT (VS LEFT), RIGHT (VS WRONG), RITE. In this case, the child will be aware of a need for a new semantic representation, but not for a new phonological representation or, consequently, for a new motor program.

Input deficits were revealed in the case of N, an American boy of CA 4;6, who had pervasive difficulties producing target fricatives and affricates: in all positions in the word he used [θ] for /θ/, /s/, /ʃ/, /f/, /ʧ/ and [ð] for /ð/, /z/, /ʒ/, /v/, /ʤ/ (McGregor and Schwartz, 1992). He also had difficulties with target /l/, /w/, /r/, for example replacing /l/ by /h/ in initial position, by /w/ in medial position, and omitting it in final position. McGregor and Schwartz used two auditory discrimination tests of the type described by Locke (1980a,b) to examine N's ability to perceive differences between the adult form and his own pronunciation of the targets that he was confusing in his speech output (see also Chapter 2 of this volume). They found that N had no problems with the affricates, or with /ʃ/, /ʒ/, /z/, but for the remaining targets, there was perceptual confusion between the target form and his own production, at least at some places in the word. This suggests that for many words containing the target consonants /θ/, /s/, /f/, /v/, /l/, /w/, /r/, N's phonological representations were inaccurate and that this was giving rise to a systematic simplification of his speech output.

In addition to the perceptual skills needed to establish accurate phonological representations, the child has to have the motor skills to produce a distinctive motor program, and preferably one that is distinctive in a way that corresponds to the adult motor program. Thus, in order to move beyond a pattern of velar fronting, the child has to be capable of producing a more back (velar) tongue contact in a position preceding a vowel. Without this ability, the production of KEY and TEA could well be homophonous, even though the child is aware that they are phonologically different.

Some older children present with this type of problem. A group of children who all fronted velar targets in their own speech were able to sort pictures correctly according to whether the label for the object depicted began with /t/ or /k/, even though they themselves consistently pronounced the target initial /k/ words with [t] (Brett, Chiat and Pilcher, 1987). In this latter case, where the child still has a motor program for KEY that produces something like [ti], it can be expected that later his/her motor programming system will develop the ability to produce [k] followed by a vowel, perhaps with the aid of speech and language therapy when progress is delayed.

Some children may not be able to perform such a sorting task, however. Thomas was one of these (Stackhouse, 1996). He had had a history of speech and language delay, specific expressive language difficulties and severe verbal dyspraxia, and at CA 8;6 presented with specific problems in spelling. By now his speech was intelligible, though it still sounded unusual because of rhythm and vowel difficulties. One pattern of consonantal errors in particular seemed to be reflected in his spelling. He realized the /ʃ/, /tʃ/ and /s/ sounds as [θ], e.g. SHADOW → [θædəʊ]; and /z/ as [ð] e.g. MAGAZINE → [mægəðin]. However, when the target sound in a word was /θ/ or /ð/ he pronounced it as [f] and [v] respectively, e.g. THUMB → [fʌm] and WITH → [wɪv]. As he could produce the sounds, his errors could not be explained by poor articulatory skills alone. When spelling, /ʃ/ was transcribed as ‹ch›, so for example SHADOW, pronounced [θædəʊ]) was written as ‹chadow› and MEMBERSHIP, pronounced [mɛmbəθɪp] as ‹memberchip›. /ʃ/ and /tʃ/ were also transcribed as ‹s› in REFRESHMENT → ‹refresment›, MACHINERY → ‹misnery›, POLITICIAN → ‹polltisn› and ADVENTURE → ‹edvenser›.

The specific confusion of fricative and affricate sounds in speech and spelling was investigated further in two ways. Firstly, Thomas was presented with a series of spoken words beginning or ending with /ʃ/, /tʃ/ and /ʤ/ and asked to decide which words began or ended with these sounds. He confused /tʃ/ and /ʃ/ on this task, for example he thought that CHEAP and CHAIR began with /ʃ/ and that MASH ended with /tʃ/. Secondly, he was presented with a series of pictures depicting words beginning with /ʃ/, /tʃ/ and /ʤ/ to sort into piles of the same onsets. There were slightly more confusions on this task, where he had to generate the word himself from his own representations, compared to the first task, where the words were spoken for him by the tester. He classified CHAIN, CHICKEN and JUMPER as beginning with /ʃ/ and SHORTS and SHE as beginning with /tʃ/. Subsequent therapy was aimed at sharpening up his phonological representations of items beginning with these consonants. It paid dividends in both speech and spelling: by the age of 9 years Thomas had no difficulties in producing or transcribing fricative and affricate sounds.

False neutralizations in speech output

Descriptions of children's speech simplifications often imply that the child is simply replacing one target sound by another, for example in the case of velar fronting, that the /k/ of KEY is replaced by [t] as in TEA. If such patterns are analysed, as we have suggested, in terms of motor programming limitations, the implication is that the child has a single motor program, which is pressed into service for two different lexical items , i.e. KEY and TEA. However, even though listeners may hear the child's production of the two words as identical, research has shown that in many cases the child is in fact systematically differentiating them. Thus in the case study of N, by McGregor and Schwartz (1992), discussed earlier in this section, spectrographic analysis showed that N's productions of [θ] for target /s/ were in fact consistently different from his productions of [θ] for the other target voiceless fricatives /θ/, /ʃ/, /f/, even though they sounded the same under normal listening conditions. In terms of our model, this indicates that N did after all have a distinct motor program for words containing target /s/, even though it did not correspond to the adult motor program.

Evidence of distinct motor programs for two words that listeners hear as identical has also been provided, and in a more direct way, by the technique of electropalatography (EPG). Gibbon (1990) reports a study of a girl MB (CA 4;10), who could not reliably imitate alveolar sounds in words or in isolation. Six productions of the target syllables /daː/ and /gaː/ were recorded and transcribed by a phonetician and a speech and language therapist. All were transcribed as [gaː]. The same production task was given to a normally-developing child who acted as a control; her versions were transcribed as being appropriate for the target. While producing the syllables, the two girls' tongue contacts against the roof of the mouth were recorded using an electropalatograph, which consists of an artificial plate fitted with 64 electrodes linked to a computer.

Plosive consonants such as [t], [d], [k], [g], are described from an articulatory point of view as having three phases: an approach phase, in which the tongue moves towards the roof of the mouth; a hold phase, in which contact is maintained between a part of the tongue (e.g. tip, blade, back) and a point on the roof of the mouth (e.g. alveolar ridge, hard palate, soft palate); and a release phase, in which that contact is released. It is the place of contact during the hold phase that is commonly used to define the articulation of a plosive, i.e. as 'alveolar', 'palatal' or 'velar'. In Gibbon's study, the electropalatographic data showed that both children used a very similar place of articulation for their realizations of target /gaː/: contact was in the velar (soft palate) region. Turning to the realisations of target /daː/, the control child had tongue contact at the alveolar ridge and sides only, as would be expected. For MB, whose realization of /daː/ was heard as [gaː] , the tongue contact was over the whole of the roof of the mouth during the hold phase. This was thus different not only from the control speaker's articulation for target /daː/, but also from MB's own articulation for target /gaː/. This closure pattern would not of itself necessarily result in a pronunciation heard as [gaː]; however, in the release phase of MB's target /daː/ (i.e. the pattern of tongue contacts just prior to the tongue being moved away from the roof of the mouth), the front of the tongue was released first and as a result, the last contacts to be released were at the sides (lateral) and at the back (velar), resulting in a syllable heard as [gaː].

By referring to the electropalatographic evidence, Gibbon was able to show that the two different targets /da:/ and /ga:/ produced by MB, both heard as [gaː], had very different articulations. MB's place of articulation for target /ga:/ was very similar to the normal speaker's, at the hold and release phases of production; but MB's place of articulation for target /da:/ was quite different from her target /ga:/ at both phases: there was more widespread closure at the point of maximum stable contact in the hold phase, and prior to release there was considerable lateral as well as velar closure.

So we can see that it is not possible to infer that a child is using the same motor program for two different targets simply because we do not hear a difference. From her side, MB makes two consistently different articulations for targets /d/ and /g/ and the inability of listeners to detect a difference does not alter this fact. Untrained listeners, in particular, have great difficulty in becoming aware of subtle phonetic differences that fall within the bounds of a single phonological category in their native language. Studies such as those of Gibbon (1990) and McGregor and Schwartz (1992) point to the usefulness of careful analysis of the child's speech output, using instrumental techniques, when attempting to pinpoint the locus of deficit in the child's speech processing system. Techniques such as electropalatography also have an important role as feedback devices for therapy, providing a method of displaying the child's own speech patterns as well as the target patterns (Gibbon, Dent and Hardcastle, 1993).

Updating the lexicon

Having developed the motor programming abilities necessary to reverse the systematic simplifying patterns they have been using, children then have to become aware that there are words already in the lexicon containing the same target sound, for which the motor program has to be revised and updated. This process does not always occur: some children have been reported who incorporate new motor patterns in their new words, but who do not apply them to words acquired earlier. In the context of normal development, a celebrated example was provided by Smith (1973), whose son Amahl, from CA 2;6 to 3;6, produced [pʌdəl] for PUZZLE, but did not use this pronunciation where it should properly occur: instead, he pronounced PUDDLE as [pʌgəl]. At this point, Amahl had not revised his existing vocabulary to take account of the motor programs he was capable of producing. The motor programs for such words have thus become temporarily 'frozen'.

More long-term instances of this behaviour are cause for concern. For instance, Bryan and Howard (1992) describe the case of a boy, DF, from Essex in the south east of England, who at CA 5;1 displayed severe speech problems in spontaneous speech, picture description activities and real word repetition. However, his repetition of matched nonwords was considerably better, as the following examples show (RW, real Word; NW, Nonword):

RW target	*RW repetition*	*RW naming*	*NW target*	*NW repetition*
SOAP	[dəʊʔ]	[dəʊʔ]	/sæp/	[sæp]
BAG	[baɪ]	[baɪt]	/bɔg/	[bɔk]
PAPER	[baɪ]	[baɪs]	/peɪpɔ/	[beɪbɔ]
WATER	[ɸɪt]	[vɜz]	/wɑtə/	[wɑdə]
TABLE	[daɪt]	[daɪn]	/tɒɪbu/	[dɒbu]
ELEPHANT	[eɪɬ]	[eɪvə]	/ʌlɪfɒnt/	[ʌlɪfɒʔ]

This pattern of performance indicates that DF's speech output skills were in fact greater than his production of real words would lead us to believe: he had acquired new motor programming skills that had not been applied to the words within his vocabulary. Following this assessment, DF had therapy which focused initially on using nonwords to heighten his awareness of phonological structure and the relationship between input and output phonology. This enabled DF to update his motor programs for real words already in his lexicon, so that after therapy, not only had his nonwords improved, but the real words had caught up with them, as was evident from his production of the same set of target words:

RW target	*RW repetition*	*RW naming*	*NW target*	*NW repetition*
SOAP	[səʊp]	[səʊp]	/sæp/	[sæp]
BAG	[bæg]	[bæg]	/bɔg/	[bɔg]

PAPER	[peɪpə]	[pɛpɜ]	/peɪpɔ/	[peɪpɔ]
WATER	[wɔsə]	[wɔtə]	/wɑtə/	[wɑsə]
TABLE	[teɪpu]	[dɛbu]	/tɒɪbu/	[dubu]
ELEPHANT	[eɪfəfənt]	[elɪvɪv]	/ʌlɪfɒnt/	[ʌdɪvɒŋk]

Children such as DF illustrate that to pass successfully through the phase of Systematic Simplification, it is necessary not only to develop sufficient perceptual and motor skills, but also to update the already existing lexical representations, and particularly the motor programs.

We have seen that the simplifying patterns described in the child phonology literature, and which are used by many therapists as the basis for assessing a child's speech, can be attributed to a range of possible factors. Child phonologists have described in detail the patterns of correspondence between child and adult forms, elucidating the complex and subtle systematicities in this period of development (e.g. Smith, 1973; Vihman, 1996). These studies show that individual children find different paths towards the adult system, while in general being constrained by some overall limitations. Within the framework and model presented here, we can view similarities across children as arising from the general characteristics of motor, perceptual and cognitive development; while the differences between children's particular paths can be attributed to their problem-solving attempts to reconcile limited but developing motor ability (itself developing somewhat differently from child to child) with awareness of the need for more distinct phonological representations, so that new vocabulary can be added. In respect of the new vocabulary, the input to each child will be different, in terms of the accents and indeed languages, to which each is exposed, as well as frequency of particular vocabulary items. This will inevitably have an impact on the details of how the phonological representations develop. From a clinical perspective, children's speech development can be arrested at the Systematic Simplification Phase, as the examples given have demonstrated; this arrest can manifest in different ways, depending on the level of processing involved.

Summary

In this chapter we have proposed that:

- In normal speech development there is a progression through identifiable phases.
- Children with speech difficulties may be viewed as having arrested, troublesome or slow development through these phases.
- In the first year of life, the various components of the speech processing system come together in the Prelexical Phase.

- Children with prelingual deafness or with abnormality of the oral structure and/or function will experience difficulties with the Prelexical Phase of speech development.
- The subsequent development of speech can be described in terms of two further phases: the Whole Word Phase and the Systematic Simplification Phase.
- The speech difficulties of children with developmental verbal dyspraxia and word-finding problems may have their origins in the Whole Word Phase.
- Children described as having phonological delay or phonological impairment have problems progressing through the Systematic Simplification Phase of speech development.

KEY TO ACTIVITY 7.1

The neonate

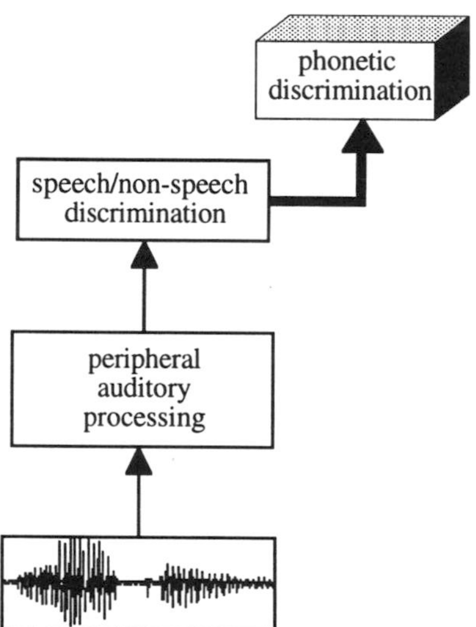

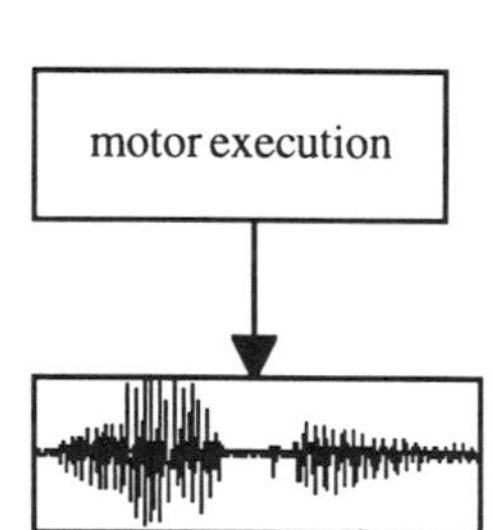

KEY TO ACTIVITY 7.2
The child at 6 months

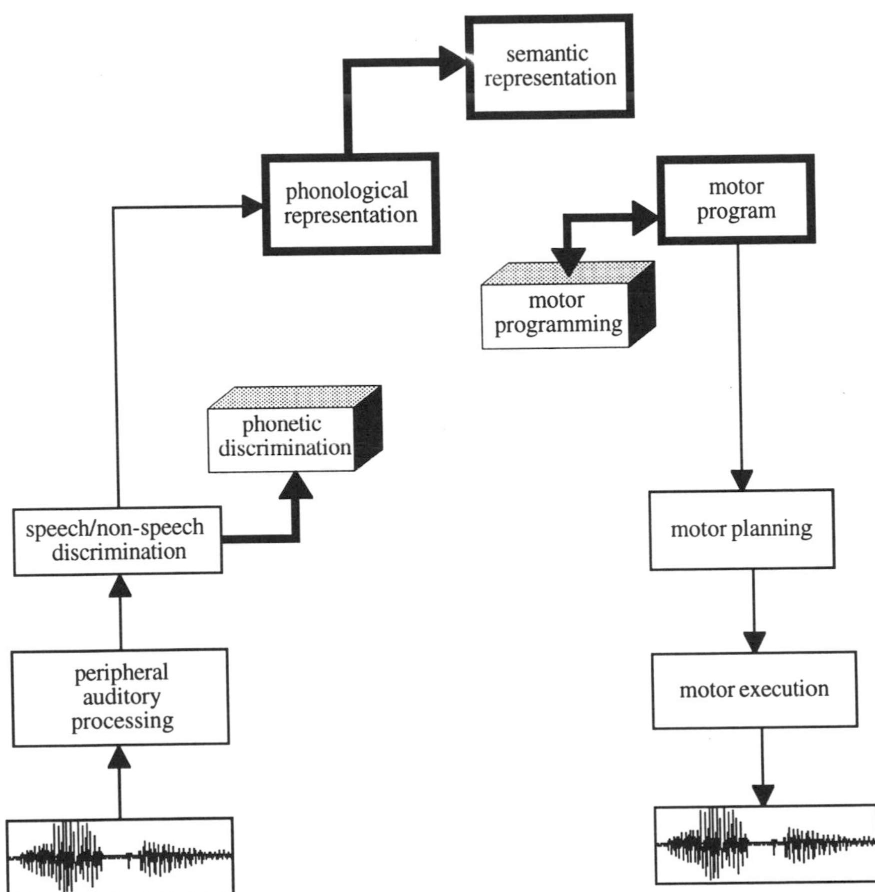

KEY TO ACTIVITY 7.3
The child at 9 months

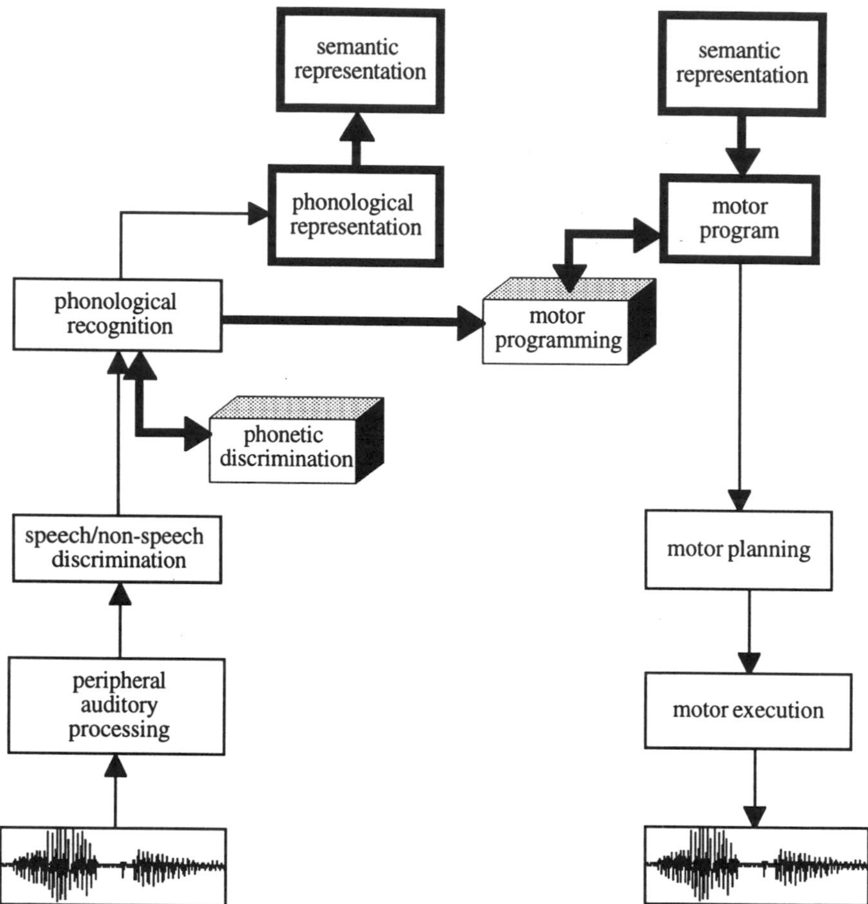

KEY TO ACTIVITY 7.4
Patrick's simplification patterns

You may have identified the following patterns. (The target words that conform to each pattern are given in parentheses.)

(1) In all consonant clusters, and also affricates, at onset position, only the plosive element is retained (PLANE, STAMP, PRAM, PLUM, PLATE, TRUCK, STICK, CHIN, JUG).

(2) All target voiceless consonants at onset position are realized as voiced (PLANE, STAMP, PRAM, PLUM, CHIN, PIP, CUP, PLATE, TRUCK, STICK, CART, CAKE, CRAB).

(3) All target voiced consonants other than nasals, in coda position, are realized as voiceless (BIB, JUG, CRAB).

(4) Where the target coda consonant is velar, the onset consonant is also realized as velar (TRUCK, JUG, STICK, CAKE).

(5) Where the target coda consonant is bilabial, the onset consonant is also realized as bilabial (STAMP, CUP).

(6) Where the target coda consonant is alveolar, it is realized with the same place of articulation as the onset consonant (PLANE, DOWN, CHIN, PLATE, CART).

CRAB is anomalous, because it does not conform to (5). If it did, it would be pronounced [bæp].

The patterns described exemplify some of the most common simplification 'processes' that have been described for child speech. (1) Is an instance of cluster reduction; (2) and (3) illustrate context-sensitive voicing; (4), (5) and (6) are all cases of consonant harmony. See text for further discussion.

Chapter 8
Phases of Development II – From Speech to Literacy

In Chapter 7, the development of speech processing in children was described up to the end of the Systematic Simplification Phase. Most children deemed to have phonological or articulatory difficulties show the characteristics either of that phase or of the previous Whole Word Phase. Most studies of normal phonological development are also concerned with these early phases of development, in which children's pronunciations of individual sounds and words deviate in various ways from the adult forms that they are meant to be acquiring. There has been less interest, from researchers into phonological development and from speech and language therapists, in the subsequent developments in children's speech and phonological processing. The aim of this chapter is to pursue the story further, tracing important developmental changes that follow the end of the Systematic Simplification Phase. In particular, we will highlight how these developments foreshadow the acquisiton of reading and spelling skills.

The Assembly Phase

Many children in their fourth year continue to show some patterns of simplification, even though the classic systemic patterns, e.g. fronting of velars (KEY → [ti]) and stopping of fricatives (ZOO → [du]), have normally disappeared by then. Persisting sources of trouble include single consonants that are articulatorily quite complex, and / or which are perceptually easily confused with another consonant. Examples include target /r/, often confused perceptually by children at this age with [w], e.g. RIGHT and WHITE; and [θ], confused with [f], e.g. THIN and FIN. The other main area of difficulty is presented by more complex articulatory sequences, such as consonant clusters, where the child has to perform rapid articulatory adjustments, e.g. STRAW, LENGTHS. Many English-speaking children also continue to experience difficulty with the production of post-alveolar affricates, as in CHURCH [ʧɜʧ], JUDGE [ʤʌʤ], which are similar to clusters in that they require sequential co-ordination of gestures for a stop followed by a fricative at the same place of articulation. In terms of our model, the persisting challenge posed by affricates and consonantal sequences can be seen as evidence that motor abilities are still developing.

Fluency

Developing the ability to produce consonantal sequences is one aspect of what we term the Assembly Phase. More generally, this phase is characterized by attempts to master the phonetic and phonological aspects of complex utterances, which the child is now attempting to produce as a result of major developments in syntax and morphology. By the fourth year, the child is attempting to produce sentences with a wide range of clause, phrase and word (morphological) structures, even if their form and meaning are not always accurately expressed. Thus Sophie, at CA 3;0, produced sentences such as the following (Fletcher, 1985):

> "mc going to watch you doing your riding lesson
> why did you give to her when her been flu"

and at CA 3;5:

> "I want to ring up somebody and her won't be there tomorrow
> when her's at school I'll buy some sweeties"

Attempts at longer, syntactically and semantically complex sentences such as these are often accompanied by a level of dysfluency noticeably greater than is habitually found in adults or older children. Such dysfluency can take the form of pauses, reformulations and word searches. Thus Sophie at CA 3;0:

> "ˋwhy did --- ˋwhy did -- Mummy ˋwhy -- ˋwhy did --- ˈHester be fast aslèep mummy"
>
> Fletcher (1985, p.92)

> "ˋwhy – ˋwhy do – me [dɪ] – ˋwhy didn't ˈme get flu éver"
>
> Fletcher (1985, p.93)

From the point of view of the child's speech output, the result is disruption to the rhythmic and intonational frame of the utterance. In terms of the speech processing model, these difficulties can be located in motor planning, where a motor pattern for the utterance is assembled on the basis of the lexical and syntactic selection that has already taken place. Studies of non-fluency in normally-developing children (as opposed to stammerers) indicate that 3-year-old children have significantly more non-fluencies than older children, and that non-fluency is associated with syntactic complexity (Gordon and Luper, 1989). Children at this age also differ from older children in the type of dysfluency: repetitions (of words, part-words and phrases, as in the above examples) are dominant, whereas older children, like adults, have more pauses at expected grammatical boundaries (Gordon, 1995).

From a clinical point of view, it is likely that there is a relationship between the non-fluency that is predominant in most children at this phase, and the onset of stuttering in some. The fourth year has been reported to be the most likely age for stuttering to begin in preschool children (Haege, 1995). Stuttering children tend to be dysfluent at the beginning of utterances or major syntactic constituents (Bernstein Ratner, 1994), which suggests that planning the utterance is involved in inducing the stutter. The examples of dysfluency above from Sophie, who is not a stutterer, conform to this pattern. Many stutterers, like normally-developing 3-year-olds, seem to have particular difficulties with assembling the utterance, and it therefore seems probable that the onset of stammering in some children is associated with the Assembly Phase.

Intonation

Apart from dysfluency, there are other ways in which the demands of the Assembly Phase can impact upon a child's speech output. As the child's utterances become longer and more complex, there is a requirement to get to grips with the intonational systems of the language, since these have an important function in, for example, signalling the ends of a speaker's turn in conversation, and in highlighting the key word or words in the utterance. Thus, in English speakers routinely draw attention to important or new information by emphasizing it, and the means of emphasis is pitch prominence, with extra loudness and lengthening. This is often referred to as the system of tonic or nuclear prominence, and the child has to learn how to use it. How this system develops has not been well researched, but there is some evidence to suggest that it becomes fully established around the beginning of the fourth year. This was the case for Sophie, examples of whose language were given earlier (Fletcher, 1985). A study of the location of the tonic on all utterances of two or more words produced in recordings taken at different ages showed that at 2;4, Sophie was operating with a strategy of making the final word prominent, with little regard for the requirements of information focus: there are only six out of 131 utterances (of two or more words) with the tonic in non-final position (for further details, see Wells and Local, 1993). The following is a typical example (an accent mark over the syllable indicates tonic prominence):

Sophie: ˈyou take a bíssy
Mother: ˈcos I was hùngry
Sophie: ˈme want a bîssy

Fletcher (1985, p.59)

When Sophie mentions 'bissy' (= BISCUIT) for the second time, it is no longer new information, and therefore would not normally be made prominent in adult English. Instead the new information would be highlighted: "Î want a biscuit". At this point, Sophie has not yet mastered the adult system. By the time Sophie is 3;0, there is a marked difference: a third of utterances have a non-final tonic, with almost identical proportions in samples from age 3;5 and 3;11 (Wells and Local, 1993). These data suggest that by 3;0, Sophie had developed the basic system of information focus / tonicity, but that at 2;4 this was not yet established. The implication is that children have to learn this aspect of English phonology, just as they have to learn to produce consonant clusters, for example. This raises the possibility of children having difficulty with acquiring these intonational systems, and thus being developmentally arrested at the Assembly Phase. Such a case is explored in Activity 8.1.

ACTIVITY 8.1

Aim: To identify an atypical intonation system, and its communicative consequences.

David is from Sandwell in the English West Midlands (Wells and Local, 1993). The following extract is taken fom a recording made when David was aged 5;4. At the time, he was having therapy on account of his severe speech and language difficulties, but tests revealed no hearing impairment. David is looking at some pictures with a speech and language therapist (T).

Study the transcript of David and his therapist (see 'Conventions' for details of prosodic notation), and answer the following questions:

(a) All David's utterances have a similar characteristic prosodic pattern. What is it?

(b) How does this pattern affect his pronunciation of compound nouns such as TEDDY BEAR, LETTER BOX, POSTMAN?

(c) How does the pattern affect his ability to signal new information, as opposed to information that has already been mentioned?

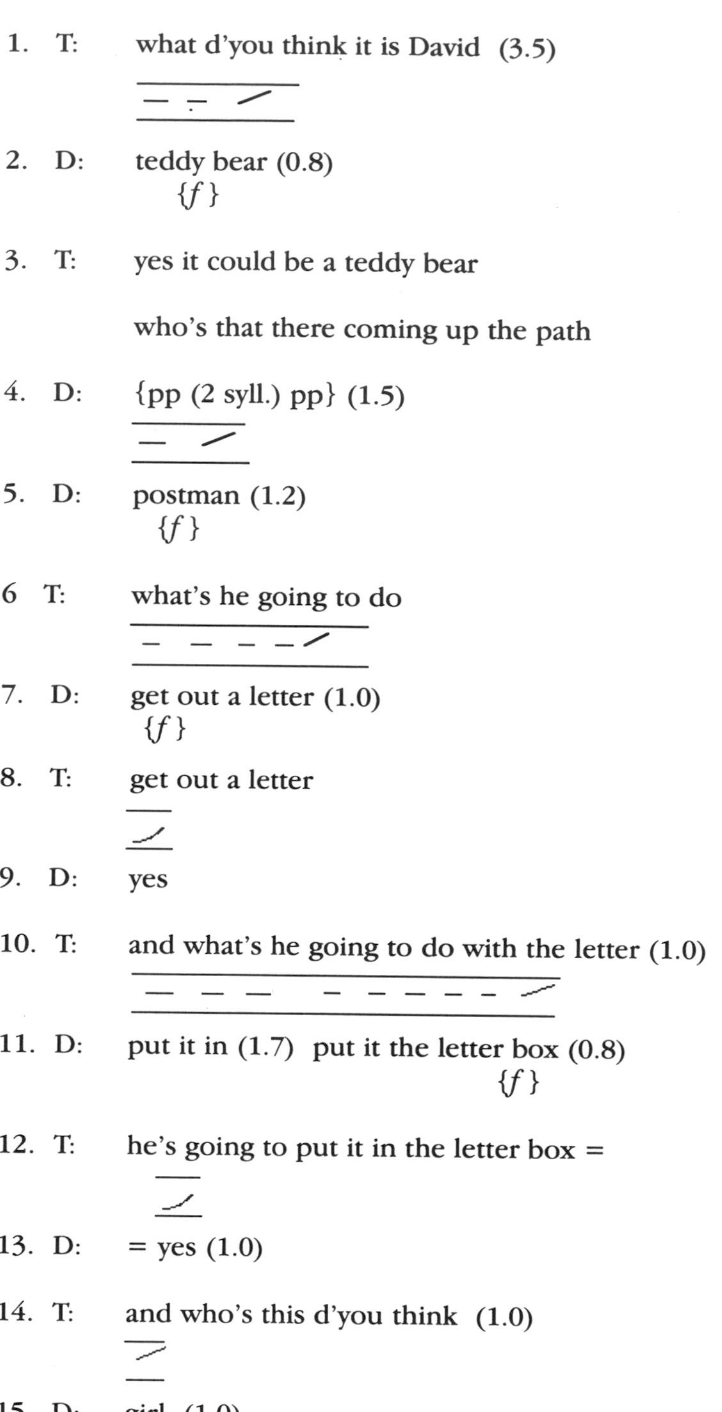
1. T: what d'you think it is David (3.5)

2. D: teddy bear (0.8)
{f}

3. T: yes it could be a teddy bear

who's that there coming up the path

4. D: {pp (2 syll.) pp} (1.5)

5. D: postman (1.2)
{f}

6 T: what's he going to do

7. D: get out a letter (1.0)
{f}

8. T: get out a letter

9. D: yes

10. T: and what's he going to do with the letter (1.0)

11. D: put it in (1.7) put it the letter box (0.8)
{f}

12. T: he's going to put it in the letter box =

13. D: = yes (1.0)

14. T: and who's this d'you think (1.0)

15. D: girl (1.0)

16. T: 's it a girl

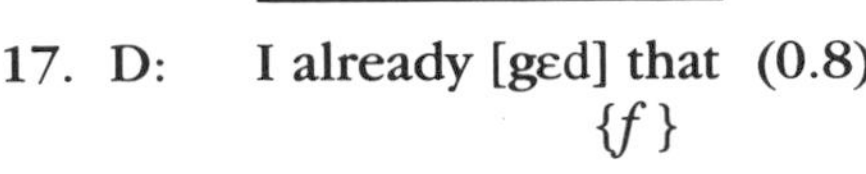

17. D: I already [gɛd] that (0.8)
{*f*}

18. T: she's already (0.5)

19. D: I already [dɛd] that (0.3) I did (5.0)
{*f*} {*f*}

20. T: see what's on the next page oh who's this again

21. D: postman
{*f*}

Compare your answer with Key to Activity 8.1 at the end of this chapter, then read the following.

The pervasive prosodic pattern of David's speech, whereby the main pitch movement regularly occurs at the end of the utterance, conforms with the descriptions of other prosodically-impaired children, and also some normally-developing children when they first begin to use two word utterances (see Wells and Local 1993, for review). The tendency to locate prosodic prominence on the final word was noted in Sophie's speech at CA 2;4. This pattern has some negative consequences for David's ability to communicate effectively. Firstly, because the main prominence occurs not merely on the final word but on the final syllable of that word, the normal pattern of lexical stress in words of more than one syllable is disrupted, as with LETTER, POSTMAN, TEDDY BEAR, LETTERBOX. This extract shows that, although David may appear to have problems with assigning word stress to the correct target syllable, his problem is not in fact with word phonology, but with utterance phonology: these words have the wrong stress pattern just because they occur in utterance final position, and *all* David's utterance final syllables bear the main accent. Thus, the incorrect stress pattern is not indicative of problems with the lexical representations of the words in question (either of the phonological representation or the motor program), but of a breakdown at the level of motor planning.

Secondly, David's prosodic pattern has consequences for his system of information focus. For example, in "I already [gɛd] that", (l.17) [gɛd], which presumably represents SAID or READ, would normally be accented at the expense of the following THAT, in order to highlight its informational importance. In David's version, it is the pronoun that is phonetically most prominent, by virtue of its utterance final position.

Even though his intonational pattern has negative consequences for the correct signalling of word stress, and for his ability to highlight the important or new information of the utterance, it nevertheless brings one big advantage: it signals very clearly to the listener that David has come to the end of his utterance. This benefit, in terms of his ability to interact more successfully in conversation, has to be weighed up against the linguistic drawbacks already described. David thus illustrates some of the pressures brought to bear by the new demands of the Assembly Phase, and one somewhat idiosyncratic response to them.

Junction

Beside these quite gross aspects of extended utterances, there are some subtle phonological features, occurring particularly around word boundaries, which are found in the speech of fluent adults and which serve to 'glue' the utterance together into a cohesive entity. In English, these include what has been termed assimilation, the way in which the final consonant of one word can accommodate to the initial consonant of the next word. For example, in most accents of English the final consonant of GREAT, in a context like GREAT ELEPHANT, is an audibly released alveolar plosive. However, in GREAT TIGER the final consonant is realized as a closure in the glottis and a silent period of contact between the tongue tip (or blade) and the teeth ridge, preceding the [t] of the second word (compare GREY TIGER). In GREAT CAT, the period of silent contact is now between the back of the tongue and the soft palate, anticipating the [k] of CAT. In GREAT BEAR the period of contact does not involve the tongue at all: instead, there is a closure of the lips, anticipating the [b] of BEAR. Such subtle adjustments at word boundaries have to be learnt by the child. There has been little developmental research into the topic, which is unfortunate since older children with speech and literacy difficulties can have trouble with these aspects of English phonology. This was the case with Richard, discussed in Chapter 5, (see also Stackhouse and Wells, 1991) and with Zoe, who will be discussed in Chapters 8 and 9 (see also Wells, 1994). In terms of the model presented in Chapter 6, we can hypothesize that the phonological representation of GREAT is not fully specified with reference to the final (coda) consonant: plosion and voicelessness are specified, but not place of articulation (Local, 1992). The accompanying motor program for the word will also contain instructions relating to degree and duration of closure and absence of vocal fold vibration, but not about where in the vocal tract the closure is to be made. That information will be gleaned at the motor planning level, when information about the following word becomes available.

Similar phonological adjustments are made when a word ends with a vowel and the next word begins with a vowel: depending on the coda vowel of the first word, a [^{w}], [^{j}] or [^{ɹ}] glide can be heard between the two words: compare TWO EGGS, THREE EGGS, FOUR EGGS. Zoe, at the age of

5;11, routinely produced much more staccato forms such as : (PUT THE) SUGAR IN [sʊ˞kəʔɪːn] rather than [ʃʊgəʴɪn]; and GO OVER [gəʊʔhəʊfə], rather than [gəʊʷəʊvə] (Wells, 1994). Some of these phonological phenomena link in to English morphology. For example, in the south of England the definite determiner THE is pronounced differently according to whether it precedes a vowel, when it is pronounced [ði] (THE ELEPHANT, THE ARMADILLO), or a consonant, when it is pronounced [ðə] (THE BABOON, THE DINOSAUR). The alternation is more obvious in the case of the indefinite determiner, where the spelling reflects the difference (AN ELEPHANT, AN ARMADILLO, VS A BABOON, A DINOSAUR). Again, the development of these aspects of phonology and morphology in children have not been studied extensively, but it has been observed that many children at this phase have not yet sorted out the alternatives. A cross-sectional study of 100 children ranging from 3;6 to 7;6 years, from the west of England (Hereford), showed a developmental trend in the children's ability to use the definite and indefinite determiner alternations accurately. By contrast, there was no difference between age groups in the use of alveolar assimilations and linking [ʷ], [ʲ] and [ʴ], suggesting that by their fourth year normally-developing children have learnt these features of connected speech (Newton, 1997).

There is another pervasive phonological feature of English connected speech that brings us back to where this section started, in the discussion of consonant sequences. There, it was mentioned that many children at this phase still have problems with words containing complex consonant clusters, in words like STRENGTH. Complex consonant sequences occur very frequently in connected speech, arising both when morphemes are affixed to the root word, e.g. the plural morpheme in LENGTHS and also when a word ending with a cluster is followed by a word beginning with a cluster, e.g. BLANK SQUARES [blæŋkskwɛəz] which contains five consonants between the vowel nucleus of the first word and the vowel nucleus of the second. In fluent colloquial speech, such sequences arise in verb phrases containing auxiliary verbs, where the auxiliaries are generally contracted to a shorter form, e.g. 's for IS, HAS, 've for HAVE, 'LL for WILL. These sequences are not always identical to the clusters found within words, and so can present new articulatory challenges to the child attempting to produce fluent utterances that incorporate more complex verb phrases, such as IT'LL'VE STOPPED BY NOW or CHRIS'S BEEN OVER.

Kelly and Local (1989, pp. 190–202) show how one girl, from the north of England coped with these demands. She was CA 5;2 and had been described as having a 'phonological disorder'. By making use of gemination (consonant lengthening) and glottal closure, rather than pronouncing each distinct articulation that made up the sequence, she managed to retain the rhythmic structure of the target (adult) forms, though at the expense of articulatory accuracy. This example demonstrates her use of gemination:

MUMMY'S WATCHING (THEM)
/mʌmɪzwɒʧɪn/ → [mʌme̠⊥w+⊥w̠⊥ɒtɕɪn]

A lengthened labial-velar articulation with close approximation is used instead of the target /zw/ sequence. While the rhythm of the target is thus preserved, the differentiation in place of articulation is lost, although Kelly and Local noted that the *secondary* articulation or resonance does in fact change, from front [w+⊥] to back [w̠⊥], during the course of the labial-velar approximant, reflecting that it represents both the /z/ of MUMMY'S and then the /w/ of WATCHING. This girl's approach to the phonological challenges presented by connected speech can be contrasted with that of Zoe, described in Chapter 9, whose speech is more staccato, but with more of the primary articulatory information preserved (cf. Wells, 1994). This is evident in the following example, where the target is pronounced with quite precise articulation, but with a pause, a prevocalic glottal stop, and lengthening of vowels and consonants, all of which contribute to a disruption of the rhythm:

SHE'S GOING UP THE STAIRS
/ʃizgəʊɪŋʌpðəstɛəz/ → [ˈʆiːjɪs̺.ˈgɵɪŋkˀʔɒ̝pː˺ˌd̺əˈˈtɛːːs]

In summary, around the fourth year of life, children's speech can be characterized as showing evidence of attempts to reconcile still immature motor skills with the phonological demands of the more complex sentences that they wish to utter. The source of resulting dysfluencies can be located in the on-line assembly of utterances, in the motor planning box on the model, while other aspects impact upon the phonological representations. Some children's speech development is arrested at this phase, as our examples have shown (see also Stackhouse 1996, pp. 24, 25).

The Metaphonological Phase

The Metaphonological Phase takes us to the child's fifth year – the year before or during which children in the UK and the USA enter school. It is characterized by the emergence of skills and behaviours that research has shown to be precursors of successful literacy development in the school years. On the input side, the majority of children at this phase are beginning to be able consciously to segment words and syllables into constituent parts. This is most evident in an ability to rhyme, which requires the ability to segment the onset from the rhyme of the stressed syllable of target word (Vance, Stackhouse and Wells, 1994); and also in the ability to play games such as I-Spy, where again the child has to be aware of the onset consonant or consonants as a unit. There is no substantial evidence that at this phase children are able to segment within the rhyme, i.e. to identify coda syllables: they find it very hard, often impossible, to think of words that *end* with a particular sound (unlike I-Spy). Nor is there much evidence that they are able to segment within the onset, when the onset consists of a cluster. The onset clusters, like the rhyme, seems to be treated as an indivisible entity (Fowler, 1991). According to two of the leading researchers in this area:

> 'Our data, together with data from illiterate adults and readers of non-alphabetic scripts...suggest that sensitivity to syllables, onsets and rimes can develop without knowledge of a writing system that represents speech at these levels'.
>
> Treiman and Zukowski (1996)

Further segmentation into phones or segments is not found without exposure to an alphabetic script, however (see Figure 3.1, Chapter 3). Laura, at CA 4;9 and not yet at school or reading, could segment the onset of the first syllable of STRAWBERRY from the rest of the word (STR + AWBERRY), but was unable to segment further within the STR cluster. Evidence that segmentation of the rhyme into nucleus and coda, and segmentation of both onset and coda into constituent consonant segments have not been achieved, or at least have not come to conscious awareness, by the end of the preschool period, is also provided by children's inability to handle allomorphic variation productively, described below, and children's earliest attempts at spelling, which are characterized by the omission of vowels and of cluster elements. Treiman (1993) has carried out several studies that support this position.

The first explicit evidence of an ability to segment phonetic input into constituent parts is, for many children, around the fifth year. Prior to this, there is no direct evidence that children have segmented words into smaller constituents, let alone into phonemes. This suggests that prior to this phase, phonological representations and motor programs for lexical items may not contain much internal phonological structure, and that what structure they have is not readily accessible to the child's conscious awareness. This has some implications for therapy and teaching activities prior to age 4: therapy activities requiring segmentation and manipulation of phonemes may be expecting too much of children who may not be progressing through these phases at the normal rate anyway.

Children's output behaviour suggests that some tacit segmentation may occur, for example the use of affixes such as -S which children appear to attach in a rule-governed way to noun roots to form plural forms. However, the experimental evidence indicates that there is a strong difference between real words and nonwords: children of 4 and above still have difficulty with attaching the correct phonological form, or allomorph, to nonwords. Berko (1958) elicited plural and past tense forms from children between from CA 4 to 7;6. The children were much more likely to use the correct allomorph for a known word than for a nonword: for example, 91 per cent of responses had [əz] for the plural of GLASS (GLASSES) but only 36 per cent for the plural of TASS. For past tense, 76 per cent of responses had [əd] for MELT (MELTED), but only 33 per cent for MOTT. Thus, although children at this phase are able to use the plural or the past tense morpheme in a productive way, they are much less proficient at attaching the correct phonological form of the morpheme to unfamiliar words. In order to come up with the 'correct' plural forms for noun nonwords, the child would need to know which particular coda consonants, not just which lexical items, require the [əz] allomorph rather than [z] as in BIRDS or [s] as in CATS. The fact that the children in Berko's famous study had problems with the nonwords suggests that children in this phase have not yet made phonological generalizations about sound classes. This casts doubt on the extent to which phonological segmentation and categorization have really occurred.

Older children with speech difficulties have been shown to have particular difficulties with the categorization of coda consonants, as required for plural formation rules. Hughes (1983) studied three children from Lancashire, in the north west of England, none of whom pronounced [s] in final position, in order to see how they handled the formation of plurals. Louise (CA 6;9) pronounced the singular forms of the following words all with final [t] or [d], even though they had different targets:

Adult: singular	*Louise: singular*	*Adult: plural*	*Louise: plural*
KNIFE	[naɪt]	/naɪvz/	[naɪt]
BED	[bɛd]	/bɛdz/	[bɛd]
BATH	[bæt]	/bæθs/	[bæt]
BUS	[bʌt]	/bʌsɪz/	[bʌt]
BRUSH	[bwʌt]	/brʌʃɪz/	[bwʌt]
CAT	[kæt]	/kæts/	[kæts]
WATCH	[wɒt]	/wɒtʃɪz/	[wɒtɪd]
MATCH	[mæt]	/mætʃɪz/	[mætɪd]
MOUSE	[maut]	/maɪs/	[mautɪd]

In terms of the target forms, the first five words illustrate the three different regular plural allomorphs of English. For Louise, they all have an aveolar plosive coda in the singular form, and retain the same form in the plural. This suggests that Louise may not even be aware of, or capable of, signalling plurality at all. However, this is belied by CAT, which has a correctly formed plural, and then by WATCH and MATCH, which show the syllabic allomorph appropriate to the target stem, even though the final consonant of the suffix is not realized accurately. These forms suggest that Louise is aware (a) that plurals are formed by adding a suffix, (b) that the suffix varies according to the final consonant of the singular form and (c) that, more specifically, sibilants in stem-final position require the syllabic allomorph. This last point is further supported by her plural form for MOUSE, which she treats as a regular noun ending in a sibilant. However, it is undermined somewhat by BUS and BRUSH, to which she gives no suffix at all, even though the target singular forms end in a sibilant too.

The cases of Louise and the other two children in Hughes' study illustrate two important points about the relationship between the speech output of children with speech difficulties, and their underlying knowledge. First, a child's own pronunciation may be a poor reflection of his/her phonological representation of the target form: all the words ending with target /s/ or /z/ were pronounced by Louise with final [t] or [d] in the singular, but she treated them in three different ways in the plural, indicating that she may be aware of three different categories of coda consonant. Thus, Louise's choice of plural form was determined not by her own (often incorrect) pronunciation of the coda, but on the basis of an underlying representation that was closer to the adult form. In terms of our model, this indicates that Louise selected a plural form on the basis of her phonological representation for the word, which, while not always completely accurate, was more adult-like than her motor program for the word, as evidenced by this pronunciation.

The second point that arises from the case of Louise is that some of the child's actual categorization may be incorrect, as evidenced by BUS and BRUSH, which Louise treated like the nouns ending in non-sibilant codas. It can be surmised that such problems, showing arrest at the Metaphonological Phase, will have consequences for literacy development, since knowledge of morphophonology is necessary for progression to the Orthographic Phase of literacy development, where the child has to identify and segment words on the basis of their morphophonological structure (Bryant and Nunes, 1997; Frith, 1985). For example, knowing that the last syllable of ADDITION, /ʃən/, is a morpheme that can be attached to other words, such as ATTENTION, and is written <tion>, is an economical strategy for reading and spelling.

In terms of our model, the Metaphonological Phase is characterized by changes on the input side in the structure of phonological representations, and on the output side in motor programming and the motor programs themselves. In Chapter 6, it was proposed that motor programming draws on a store of units for the different positions in syllable structure, each of which has a gestural realization, which can be combined to create programs for different syllables and words. In developmental terms, there is a steady progression from the Whole

Word Phase, when the motor program is co-extensive with the word. This progression consists of a gradual segmentation into smaller units:

(i) word into syllable (weak vs strong);
(ii) the syllable into onset and rhyme;
(iii) the rhyme into nucleus and coda;
(iv) both onset and coda into constituent consonant segments.

A great deal of research has emphasized the importance of phonological awareness skills, including segmentation into onset / rhyme and into phonemes, for the subsequent development of literacy skills. Recently, there has been debate over the extent to which it is phonological awareness that is crucial, or whether the tacit segmentation of input and establishing of accurate underlying phonological representations is more important, as argued by Snowling and Hulme (1994). Whatever the answer, the importance of the Metaphonological Phase as part of the normal path of phonological development for speech and literacy is evident for teachers and therapists working on pre-literacy skills.

Speech Processing and Literacy Difficulties

In Chapters 7 and 8 we have presented an account of the phases of development of speech processing, with indications as to how some kinds of developmental speech problem can be interpreted as delayed or arrested development. Two important threads now need to be made explicit: the nature of developmental speech difficulties, and the relationship with literacy development. For example, in the discussion of the Whole Word Phase, mention was made of similarities between the characteristics of very young normally-developing children at this phase of development, and some of the speech features characteristic of older children diagnosed as having developmental verbal dyspraxia. These characteristics include inconsistent speech output and sequencing difficulties. A developmental view of such children is that they have not moved through the early Whole Word Phase of speech development. They are unable to break through to the Systematic Simplification Phase, where the patterns of correspondence between target segments and the child's productions are consistent and where mis-sequencing of segments is rare. This is analogous to Frith's account of classic developmental dyslexia (see Chapter 1 of this volume for an exposition of Frith's model). Frith (1985) suggests that children with phonological dyslexia are arrested at the Logographic Phase of literacy development, where they can only read and spell words that they have learnt as a whole, but are unable to decode or spell unfamiliar words. To tackle unfamiliar material, children need to break through to the Alphabetic Phase of literacy development, which is characterized by an ability to decode unfamiliar words for reading and to segment words for spelling purposes.

An analogy has been drawn between the child with verbal dyspraxia failing to break through from the Whole Word Phase to the Systematic Simplification Phase, and the child with phonological dyslexia failing to break through from the Logographic Phase to the Alphabetic Phase. The comparison between Frith's phases of literacy development and the phases of speech development presented in this chapter shows how a developmental perspective might be used to throw light on children's speech processing difficulties. However, there is also a more substantial aspect to the analogy: namely the possibility that progressing from the Whole Word Phase to the Systematic Simplification Phase is in fact a *prerequisite* for the child subsequently to progress from the Logographic Phase to the Alphabetic Phase. By contrast to the Whole Word Phase, the Systematic Simplification Phase is characterized by stable correspondences between segments in the target form of words and the segments that make up the child's production. Thus, in simplifying patterns such as fronting of velars, e.g. KEY → [ti], there is a one-to-one correspondence betwen the place in structure of the [k] in the adult target and the place in structure of the [t] in the child's pronunciation. The same is true of the other common patterns of systemic simplification, such as stopping of fricatives (ZOO → [du]) and affricates (CHAIR → [dɛə]), fronting of postalveolars (SHOE →[su]), or gliding of liquids (ROAD →[wəʊd]). Even patterns that involve apparent deletion or coalescence of segments, such as cluster reduction, observe the phonological constituency of the syllable: thus cluster reduction affects either the onset or the coda. Simplification patterns such as consonant harmony, context sensitive voicing and reduplication, that do not observe the segmentation of the syllable into onset and rhyme or beyond, are the ones that disappear earliest (Grunwell, 1987), and for that reason were described earlier in this chapter as being transitional between the Whole Word Phase and the Systematic Simplification Phase. We suggest that stable correspondences between onsets, rhymes, nuclei and codas in the target word and the child's own pronunciation form a basis for the child's gradual segmentation of phonological representations into phonological constituents, which culminates in the Metaphonological Phase.

This developmental perspective on the early phases of speech and literacy development makes it clear why children with developmental verbal dyspraxia have such serious literacy difficulties (Stackhouse and Snowling, 1992a). Their inability to break out of the Whole Word Phase of speech development means that they do not develop the segmentation skills that are rooted in the Systematic Simplification Phase and which manifest in the Metaphonological Phase. These skills are necessary for breaking through from the Logographic to the Alphabetic Phase of literacy development. This idea will now be explored in more depth through case studies of two children, Michael and Caroline (Stackhouse, 1989).

Arrested Development at the Whole Word and Logographic Phases

The development of speech, phonological awareness, reading and spelling in Michael and Caroline was studied over a 5-year period. At the beginning of the study, Michael was aged 10;7 and Caroline was 11;0. They attended a secondary school where they were integrated into mainstream, but where they received daily remedial teaching and twice weekly speech and language therapy within a language unit attached to the school. Both were of average intelligence. On the *British Ability Scales* (Elliot, Murray and Pearson, 1983), Michael gained an estimated IQ of 100 and Caroline an IQ of 111. Their speech had been unintelligible during the preschool years and they had a persisting and obvious phonological impairment. In addition, they had serious literacy problems. Both children had a history of fluctuating hearing loss but hearing was within normal limits at the time of the study.

Speech

Clumsiness, incoordination of the vocal tract, groping for articulatory postures and inconsistent articulatory output were observed in both Michael and Caroline. Michael's speech errors comprised phonetic distortions (CRAB → [kxə'wæb]), syllable reduction (TELEVISION → [tɛ'vɪʒn̩]) and difficulties with articulatory place change (BUTTERCUP → ['kʌkə.kʌʔ]). Caroline, in particular, struggled to produce target words, making repeated attempts to get them right, e.g. TREASURE → [s st 'stɛɾə 'stɛvə 'ʤɛvə 'stɛɪə 'ʤɛlɪʃ 'ʤɛdə] .

Michael and Caroline's speech errors were compared with those from a group of younger normally-developing children matched on articulation age (measured by the *Edinburgh Articulation Test*, Anthony, Bogle, Ingram, et al., 1971). The normally-developing children were in the chronological age range of 3;3 to 5;6 and had an articulation age range of 3;0 to 5;6. The tasks presented included single word naming and imitation, a connected speech condition, and a nonword imitation task. The target words increased in syllable length, e.g. KITE, ROCKET, CARAVAN and TELEVISION and also included clusters e.g. NEST, SPIDER, STAMP.

The normally-developing children performed equally well across all the conditions. In contrast, Michael and Caroline's performance was much more variable, with particular difficulties evident on the continuous speech condition. Qualitative analysis revealed that although young normally-developing children made dyspraxic-like speech errors, these were not as frequent or in such a severe form as those from the older children with speech difficulties. Therefore, it was decided to compare the number of speech errors occurring in the target words spoken by Michael and Caroline with the normal controls. To make this comparison, the number of errors occurring in each target word was calculated, for example TREASURE realized as ['ʤɛdə] contains a total of three errors:

(1)	affrication of the cluster	['tɹɛʒə] → ['ʧɛʒə]
(2)	prevocalic voicing	['ʧɛʒə] → ['ʤɛʒə]
(3)	stopping	['ʤɛʒə]→ ['ʤɛdə]

This analysis revealed that Michael and Caroline could pronounce more words correctly than the younger children. Unlike the normally-developing children, however, when they were unable to pronounce a word they made multiple errors. Thus, Michael and Caroline either *could* or *could not* produce a word, and when they could not produce a word, it contained several errors. In contrast, the normal controls made only one or two errors per word but in a wider range of words (Stackhouse and Snowling, 1992b).

Reading and spelling

A parallel finding emerged from an analysis of Michael and Caroline's reading and spelling errors. Michael and Caroline both met the criteria for a diagnosis of phonological dyslexia. The children read words as visual wholes rather than breaking them up into their sound components. This meant that they were likely to make visual errors when reading, (e.g. <pint> read as "paint" and <organ> as "orange") and they were unable to tackle new words. They had particular difficulty when spelling. Michael's attempts to apply the phonics he had been taught were unsuccessful, as seen in these spellings of three-syllable words: CIGARETTE → ‹satersatarhaelerar›, UMBRELLA → ‹rberherrelrarlsrllles›. Although these spellings appear bizarre, they can be explained by a failure to segment the word into syllables and sounds. These nonphonetic spellings occurred as Michael transcribed his repeated attempts at segmentation. For example, the following illustrates Michael's spellings when mapped on to the words' syllable structure ($ = syllable boundary):

Target	*Spelling*
CIGARETTE	sa $ ter $ sa $ tar $ haelerar
1 2 3	1 3 1 3 2
UMBRELLA	r$ be $ rher $ re $ l $ ra $ r $ l $ sr $ lll $ es
1 2 3	2 2 2 2 3 2 2 3 ?2 3 ?

The first example shows how Michael had more success with the first and last syllables, which are the most acoustically salient. The second example reveals deletion of the first syllable which is unstressed, particular difficulty segmenting the cluster /br/ which he could not pronounce and some visual notion that the word contains more than one letter ‹l›.

Caroline's spellings also revealed segmentation difficulties but of a different kind. She had adopted a lexical strategy where she selected words she knew to represent the syllables, for example ADVENTURE → ‹andbackself›, REFRESHMENT → ‹withfirstmint›. Unlike Michael, all of her spellings included the correct number of syllables. However, like Michael, she could not segment sounds *within* the syllable for spelling purposes.

A qualitative developmental analysis revealed that neither of the children's spellings was typical of younger normally-developing children (Stackhouse and Snowling, 1992a). Just as in the speech study above, where they either could or could not pronounce words, Michael and Caroline either could or could not read and spell words. When they could not read or spell a word, they made complex errors because they did not have the phonological processing skills necessary to segment and blend the components of the target.

In both speech and literacy development, Michael and Caroline tackled each new word separately, rather than utilizing phonological processing skills to identify similarities across phonologically related words. This lexical approach to acquiring new words is typical of very young children, characteristic of the Whole Word Phase as described in Chapter 7, and parallels Frith's (1985) description of the Logographic Phase of literacy development. The indications were that Michael and Caroline were arrested in their speech and literacy development at a phase prior to the development of phonological awareness. If this were so, it could be predicted that they should be unable to perform tasks that tap phonological awareness skills, such as rhyme.

Rhyme

First, a rhyme detection task was devised in which Michael and Caroline were to select the word that rhymed with a target (e.g. CAT) from two alternatives (e.g. CAT : FISH or HAT , GOAT: BOAT or GATE). The non-rhyming target was either semantically related to the target (FISH) or an alliteration of it (GATE). To compare performance in the auditory and visual modalities, the stimuli were either spoken words or presented as pictures. Normally-developing 7-year-olds matched on reading age were at ceiling on these tasks (Stackhouse, 1989). Caroline at age 11;0 performed at ceiling in the visual modality and scored 85 per cent correct in the auditory modality, indicating that she was making connections between rhyming words. In contrast, Michael at 10;7 performed significantly less well: 70 per cent correct in the visual modality and only 60 per cent correct (i.e. at chance) in the auditory modality. He was also more likely to choose a semantically related distractor as his response.

Second, Michael and Caroline were tested on a rhyme production task. They were asked to produce rhyme strings to a series of simple words (e.g. MAP, SUN, KEY). This task requires the child to segment the stimulus into onset and rhyme (/m/+/æp/), and then either to search the lexicon for words with the same rhyme, and retrieve and produce such words, or search for different onsets while maintaining the rhyme and then reassemble new rhyming words. The first strategy results in only real words being produced, while the second explains why children often produce a mixture of real and nonwords when producing rhymes (cf. Chapter 3). On this task both Michael and Caroline could make at most only one correct rhyme response to each target.

Although their rhyme detection skills improved over time, their persisting difficulty with rhyme production was evident at follow-up when Michael's chronological age was 14;5 and Caroline's was 15;0 years. At this age, Michael was still more proficient at making semantic than phonological links in his lexicon. For example, for a rhyme with WOOL, he replied "sheep". It also became clear that the rhyming responses he made had been well taught and were not spontaneous. When asked what rhymes with DRAW, he responded rather anxiously "Miss V (his speech and language therapist) not tell me about draw!"

In contrast, Caroline's responses indicated that she had made phonological links in her lexicon and was attempting to produce rhyming words. However, persisting speech output difficulties, no longer so apparent in Michael's speech, interfered with her rhyme production by taking her further away from the target, e.g. WOOL → ['wiʊ 'wiʊl 'luʊ 'wɪl 'dɪl 'bɪl]. A similar pattern of performance was evident on other phonological awareness tasks, e.g. sound blending.

Sound blending

When Michael was asked to blend the word PRAM, presented as /pr + æ + m/, he first attempted to blend the segments, producing "prom, promp" but then gave up on this and responded "we call it a pushchair!", again indicating strong semantic links. Caroline, however, had more intrusive articulations; e.g. SANG /s + æ + ŋ/ was blended as [sæzŋ] and sometimes her distorted response led to access of the wrong lexical item, e.g. BUST, /b + ʌ + st/, was blended as "[bʌ sːːːt], basket".

The results from the phonological awareness tasks confirm that Michael and Caroline were arrested in an early stage of speech and literacy development. Michael's lexicon was not organized along phonological lines. He had not progressed to a phase in which phonologically similar words (e.g. words with a shared rhyme) are closely connected (Waterson 1981, 1987). The connections within Michael's lexicon were predominantly semantic, as evidenced in his rhyme and blending responses. In contrast, Caroline had made some progress with her phonological organization skills but her attempts to search her lexicon were undermined by her persisting speech output difficulties. Further investigation of their lexical skills was carried out.

Lexical decision

On the nonword repetition task reported earlier, Michael produced a real word response more often than did either Caroline or the normally-developing children. For example, he reproduced SLEPPER as "slipper", and DACKS as "ducks". Out of a total of 30 nonwords, the normally-developing children lexicalized on average on only 1.6 of the targets (range 1–3). Caroline lexicalized on three items (i.e. at the top of the normal range), but Michael lexicalized significantly more – seven.

Michael, in particular, also had difficulties with a nonword spelling test (cf. Campbell, 1983) where a spoken list of words was presented within which were embedded a number of nonwords, e.g. DISH, NIGHT, COAL, /brəʊl/, LADY, BOIL, /wɒɪl/. The task was for the child to stop the tester every time a nonword was heard and then to write it down. Michael accepted 81 per cent of the nonwords as real words and Caroline accepted 58 per cent of them. However, unlike Caroline, Michael was very confident that he had responded correctly and went on to define the nonwords (e.g. /jaɪt/ → "light", /tid/ → "tea").

In order to check whether this difficulty was specific to the auditory modality, Michael and Caroline were presented with a written and spoken lexical decison task (after Coltheart, 1980). They had to sort words into real word and nonword categories, e.g. real word: BLACK, nonword: BRACK. In the visual modality, Michael and Caroline did not perform significantly differently from a group of 33 normally-developing children matched on reading age. However, when the stimuli were presented auditorily, both children performed significantly less well than the controls. Michael, in particular, found this task difficult.

These results support the hypothesis that Michael may have been having more difficulty with input phonological processing than

Caroline. However, both children were more willing than reading age matched controls to accept similar sounding nonwords as real words. This indicated that their lexical representations were less precise than those of the younger normally-developing children. This lexical deficit was particularly apparent in Michael's case, and put him at a disadvantage when learning new words, which he was liable to misrepresent or falsely categorize as known words.

One hypothesis regarding the cause of Michael's and Caroline's imprecise lexical representations is that they had deficits in auditory discrimination which resulted in a failure to identify fine phonetic distinctions. This would affect their ability to construct accurate phonological representations for new lexical items. Auditory discrimination tasks were administered in order to test this hypothesis.

Auditory discrimination

Initial testing on the *Wepman Auditory Discrimination Test* (Wepman and Reynolds, 1987), which comprises simple minimal pair words, did not support the hypothesis. Michael and Caroline were able to detect when two words were the same or different perfectly well, e.g. PIN vs BIN, PIN vs PIN. A more stringent test was therefore designed. This comprised a series of complex nonwords which differed in:

(1)	place of articulation	/spəʊb/	vs	/spəʊd/
(2)	voicing	/beɪt/	vs	/peɪt/
(3)	cluster sequence	/wɛsp/	vs	/wɛps/
(4)	phoneme sequence	/ˈbɪkʌt/	vs	/ˈbɪtʌk/

The test was administered to Michael and Caroline and to 42 normally-developing children in the age range of 3;3 to 8;11. On this test, both Michael and Caroline performed less well than the controls. Although able to detect same nonword pairs 100 per cent of the time, they were only able to detect different nonword pairs at a 69 per cent accuracy level. In comparison, the controls scored 88 per cent correct on the detection of different nonword pairs.

These results indicated that while Michael and Caroline did not have an auditory discrimination problem on a simple test comprising CVC words, they did have difficulties discriminating words differing in the *sequence* of sounds, particularly if these words were new to them. This auditory discrimination task may itself be dependent on articulatory and phonological awareness skills, since when asked to make a same/different judgement on a pair of complex and unfamiliar words, a common strategy is to repeat the words while reflecting on their structure. Michael's and Caroline's variable speech production and poor segmentation skills prevented successful use of this strategy. An alternative support strategy of visualizing the written form of the word was also problematic for them: neither Michael nor Caroline could read or spell simple nonwords and therefore were not able to utilize such a strategy on this task.

This longitudinal study of Michael and Caroline, two children with severe speech output difficulties, revealed the pervasiveness of their underlying phonological processing deficits. The difficulties with input, representation and output processing resulted in poor performance on phonological awareness tasks and were directly related to their literacy problems. One of the most important findings from this study was the discovery of a similar pattern of development in both their speech and literacy skills; phonological processing skills were not developed sufficiently to tackle the next phase of development in either speech or literacy. Frith's (1985) model of literacy development explains this arrested development as a failure to pass from the Logographic to the Alphabetic Phase. In terms of the account of speech processing development given in Chapter 7, Michael and Caroline were also having great difficulty in moving beyond the Whole Word Phase.

Arrested Development at Later Phases

Children who progress without difficulty from the Whole Word Phase to the Systematic Simplification Phase create a foundation for the development of segmentation skills which can subsequently be applied to literacy. For some children the Systematic Simplification Phase may persist for longer than expected; such children are typically referred to speech and language therapy for immature or delayed speech. There are a number of reasons why this phase may continue for longer than usual, alluded to in Chapter 7. These include failure to perceive or be aware of certain phonological contrasts and therefore to incorporate this information into phonological representations; an inability to produce the required pronunciation at the level of motor execution; and a failure to extend new pronunciation abilities to words already in the child's vocabulary, i.e. to update existing motor programs. As long as there is no serious underlying speech processing deficit identifiable on the speech processing profile (see Chapter 5), there is no reason why these children should not develop literacy skills satisfactorily. Speech and language therapy that has as its main focus children's immature speech patterns can incidentally accelerate phonological awareness skills; this is particularly likely to happen where the approach to the speech problem explicitly incorporates phonological awareness activities, as in the *Metaphon* programme (Howell and Dean, 1994). Such therapy helps children to progress to the Metaphonological Phase, putting them in a good position to break through to the Alphabetic Phase of literacy development as they begin school.

Difficulties at the Assembly Phase are often described as 'residual' problems in children who have had obvious speech difficulties earlier on, i.e. at the Whole Word or Systematic Simplification Phases. Some of these may be observable within the word, for instance substitutions of [f] for /θ/, [w] for /r/, or imprecise pronunciation of consonant clusters. Others are evident in connected speech, such as with consonant sequences and other types of between-word junction, or unusual rhythm and intonation. Such speech characteristics can be viewed as warning signals that a child is not progressing in the usual way through the phases of speech development. They are often overlooked by parents and professionals because the child can by now produce all the individual segments of English. Specific problems with consonant clusters in both speech and spelling have been described in a case study of a boy with phonological dyslexia (Snowling, Hulme, Wells, et al., 1992). 'Mumbley' speech commented on by parents or teachers is often a sign of speech processing difficulties in children at risk for phonological dyslexia, as in the case of Richard who was described in Chapter 5. In terms of the speech processing model, these speech difficulties are probably indicative of motor programs for words that are not fully specified. In the case of consonant clusters, for example, the child may be able to get away with a pronunciation that makes a cluster distinct from other clusters it could potentially be confused with, while still not having mastered the precise sequence of gestures used in the adult language. However, this imprecision becomes problematic when the child needs to spell words containing clusters.

Earlier in this chapter it was suggested that for some children who stammer, the Assembly Phase may be the origin of their difficulties, and that stammering can be related to a deficit in motor planning. If this is the case, it suggests that such children should not have particular difficulties with phonological segmentation and thence phonological awareness, since these skills are to do with the analysis of lexical representations whereas motor planning happens at a lower level of processing on the output side. Thus stammering children, like children with cleft palate or dysarthria who have deficits at motor execution, should not be particularly at risk for dyslexia. Research bears out this prediction, at least in part. Some children who stammer perform just as well as controls on tasks of rhyme detection and production, for example (Forth, Stackhouse, Vance, et al., 1996). However, other children in the same study, whose stammer was no worse, had major difficulties on the rhyme tasks. This suggests that the stammer itself may indeed be independent of higher level phonological processing, and so not a predictor of literacy difficulties. At the same time, some children who stammer may also have higher level phonological processing deficits which put them at risk as far as the development of literacy skills is concerned. This reflects the fact that many children who stammer, perhaps 30–40 per cent, also have segmental phonological problems – a much higher proportion than in the population at large (Louko, 1995; Conture, Yaruss and Edwards, 1995). The possibility of both association and dissociation, in different children, of stammering and phonological processing deficits points to the importance of individual profiling of the child in order to arrive at an assessment that can provide a sound basis for intervention.

Finally, the Metaphonological Phase marks children's successful passage through the phases of speech development to the point where they are ready to take on literacy instruction when they start school. During this phase it is likely that children will already be able to recognize the written form of some familiar words: they are thus simultaneously in the Logographic Phase of literacy development. It is during this phase that they will be building up the phonological awareness skills that are prerequisite for breaking through to the Alphabetic Phase of literacy development, and also the morphophonological knowledge that will permit progression to the Orthographic Phase. Although there are aspects of speech production that are not yet adult-like, most children will not be carrying with them the 'baggage' of the earlier phases of speech development when they start school. If, however, some of the characteristics of earlier phases are still salient in the child's speech, it is possible that underlying speech processing problems will interfere with literacy development.

Summary

In this chapter it has been proposed that our perspective on speech and literacy problems needs to be not only psycholinguistic but also developmental. In Chapters 9 and 10, we will illustrate in some detail how these developmental phases can be used, in conjunction with the assessment framework of Chapters 4 and 5 and the processing model from Chapter 6, to throw light on the unfolding speech and literacy difficulties of one child.

The main points arising from Chapter 8 are as follows:

- In normal speech development children progress through two further identifiable phases, giving five in all:

  The Prelexical Phase
  The Whole Word Phase
  The Systematic Simplification Phase
  The Assembly Phase
  The Metaphonological Phase.

- The nature of a child's speech difficulty is related to the developmental phase (or phases) that s/he finds particularly troublesome.
- The development of literacy skills can also be viewed as a progression through identifiable phases, following Frith (1985):

  The Logographic Phase
  The Alphabetic Phase
  The Orthographic Phase.

- Progress through the phases of literacy development is dependent on successful progress through the phases of speech processing development.
- Children with speech and literacy difficulties may be viewed as having arrested, problematic or slow development through the phases of speech and literacy development.
- The same pattern of difficulty can be present in both speech and literacy development.
- Arrested development at the Logographic Phase of literacy development can be linked to arrested development at the Whole Word Phase of speech development.
- Progress through the Systematic Simplification Phase of speech development is a necessary prerequisite for the normal development of phonological awareness skills.
- Problems at the Assembly Phase of speech development may be indicative of underlying motor programming or motor planning difficulties, which may be reflected in a child's spelling of consonant clusters for example.
- Children need to have entered the Metaphonological Phase of speech development in order to make sense of literacy instruction at school.

KEY TO ACTIVITY 8.1
David's intonation system

(a) The main pitch movement invariably occurs on the final syllable of the utterance, is rising, and is accompanied by slowing of tempo and increased loudness.

(b) Because the main prominence occurs not merely on the final word but on the final syllable of that word, the normal pattern of lexical stress in words of more than one syllable is disrupted. This can be seen on LETTER, POSTMAN, TEDDY BEAR, LETTERBOX, which are normally accented on the first syllable. In David's speech in this extract, the main prominence is instead on the last syllable (n.b. these words only occur in utterance final position in this extract).

(c) David's prosodic pattern has consequences for his system of information focus or emphasis. For example, in "I already [gɛd] that", (l.17) [gɛd], which presumably represents SAID or READ, would normally be accented at the expense of the following "that", in order to highlight its informational importance. In David's version, the pronoun "that" is phonetically most prominent, by virtue of its utterance final position: see (a) above.

Chapter 9
The Unfolding Deficit I – Barriers to Speech

So far we have outlined a psycholinguistic approach to the investigation of developmental speech and literacy disorders, which has been formalized in terms of an assessment framework in Chapter 4 and illustrated with profiles of two contrasting case studies in Chapter 5. The underlying psycholinguistic assumptions of the approach have been made explicit in terms of a speech processing model in Chapter 6, and have been presented from a developmental perspective in Chapters 7 and 8. In this chapter and the next, the various strands will be pulled together through a case study of one child, Zoe. One aim of this case study is to show how a profile of assessment findings can be interpreted in terms of a model of speech processing. A second aim is to suggest how the developmental phases outlined in Chapters 7 and 8 might offer insights into how speech processing deficits can unfold through childhood, with particular reference to the development of reading and spelling. 'Snapshots' will be presented of Zoe's speech and literacy development at three points, CA 3;9, 5;11 and 9;8, which catch her in the preschool period, after a year of primary school, and in the later phases of her primary education. For each point in time, a speech processing profile will be presented on the basis of the data that are available from clinical records and from the more specific psycholinguistic investigations carried out at the latter two points in time. Each profile will be interpreted in terms of the model of speech processing presented earlier. Finally, Zoe's unfolding difficulties in speech and literacy will be interpreted in terms of phases of development of speech processing. This chapter is mainly concerned with Zoe's speech, and focuses on the period up to 5;11, while in Chapter 10 the implications of her speech processing deficits for literacy development are considered.

Zoe's Early Development

There had been no medical problems at Zoe's birth, and her health was good. Zoe's co-ordination and motor skills were age-appropriate throughout. She had no chewing or feeding problems. It was reported that she babbled normally, and that her first word was at CA 0;11. Zoe had no problems apart from her speech and language, about which her mother became concerned when Zoe was 16 months old. She first had speech therapy when she was 2;10. There is no family history of speech and language problems, but her younger brother was subsequently referred for therapy.

Her verbal comprehension was tested on the *Reynell Developmental Language Scales* (Reynell and Huntley, 1985) at CA 2;10, when she scored at an age appropriate level (raw score: 37; standard score: 0,4; age equivalent: 2;11). She was given the *Symbolic Play Test* (Lowe and Costello, 1988) at CA 3;1, and was at ceiling (raw score 23, age equivalent 3;0). She attended a preschool language group from CA 2;10 to 3;0, during which her listening and attention improved greatly. She attended an intensive language course at C.A. 3;1. She had good comprehension but mixed auditory discrimination skills. Expressive language was still found to be well behind receptive skills. She had a good range of tongue and lip movements and imitation of consonants and vowels was described as 'fairly good'; however, she exhibited groping oral movements before vocalization and sounds were 'inconsistent and deviant'. She had a very poor diadochokinetic rate and was aware of her mistakes. It was concluded by her speech and language therapist that she showed the signs of developmental verbal dyspraxia.

Following this, she had weekly therapy from CA 3;2 to 3;6, using the *Nuffield Dyspraxia Programme* (Connery, 1992), working on different sound classes, using the picture symbols from the Nuffield Programme with the aim of producing voiceless plosives [p t k], nasals [m n], vowels, then voiced plosives [b d g] and fricatives [f v s z ʃ], followed by CV sequences. Auditory discrimination was also practised, and there was work on tongue and lip movement. Initially in this phase, all her spontaneous utterances were reduplicated single words, e.g. DOG → ['wɔwɔ], CAR → ['gɑgɑ], but this gradually reduced, e.g. CAR → [gɑ]. From CA 3;7 to 3;8 she attended a therapy group for children with dyspraxia, with two other children. She could now produce and discriminate sounds using the Nuffield symbols but there had been no increase in her expressive language. Hearing and vision were satisfactory when tested at CA 3;7, hearing having been assessed by an ear, nose and throat specialist.

Zoe at CA 3;9

At CA 3;9, Zoe presented as a neat girl, with well-developed gross and fine motor skills. Her visuo-motor and visuo-perceptual skills were age appropriate, on tasks such as colour matching and copying with bricks. She seemed quiet, with a limited expressive vocabulary used solely for object labelling and was mostly unintelligible, though she seemed able to understand others. She had good eye contact, communicated her needs using simple gesture, but very rarely initiated communication.

Assessment results at CA 3;9

Receptive language

On a test of receptive vocabulary, the *British Picture Vocabulary Scales (Long form)* (Dunn, Dunn Whetton, et al., 1982), Zoe scored at the 42nd centile, giving an age equivalence of CA 3;5, with a confidence band of 3;0 to 3;10. Thus, receptive vocabulary was not a particular cause for concern. Her language comprehension was not formally tested again at this phase, but through informal assessment it was established that Zoe was able to understand sentences containing up to three information-carrying words, e.g. "Put teddy on the chair".

Auditory discrimination

Thirty-eight pairs of picture cards were presented, depicting pairs of CV or CVC words that were minimally contrastive, e.g. CART ~ TART, DIG ~ DOG, BIB ~ BIG. One of the two words was spoken by the tester and Zoe was asked to point to the word she heard. Zoe scored 33/38 correct. Three of her errors involved the voice ~ voiceless contrast: LOCK ~ LOG, TEAR ~ DEER, ROBE ~ ROPE.

In order to investigate Zoe's oral and articulatory skills, the *Nuffield Dyspraxia Assessment* was administered (Connery, 1992).

Oral examination

Zoe demonstrated a good range and rate of lip and tongue movements. There was some groping behaviour. She blew and sucked strongly with good lip seal. There was no nasal escape.

Imitation of single sounds.

Zoe imitated plosives, nasals and approximants quite accurately. Fricatives were mainly devoiced and / or lateralized: [f, v] → [f]; [θ, ð]

→ [θ]; [s] → [ɬ]; [z, ʒ] → [ɮ]; [ʃ] → [s]. Affricates were fronted / stopped: [ʧ] → [tʰi]; [ʤ] → [djə]. There were minor distortions of some vowels.

Sequencing of sounds

With one place of articulation, e.g. [t t t t], Zoe would attempt three to five sounds in a row, but the rhythm was irregular. She found changing place of articulation very difficult, and was reluctant to attempt sequences such as [p t p t p t] .

Contrasting of CV structures

She scored 2/7 on this section, e.g. BEE ME, but was inaccurate on any that involved a change of place of articulation, e.g. TAR CAR → [gɑ di].

Sequencing in words

In this task, the child has to name, then imitate, real words that have increasingly complex phonological structures: CV (e.g. BEE), CVC (e.g. TAP) CVCV (e.g. BABY, PARTY). Zoe could only name accurately 6/18 words attempted. Her attempts were characterized by a limited range of phones and a tendency to total or partial reduplication (see Table 9.1). As for repetition, she only repeated completely accurately 6/70 words attempted. A sample of her attempts at single word repetition is discussed in more detail in the next section.

Table 9.1: Sample of Zoe's naming responses at CA 3;9

Target structure	*Target word*	*Response*
CV	ME	mi mɪ
	CHAIR	dɛə
	TEA	di
	TWO	du
	FOUR	fɔ
	BYE	bæ
	KEY	keiki
	CAR	gaga
CVC	CAT	jaujau
	DOG	wauwau
	BATH	bɑs
	ONE	wʌ
	TAP	tijə

Table 9.1: continued

CCVC	SCHOOL	gul
CVCV	BABY	beɪbi bɛbi
	MUMMY	mʌmə
	DADDY	dædə
	WEEWEE	wiwi
CVCCV	BIRTHDAY	bʌbə
CVCVC	TABLE	gɛti

Prosodic features

The following prosodic features were noted in Zoe's connected speech and on the above speech tasks: low pitch, quiet volume; disjointed and irregular rhythm during sequencing tasks; rather flat intonation; rough voice quality, though normal resonance.

ACTIVITY 9.1.

Aim: To draw up Zoe's speech processing profile at age 3;9.

Drawing on the assessment results just presented, fill in a speech processing profile for Zoe at 3;9, using the profile sheet in Figure 9.1.

Compare your profile with the one given in Key to Activity 9.1 at the end of this chapter, then read the following.

The profile in Key to Activity 9.1 is based on the following observations:

Auditory discrimination

On the profile, the auditory discrimination test comprising minimal pair picture cards addresses question E: *Are the child's phonological representations accurate?* The answer is yes, for all pairs except those involving the voicing distinction.

Imitation of single sounds and sequencing of sounds

These address question K: *Does the child have adequate sound production skills?* With regard to single sounds, the answer is only in part, as there are difficulties with affricates, fricatives and some vowels. With regard to sound sequencing, the answer is negative, as Zoe was unable to produce sequences such as [pətəkə].

SPEECH PROCESSING PROFILE

Name: Zoe

Age: 3;9 d.o.b:

Date:

Profiler:

Comments:

INPUT

F Is the child aware of the internal structure of phonological representations?

E Are the child's phonological representations accurate?

D Can the child discriminate between real words?

C Does the child have language-specific representations of word structures?

B Can the child discriminate speech sounds without reference to lexical representations?

A Does the child have adequate auditory perception?

OUTPUT

G Can the child access accurate motor programs?

H Can the child manipulate phonological units?

I Can the child articulate real words accurately?

J Can the child articulate speech without reference to lexical representations?

K Does the child have adequate sound production skills?

L Does the child reject his/her own erroneous forms?

Figure 9.1: Blank profile for Activity 9.1

Contrasting of CV structures and sequencing in words (repetition)

These involve repetition of real words, with one real word on its own or two real words presented in sequence for repetition. As such the tasks address question I. *Can the child articulate real words accurately?* Again, the answer is negative on both tasks.

Naming and sequencing in words

The naming task addresses question G: *Can the child access accurate motor programs?* Zoe was only able to name a handful of items accurately. Her productions were characterized by simplifying patterns such as reduplication of monosyllables, which normally occur very early: Grunwell (1987) indicates that it has normally disappeared by the second birthday. There are also some developmentally unusual pronunciations, e.g. TAP → [tijə].

Summary of Zoe's speech processing profile at 3;9

The data available pertained mainly to the output side of the profile, and indicated pervasive deficits at all levels tested, although on a more positive note, oral motor skills were relatively strong, and there was no structural abnormality. No data were available on phonological awareness tasks such as rhyme, but it was anyway most unlikely that Zoe, at 3;9, would have had any success on these, since most normally developing 3-year-olds are unable to perform such tasks (Vance, Stackhouse and Wells, 1994). On the input side, at the most peripheral level, again there was a strength, in that there was no hearing impairment. Higher up, auditory discrimination tapping into phonological representations was also strong, with the possible exception of the voiced-voiceless contrast. In conclusion, the profile indicated relatively intact input skills – an interpretation which was supported by her age-appropriate linguistic comprehension performance, including receptive vocabulary. On the output side, by contrast, there were pervasive deficits which did not appear to result from obvious physical causes.

Zoe's speech output at 3;9

The severity and pervasiveness of Zoe's speech difficulties warranted more detailed phonological analysis of her speech output, since this could suggest more specific hypotheses about the nature of the output deficits. In free play, it was observed that Zoe's vocalizations consisted mainly of the consonants [g] and [d] with different vowels, repeated in a CVCV pattern. A wide range of pitch was used. It was possible to collect only a very small sample of utterances in a picture-labelling situation (see Table 9.1).

Although the sample is small, some indications of recurrent features or patterns can be noted. In terms of syllable and word structure, all Zoe's words were either CV or CVCV, apart from two examples of CVC:

BATH → [bɑs], SCHOOL →[gul]. There were two cases where target monosyllables are reduplicated in full or in part: CAR → [gɑgɑ], KEY → [keiki]. Partial reduplication of the first syllable was also found for some target bisyllabic words: BIRTHDAY → [bʌbə] and possibly MUMMY → [mʌmə] and DADDY → [dædə]. Bilabial [b], alveolar [t], [d] and velar [k], [g] plosives were all found in syllable initial position, as were [m], [f], [j], [w]: FOUR →[fɔ], CAT →[jaujau], DOG →[wauwau]. [s] and [l], by contrast, were only found in final position: BATH → [bɑs], SCHOOL →[gul]. Some target voiceless consonants were voiced in initial position: CHAIR → [dɛə], TEA → [di], TWO → [du], CAR → [gɑgɑ]; but this was not always the case: KEY → [keiki], TAP → [tijə], FOUR → [fɔ].

Repetition data

Zoe's repetitions of approximately 70 words were transcribed, of which the majority are presented in Table 9.2.

Table 9.2: Sample of Zoe's repetitions at CA 3;9

Target structure	*Target word*	*Response*
CV	PIE	bai
	PEA	pi bi
	BEE	bi
	TIE	dai
	TWO	ti
	CAR	gɑ
	COW	gau
	FOUR	fɑ fu
	SAW	ɔːs
	SO	auʃ
	SIGH	aisʲ
	SUE	ɪz
	SHOE	uʃ
	CHAIR	tɛəs
CCV	TREE	diːʃ
VC	AT	æs
	OUT	ausʲ
	ADD	æʃ
	IF	ɪs
	ASH	auʃ
	ARCH	ɑz
	EACH	is
	ARM	ai
CVC	POP	bæ
	PIPE	paiji
	BED	bais

	BIKE	bai
	TART	tijə
	TAP	tijə
	DOG	geis
	CAT	tiːs
	CAKE	geis
	HOUSE	haus
CCVC	STAR'S	taiːs
CVCV	PARTY	bɑti
	BUTTER	tætisʲ
	BUNNY	bʌpɔ
	TEDDY	tɛdi
	TURKEY	tɛt̚i
	DINNER	dædi
	DIRTY	dɜti
	KEEPER	bæbə
	COOKER	kʊgə
	MONEY	mʌmi
	LOLLY	hædi
CVCVC	BOTTLE	gɒgi
	TABLE	gɛgi
	DIGGING	gɪgi
	COTTON	kɛti
	GARDEN	gɑkə
	CHICKEN	di
CCVCVC	SNOWMAN	nɔnə
CVCCVC	DONKEY	gɪgi
	MONKEY	gəgi
	SAUCEPAN	gəgu
CCVCCV	TRACTOR	dɔdi

Some of the observations made about Zoe's spontaneous speech were confirmed by this bigger sample. The voicing of initial consonants is unstable, with target voiceless consonants frequently being realized as voiced, but not always: e.g. TIE ⟶ [dai] CAR ⟶ [gɑ], COW ⟶ [gau] TREE ⟶ [diʃ], POP ⟶ [bæ] vs CAT ⟶ [tis], TAP ⟶ [tijə], PIPE ⟶ [paiji], with PEA showing both forms: [pi], [bi].

The partial reduplication of bisyllabic target words is again evident, though this could be interpreted as consonant harmony: see KEEPER, BUNNY, MONEY (bilabial harmony); GARDEN, DIGGING, BOTTLE, TABLE, MONKEY,

DONKEY, SAUCEPAN (velar harmony); TRACTOR, SNOWMAN, TURKEY, BUTTER (alveolar harmony). It is not clear from this sample whether there was any consistency about which consonant in the target determines the place of articulation that Zoe used. It looks as though she was treating the target in a parametric way (cf. Chapter 7), latching on to one place of articulation which was salient for her, and using it for syllable initial consonants through the word. Only three bisyllabic target words did not display the harmony pattern: PARTY, DIRTY, COTTON, perhaps indicating progress towards an adult-like structure.

There was no evidence of Zoe using reduplicated forms for target monosyllabic words, though two examples of this had been noted in the naming sample. This may also indicate progress: when accessing words stored in her own lexicon (in picture naming) she used more immature, reduplicated forms; but when the adult form was modelled for her (in repetition) she produced a form that was monosyllabic. In terms of the model presented in Chapter 6, this suggests that she had developed the motor programming capacity to produce more advanced forms, but that she had not yet updated the motor programs for individual words already stored in her lexicon: compare spontaneous CAR → [gɑgɑ] with repeated CAR → [gɑ].

In her realizations of target monosyllables that have final consonants, she generally marked the final consonant – such words were not subject to final consonant deletion. However, the way she marked the target final consonant was unusual: most often it was with a lingual fricative, either alveolar, palatalized alveolar, or postalveolar, even when the target final consonant was a plosive, e.g. OUT → [ausʲ], ADD → [æʃ], BED→ [bais]. In fact, she never had plosives in final position, only fricatives. Even more unusual was her treatment of target words with lingual fricatives at onset position, such as SAW, SHOE, SIGH, SO. In Zoe's pronunciation of these words, the fricative appeared in coda position, rather than at onset as in the target: [ɔːs] , [uʃ], [aisʲ], [auʃ].

This suggests that Zoe was able to perceive and latch on to the fricative portion of the stimulus, but was unable to realize it herself at the correct place – possibly for motor reasons, since the production of lingual fricatives such as [s] or [ʃ] in initial position may require a greater degree of fine control over tongue position, and co-ordination with breathing, than is the case in final position. This behaviour again suggests that Zoe had a parametric approach to the phonetic 'ingredients' of the target: she lacked the motor ability to sequence the phonetic ingredients in the adult way, but nevertheless signalled them within the constraints of her own motor capabilities. At the same time, the pattern was relatively consistent, extending to target initial affricates, where the fricative portion migrated to the coda, while the onset consonant was realized as a plosive: CHAIR → [tɛəs] ; TREE → [diːʃ]. Another very unusual pattern is found in her realization of some CVC targets: TART → [tijə];

PIPE → [paiji]; and TAP → [tijə], the last in spontaneous naming as well as repetition. This seemed to be another way of signalling a target con-son- ant within the limited phonetic resources available to her in final position, though here it involved the creation of a further syllable and, in two cases, alteration of the vowel.

From profile to model: Zoe at 3;9

Having analysed Zoe's speech patterns in some detail, we can now attempt to relate this analysis and her speech processing profile to our speech processing model (presented in Chapter 6), in order to make more specific hypotheses about the locus or loci of deficit that were giving rise to her difficulties.

ACTIVITY 9.2

Aim: To map the results from Zoe's speech processing profile on to the speech processing model described in Chapter 6.

On the speech processing model presented in Chapter 6, reproduced here as Figure 9.2, attempt to locate the deficits that you think might be responsible for Zoe's speech difficulties, using the speech processing profile given in the Key to Activity 9.1. For example, the profile suggests that Zoe had some difficulty with non-linguistic sound production. On this basis you might locate a deficit in the motor execution box on the model. Consider in turn the different types of error that Zoe made (with the voice / voiceless contrast, affricates, the unusual use of fricatives in coda position etc.). Is it possible that the loci of deficit responsible for them may differ?

Compare your answer with the model presented in Key to Activity 9.2 at the end of this chapter, then read the following.

Voicing

The difficulties of transcribing the voicing parameter accurately are well known, as a continuum is involved, rather than articulatorily identifiable categories. Nevertheless, it appears that Zoe did not use distinctions either in voice onset time or in articulatory strength to signal the target phonological opposition between lenis (voiced) and fortis (voiceless) consonants. Given Zoe's inconsistent realizations of the target fortis ~ lenis categories, it could be hypothesized that she lacked the ability to co-ordinate precisely the onset of vocal fold vibration with supralaryngeal articulatory gestures, such as approach and release of the tongue or lower lip to the passive articulator (cf. Chiat, (1983) and

Brett, Chiat and Pilcher (1987) for such an account of voicing errors in phonologically-disordered children). This interpretation is supported by the fact that she sometimes devoiced target voiced fricatives in the test of imitation of single sounds.

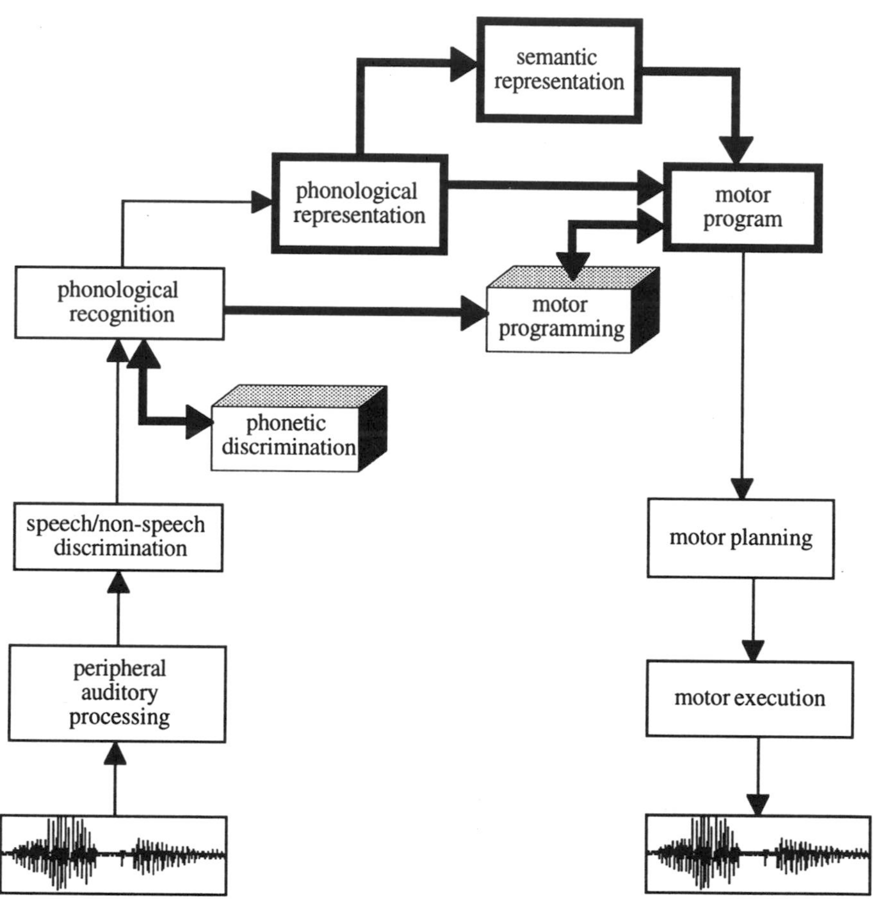

Figure 9.2: Speech processing model for Activity 9.2.

However, an alternative hypothesis would be that Zoe could not perceive the distinction between voiced and voiceless consonants in input; as a result the distinction was not encoded in her internal phonological representations, and so she had no basis for signalling it in her output. The latter hypothesis is supported by the fact that three of the five errors that Zoe made on the test of auditory discrimination involved the voice ~ voiceless opposition (this opposition was tested 10 times). On our model, we can hypothetically locate the deficit giving rise to inconsistent voicing errors both at phonological representations and at motor execution (see Key to Activity 9.2).

Fricatives, affricates and plosives

Other features of Zoe's speech patterns could also be attributed to low level difficulties with motor execution. These include her problems with affricates, which she could not imitate in isolation in a test of single sound production; on this test she also distorted lingual fricatives, producing lateral friction for /z/ and /s/ and an alveolar articulation for /ʃ/. This may help explain why Zoe did not produce target lingual fricatives and affricates in onset position. However, it does not account for why she did use final lingual fricatives so much in coda position, often for plosive targets. It appears that Zoe was unable to close a syllable with a plosive. If a plosive did follow the first vowel, in Zoe's speech it had to be followed by a further vowel, as in the reduplicated forms. Alternatively, if the syllable was to be produced as CVC, the coda had to be a lingual fricative (Figure 9.3). In terms of the model, these pervasive constraints on syllable type in Zoe's output are regarded as limitations of motor programming: at this point in her development, Zoe was capable of creating only a very restricted set of motor programs.

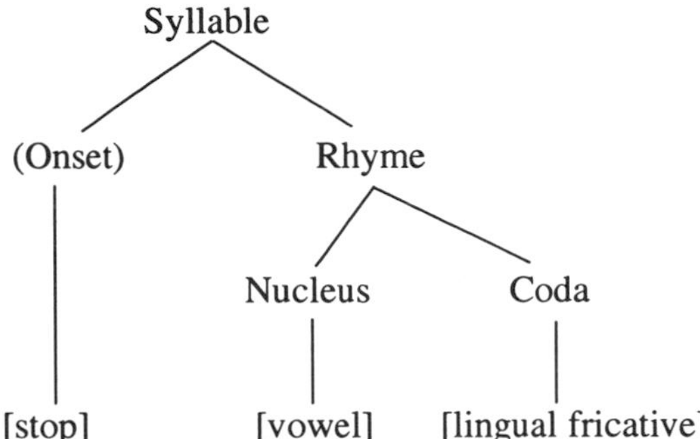

Figure 9.3: Template for Zoe's (C)VC words, at CA 3;9.

Consonant harmony

Another restriction on Zoe's motor programming capacity was that it could only produce programs for bisyllabic words where both consonants were stops and shared the same place of articulation, e.g. BOTTLE → [gɒgi] , GARDEN → [gɑkə] , TURKEY → [tɛt̚i]. This constituted a second template. Templates such as this can be set up without reference to the phonology of the target word. Any word that Zoe spoke had to conform to one of them, irrespective of its adult form. Thus consonant harmony, and also the obligatory fricative codas, can be located in motor programming.

As noted earlier, there are three exceptions to the consonant harmony constraint (COTTON → [kɛti], DIRTY → [dɜti], PARTY → [bɑti]), which may indicate that this constraint was beginning to be relaxed, i.e. that Zoe's motor programming capacity had developed to the point of being able to create programs for bisyllabic words with different consonantal places of articulation. Once motor programming has developed in this way, there should be an updating of the motor programs of existing lexical items, to bring them into line. This clearly had not yet happened for the large majority of bisyllabic words produced by Zoe. It can therefore be inferred that there was also a deficit in the updating process, i.e. the arrow between motor programming and the motor program in the lexical representations (see Key to Activity 9.2).

To summarize, we have suggested that Zoe's restricted speech patterns can be accounted for in terms of limitations in motor execution and motor programming, which resulted in a restricted set of motor programs. There were difficulties with the process of updating motor programs; and possibly some deficits in phonological representations that related specifically to the voice ~ voiceless contrast (Key to Activity 9.2).

The developmental perspective on Zoe at 3;9

So far, we have drawn up a speech processing profile for Zoe, in the way described in Chapter 5, and we have interpreted the profile in terms of the speech processing model outlined in Chapter 6. We can now consider how this pattern of deficits can be related to the five phases of speech development proposed in Chapters 7 and 8, which very roughly coincide respectively with the first 5 years of life in normally-developing children: Prelexical; Whole Word; Systematic Simplification; Assembly; Metaphonological.

ACTIVITY 9.3

Aim: To interpret data about a child's speech development in terms of the five developmental phases of speech processing.

On the basis of the data presented earlier, which phases of development do you consider Zoe (a) to have passed through (b) not yet to have entered? From your answer, what can you conclude about her speech development at the age of 3;9?

Check your answer with Key to Activity 9.3 at the end of this chapter, then read the following.

Some of Zoe's speech patterns are suggestive of the Whole Word Phase. The 'parametric' aspect of this phase is suggested by the way in which Zoe seemed to latch on to the phonetic ingredients of the target word she was aiming for, yet in many instances reassorted these ingredients in a different sequence. One example is the realization of target onset fricatives in coda position. Another example is the pervasive use of consonant harmony and sometimes reduplication, where Zoe picked on a salient place feature from the target and reproduced it throughout the word. Such features are reminiscent of the behaviour of very young children such as Patrick, described in Chapter 7. The 'gestalt' or Whole Word aspect of this phase is indicated by the fact that Zoe was still using single word utterances exclusively.

However, other aspects of Zoe's speech are more indicative of the Systematic Simplification Phase, in particular the fairly high degree of consistency with which she treated words of a similar pattern. For example, the pattern of realizing target coda plosives as [s] was a consistent one in the repetition data, as was the pattern of placing target onset lingual fricatives in coda position. The regularity with which these patterns were used suggests a systematic treatment of target sound types, rather than the variability that is more characteristic of the earlier Whole Word Phase. These patterns are not instances of the so-called 'natural processes' commonly observed, (though for a quite similar pattern, recall from Chapter 7 the case of W, a girl of CA 2;9, described by Leonard and McGregor, 1991). On these grounds, it is proposed that Zoe, at CA 3;9, may have been at a transitional point between the Whole Word Phase and the Systematic Simplification Phase – a point which most children with normally-developing speech reach soon after their second birthday.

Zoe at CA 5;11

The second snapshot is taken 2 years later, when Zoe was attending a local school with a language unit, at which she received regular speech and language therapy. Educational psychologists' reports made at CA 5;0 suggested that Zoe had academic potential within the average range. On the *British Ability Scales* (Elliott, Murray and Pearson, 1983) she performed significantly better on visual tasks (IQ 96) than on verbal tasks (IQ 71) when tested at CA 5;0. She scored poorly on the test of short-term auditory memory, as assessed by digit span (percentile score = 3). The scatter of scores suggested that she had a specific expressive verbal difficulty. In the two years since our previous snapshot, it had become apparent that her difficulties affected her expressive language as well as her speech. Results of assessments carried out over the previous few months are presented in Table 9.3.

Table 9.3: Zoe at CA 5;11, language assessments

Assessment	Age (years; months)	Results
Receptive vocabulary		
British Picture Vocabulary Scales (Long Form)	5;9	40th centile AE 5;3
Expressive vocabulary		
Renfrew Word Finding Vocabulary Scale	5;5	Raw score: 34 AE 5;4
Receptive language		
Test of Reception of Grammar	5;9	8 blocks; AE 4;9
Reynell Developmental Language Scales	5;5	Standard score: 0.4 AE 6;0–6;5
Expressive language		
LARSP	5;10	Clause: Phase III–IV (AE 2–3) Phrase: Phase II-III (AE 1;6–2;6)
Renfrew Action Picture Test	5;9	Information: 34.5 AE 6;6–7;0 Grammar: 11 AE 3;6–3;11

AE, Age equivalent.

The results of the *British Picture Vocabulary Scales* (Dunn, Dunn, Whetton, et al., 1982) and the *Renfrew Word Finding Vocabulary Scales* (Renfrew, 1972) indicated that Zoe was at the lower end of the normal range of performance on both receptive and expressive vocabulary. Although there was a delay in grammatical comprehension as measured by the *Test of Reception of Grammar* (Bishop 1989), there was a relatively high level of vocabulary and receptive language development on the *Reynell Developmental Language Scales* (Reynell and Huntley, 1985). This was in contrast to her performance on the *Renfrew Action Picture Test* (Renfrew, 1989) and the *Language Assessment, Remediation and Screening Procedure – LARSP*, (Crystal, Fletcher and Garman 1989) where her expressive grammatical development was delayed by as much as 2 or 3 years. The LARSP analysis indicated that Zoe made very little use of complex sentence structures such as subordination and clausal or phrasal postmodification. In a 3-hour assessment session recorded at age 5;11, the most complex clause structure she produced was: "and he waiting ambulance come".

Assessment of speech processing at CA 5;11

Auditory discrimination

At 5;11, Zoe was given *The Auditory Discrimination and Attention Test* (MorganBarry, 1988), which involves choosing a picture from a pair of minimally contrasting pictures (e.g. LOG ~ LOCK), on hearing one of the two words spoken by the tester (cf. Chapter 2 of this volume). The test includes minimal pairs targeting various consonantal oppositions (place, manner, voicing) in singleton consonants and clusters. Each minimal pair of words was tested 12 times. Most of Zoe's errors were with the voicing contrast: she failed consistently on all four pairs that tested it. The only other contrasts that were confused more than twice were /r/ ~ /w/ and /m/ ~ /b/.

Rhyme detection

Zoe's ability to detect rhyme was tested using a silent rhyme detection task. This is a picture-pointing task, which does not require any verbal output from the child. After practice and explanation of the concept of rhyme, the child is asked: "Which of these two pictures rhymes with the target picture?" (Stackhouse, 1989). Neither the stimulus nor the target word is pronounced by the tester. In each item, the non-rhyming word is either a semantic or an alliterative distractor, for example:

Rhyme target:		CAT			GOAT	
Choice:	FISH	or	MAT	GATE	or	BOAT

Zoe scored 6/10 correct on this test (not significantly better than chance). Her performance was comparable to that of the worst performing children in a group of younger pre-readers (CA 4;1–5;8, mean 4;9), who were also tested on these items (Stackhouse, 1989). Three of her errors were sound based (alliterative), e.g. she selected GATE as a rhyme with GOAT, PIG to rhyme with PEG, and COW with KEY. One of her errors was semantic: she paired SPOON with KNIFE.

Rhyme production

Zoe was asked to produce as many words as she could think of that rhymed with a target word spoken by the tester, e.g. LOG, KEY

(Stackhouse, 1989). Zoe was unable to produce rhyming words to six targets presented orally. Normally-developing 5-year-old children, on a similar test, were on average able to produce at least one rhyming response to each item presented (Vance, Stackhouse and Wells, 1994). Zoe made three semantically related initial responses, of which two were also alliterations:

Target	*Response*
KEY	"key lock"
HAT	"hair"
FOUR	"five"

She also produced isolated sounds, for example for the target KEY and LOG:

Target	*Response*
KEY	"key lock [ga] [jə] [wə] [nə]"
LOG	"[lə] [wə]"

Real word repetition

No formal test of real word repetition was carried out on this occasion. However, Zoe was asked to repeat following a model on numerous occasions, as exemplified here:

Target		*Realization*
HEAD	→	[het]
COAT	→	[gout]
BROTHER	→	[bufə]
BRIDGE	→	[bitʃ]
BRUSHING	→	[bʌʃiŋ]
FRUIT	→	[fut]

The following are examples of items that were named spontaneously and subsequently repeated following a model:

Target		*Naming*	*Repetition*
GOAT	→	[gou]	[gout]
FAN	→	[fac]	[fan]
THROW	→	[fəu]	[fʊəu]

Here we can see some improvements on repetition: in GOAT, the final consonant was realized; in FAN, the place and manner of articulation of the final consonant were realized more accurately and in THROW the second element of the cluster appeared. Thus, having a spoken model sometimes facilitated her speech performance.

Nonword repetition

No formal test was carried out. However, there were a few instances where Zoe attempted to repeat what was clearly a completely new word for her, i.e. effectively a nonword, e.g. PUMPKIN, which was repeated in three different ways: [pʊɲpoiɲc], [pʊŋkiŋ] , [pəiɲciŋ].

Phonological analysis

To obtain detailed information relating to the output side of the profile, a phonological analysis of Zoe's speech was required. At the phonological level, Zoe had problems that were immediately obvious to the listener, who would have difficulty in following what she is saying. Phonological analysis of a speech sample enables us to identify the parts of the target phonological system that the child has not yet mastered (Grunwell, 1987). The sample on this occasion included spontaneous picture naming and repetition (Weiner, 1979; MorganBarry, 1988), as well as some spontaneous speech and description of picture sequences. No formal naming test was administered, though extensive confrontation naming data was collected using the pictures in Weiner (1979), which target common simplification processes. For reasons of space, the results of this analysis are not given here in full; instead, some phonetic data are presented in order to illustrate certain aspects of Zoe's phonology that can be interpreted within the psycholinguistic framework.

Phonotactic structures

Zoe demonstrated a range of phonotactic structures in connected speech and in isolated words:

Target structure	*Example*		*Zoe's realization*
CV	TIE	→	[t̄ai]
CVC	MOON	→	[mʉn]
CCVC	DRESS	→	[dʋɛs]
CVCC	KICKED	→	[k⁻ɪʔ͜kt]
CVCVC	CARROT	→	[ɟɛʋət]
CVC.CVC	PUMPKIN	→	[pʊŋkiŋ]
			[pəiɲciŋ]

Thus, Zoe had the potential to realize many of the phonotactic structures found in English. However, at this time there were limitations on the combinations of phones that could occur within these structures. For example, clusters occurring at syllable initial position were highly restricted.

Singleton consonants

Place of articulation was generally quite accurate in Zoe's speech, with the exception of postalveolar targets /ʃ ʧ ʤ ɹ/. Manner of articulation too was generally accurate, with the exception of affricates. These two problem areas are illustrated in the following spontaneous productions:

Target		*Realization*
WASHING	→	[wɒçiŋ]
CHICKEN	→	[hikin]
JUMPING	→	[dʑʊmpɪn]
READY	→	[ʋɛʔti]

Postalveolars and affricates are often late to be acquired in normal development (Grunwell, 1987).

Consonant clusters

In order to illustrate certain aspects of Zoe's realization of consonant clusters at this point in her development, we will consider her realization of some words that begin with clusters where, in the target words as pronounced in this part of England, the first element is a plosive (e.g. [b], [t], [d], [g],) or a fricative (e.g. [f], [θ]) and the second is a postalveolar median approximant [ɹ]:

Target		*Realization*
BROTHER	→	['bufə]
BRIDGE	→	[bitʃ]
BRUSHING	→	['bʌʃiŋ]
FRUIT	→	[fəʉt]
TRAIN	→	[tʋen], [də'ʋein]
TREE	→	[də'wi]
TRUCK	→	[tə'ʋʊk]
DRESS	→	[dʋɛs]
GRASS	→	[[gə'ʋas]
THROW	→	[fʋəu], [fəu]

Some of Zoe's realizations involved the omission of the target approximant /ɹ/. In these cases, the target began with a consonant that involves the lips in closure of some kind: /b/, /f/, e.g. BRUSHING, FRUIT. On other occasions, when the target initial consonant involved closure between the tongue and the roof of the mouth, the target /ɹ/ was realized as an approximant, but at a different place of articulation – one that involved the lips. This was either labiodental [ʋ] or labial-velar [w]. Sometimes, the cluster was broken up by a short central vowel [ə], e.g. TRUCK, TREE, GRASS. The target word THROW was treated according to both patterns on different occasions. This may reflect its intermediate position in terms of articulatory placement: the active articulator for initial dental fricative /θ/ in the target THROW is the tip or blade of the tongue, as for /t/ or /d/, but the passive articulator is the teeth, making it more like /f/.

Fortis ~ lenis consonants

We will now consider Zoe's handling of target voiceless (fortis) vs voiced (lenis) consonants, since this had been noted as a problematic area in Zoe's speech output at CA 3;9. A difficulty with the auditory discrimination of this opposition at 5;11 was also noted (see above). Minimal pairs involving the fortis ~ lenis opposition were elicited using the pictures in MorganBarry (1988), as a preliminary to administering the auditory discrimination test. Zoe's pronunciation of these words is presented here to illustrate her realization of these target consonants more generally:

Target		*Realization*
PEAR	→	[p˭ɛː]
BEAR	→	[bɛː]
COAT	→	[k˭out]
GOAT	→	[gout]
LOCK	→	[lɐ.kxə], [lɐk]
LOG	→	[lɐ.kh]
FAN	→	[faʔc]
VAN	→	[fan]

The following patterns can be identified:

(1) target fortis plosives were realized as unaspirated when word initial (PEAR, COAT);
(2) target lenis plosives were realized as voiceless when word final (LOG);
(3) target lenis fricatives were realized as voiceless when word initial (VAN).

It is difficult to transcribe the voicing parameter reliably as a continuum is involved, rather than articulatorily identifiable categories. Nevertheless, it was apparent, both from listening to Zoe's speech and from measurements of voice onset time in tokens of target voiced and voiceless consonants, that Zoe did not use distinctions either in voice onset time or in articulatory strength to signal consistently the phonological opposition between target lenis and fortis consonants.

Connected speech

Zoe's speech was quite unusual in its patterns of pitch and loudness prominence, slow and disjointed in rhythm, with a deep, intermit tently creaky and harsh voice quality. These and other prosodic features are now considered in more detail. Although no formal test was administered, a sample of connected speech data was transcribed and analysed, including Zoe's responses to 'Verb Tense' pictures. These consist of sets of three pictures; in each set the first depicts what is going to happen, the second what is happening and the third what has happened. In the first examples, picture (i) shows a girl with wet hair, picture (ii) the girl drying her hair and (iii) the girl brushing her hair:

(i) "she been washing her hair"

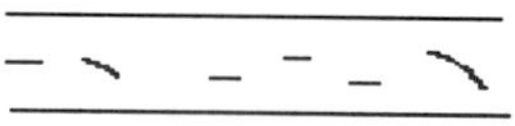

ɕi.ˈbint.ˈwɒˌçɪŋ.ˈɕis.ˈˈhɛːː

(ii) "now she drying her hair"

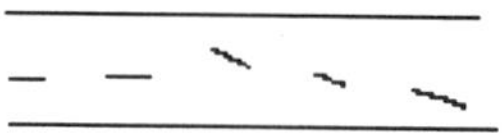

ˌnɑu.ˌʃːi..ˈˈdəŋk ˌɕis ˈhɛːː

(iii) "and she finished drying her hair"

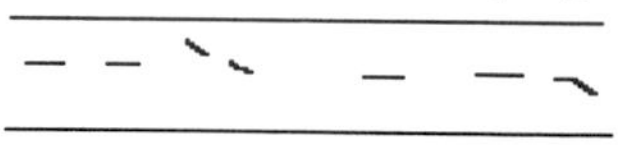

ˌən.ˌʃːi.ˈfɪˌnɪʃ...ˌdəŋk ˌɕis ˌhɛːː

In (iv) a girl is about to walk up the stairs, and in (v) she is walking up the stairs:

(iv) "she is going up the stairs"

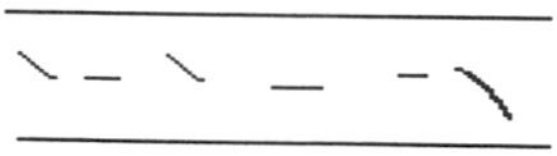

ˈʆiːˌjɪs̪.ˈgɵɪŋkˈʔo̞pː˺ˌd̪əˈˈtɛːːs

(v) "she <u>up</u> the stairs"

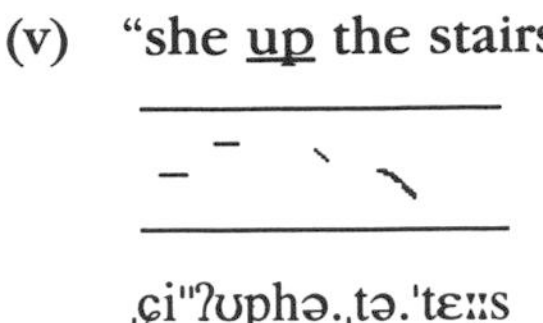

ˌɕi''ʔʊphə̥.ˌtə.ˈtɛ̥ːːs

These examples of Zoe's connected speech show that she delivered utterances in a staccato manner, that was attributable to the frequent occurrence of a pause at the end of a word, as in (i); to the prevalence of glottal stops before words beginning with a vowel, as before UP in (iv) and (v); to the undifferentiated rhythm that resulted from the presence of stress on syllables or words that would be unstressed in adult English, as in (i); and finally to the overall slowness of delivery and unusual lengthening on the final syllable of each utterance, though the latter feature did contribute to the signalling of the end of the utterance. She also signalled effectively the new or important information of the utterance, by means of pitch prominence, loudness and some of the temporal features just mentioned that made her speech seem disjointed: see the emphasis on DRYING in (ii), FINISHED in (iii) and UP in (v). For further details see Wells, (1994).

ACTIVITY 9.4.

Aim: To draw up Zoe's speech processing profile at age 5;11.

Drawing on the assessment results just presented, fill in a speech processing profile for Zoe at 5;11, using the profile sheet in Figure 9.4.

Compare your profile with the one given in Key to Activity 9.4 at the end of this chapter, then read the following.

The profile in Key to Activity 9.4 is based on the following observations.

Auditory discrimination

Zoe's performance on the picture-pointing auditory discrimination task suggested that there might be confusions in her lexical representations of some words. This was particularly the case with the voicing contrast. Thus, a cross is warranted against question E: *Are the child's phonological representations accurate*?

Rhyme detection

Zoe's performance on silent rhyme detection was not above chance level, and was well below what would be expected for her age (Stackhouse, 1989). On the profile, this task addresses question F: *Is the child aware of the internal structure of phonological representations?* since it involves the segmentation of words already in the child's lexicon into onset and rhyme constituents. It can therefore be inferred that

SPEECH PROCESSING PROFILE

Name: Zoe

Age: 5;11 d.o.b:

Date:

Profiler:

Comments:

INPUT

F Is the child aware of the internal structure of phonological representations?

E Are the child's phonological representations accurate?

D Can the child discriminate between real words?

C Does the child have language-specific representations of word structures?

B Can the child discriminate speech sounds without reference to lexical representations?

A Does the child have adequate auditory perception?

OUTPUT

G Can the child access accurate motor programs?

H Can the child manipulate phonological units?

I Can the child articulate real words accurately?

J Can the child articulate speech without reference to lexical representations?

K Does the child have adequate sound production skills?

L Does the child reject his/her own erroneous forms?

Figure 9.4: Blank profile for Activity 9.4

Zoe did not yet have this level of metaphonological awareness. The fact that more of her errors were sound-based than semantic may indicate that she had some awareness of sound similarity.

Rhyme production

Zoe's performance on rhyme production was well below that of her peers. She was unable to produce any rhyming responses, whereas normally-developing 5-year-old children, on a similar test, were on average able to produce at least one rhyming response to each item (Vance, Stackhouse and Wells, 1994). The task addresses question H: *Can the child manipulate phonological units?* Zoe's performance suggested that she did not yet have this ability.

Naming

The analysis of Zoe's spontaneous speech allows us to address question G: *Can the child access accurate motor programs?* In the case of the words with initial consonant clusters presented earlier, there was little evidence to suggest that the phonological representations themselves were inaccurate (question E), since on the test of auditory discrimination, Zoe did not seem to have particular problems with words such as GRASS vs GLASS. It seems more likely that the origin of Zoe's inaccurate realizations of these words was on the output side of the processing chain. At the same time, the patterns of realization were relatively systematic: cluster reduction occurred with target clusters starting with bilabial plosives [b, p] and labiodental fricatives [f], but not with alveolars or velars. This consistency and the systematic but different ways in which the two classes of cluster were treated by Zoe suggest that her realizations were the result of stored patterns, i.e. simplified motor programs, rather than a general lack of motor control or articulatory precision. This suggests that, for this type of cluster, we should put a cross against question G.

As in the case of consonant clusters, the phonological analysis of voicing, i.e. of target fortis ~ lenis consonants, can be used to generate hypotheses about the level of breakdown or deficit that was responsible for Zoe's inaccurate speech output. Given that Zoe's realizations of the target fortis ~ lenis categories overlapped, it could be hypothesized that she lacked the ability to co-ordinate precisely the onset of vocal fold vibration with supralaryngeal articulatory gestures, such as approach and release of the tongue or lower lip to the passive articulator. This point was discussed above, in relation to Zoe's profile at 3;9. To reflect this, we have put a cross against question K: *Does the child have adequate sound production skills?*

An alternative hypothesis is that Zoe could not perceive the distinction between voiced and voiceless consonants in input; as a result, the distinction was not encoded in her internal phonological representations, and so she had no basis for signalling it in her output. This is captured by the cross that has already been entered under question E:

Are the child's phonological representations accurate? on the basis of Zoe's poor performance on voicing in the auditory discrimination task. In fact, there is no reason why deficits might not exist at both levels, and indeed be related: inaccurate feedback arising from inconsistent articulation may have made it difficult for Zoe to establish a clearly defined phonological opposition in her representations.

Real word repetition

This addresses question I: *Can the child articulate real words accurately?* The repetition data presented earlier, which contained inaccurate productions particularly in respect of the two areas already discussed (voicing and initial clusters) suggest that the answer to question I is negative, and that there should therefore be a cross under I. At the same time, some improvements from spontaneous speech to repetition was noted, indicating that, at least for some aspects of phonology, repetition was superior to spontaneous production. This suggests that Zoe may have had some imprecise phonological representations and/or motor programs that she was able to revise and update when the adult form was modelled for her.

Nonword repetition

On the profile, nonword repetition data help to address question J: *Can the child articulate speech without reference to lexical representations?* This was not addressed formally through a test of nonword repetition, but some data were presented from Zoe's treatment of new words, e.g. PUMPKIN, which showed inaccurate realizations and considerable variability. Such examples suggest that Zoe has difficulty in establishing a motor program for new multisyllabic words. The available evidence indicates that the answer to J is negative.

Zoe's inability to produce accurate pronunciations of postalveolar and affricate singleton consonants is suggestive of motor immaturity, since the postalveolars and affricates are often late to be acquired in normal development. On the profile, this suggests some, albeit residual, problems with motor execution, meriting a cross under question K *Does the child have adequate sound production skills?*

At this session there was no evidence that Zoe was spontaneously attempting to repair her own erroneous forms (question L: *Does the child reject his/her own erroneous forms?*). It is true that her pronunciation of some target words could vary considerably from one occasion to the next, but there was no evidence that she was treating one form as superior to another. The repetitions of PUMPKIN just described were produced 'to order': Zoe was asked to say the word three times by the tester. Therefore the answer to question L is also negative.

From profile to model: Zoe at 5;11

If we compare this profile to the one drawn up for Zoe at CA 3;9, we can see a less pronounced deficit in the production of real words, reflecting the fact that Zoe's single word production, though not age appropriate, nevertheless was adequate in signalling many of the necessary phonological contrasts. However, there were new deficits on areas not tested earlier, notably those tapping metaphonological skills, and also in connected speech. The possibility of an input deficit, raised at 3;9, was confirmed.

We can now relate Zoe's performance at CA 5;11 to the speech processing model presented in Chapter 6, in order to be more specific about the loci of deficits responsible for her difficulties.

ACTIVITY 9.5

Aim: To map the results from Zoe's speech processing profile at 5;11 on to the speech processing model described in Chapter 6.

Repeat the 'profile to model' exercise that you did for Zoe at CA 3;9. On the speech processing model presented in Chapter 6, reproduced here

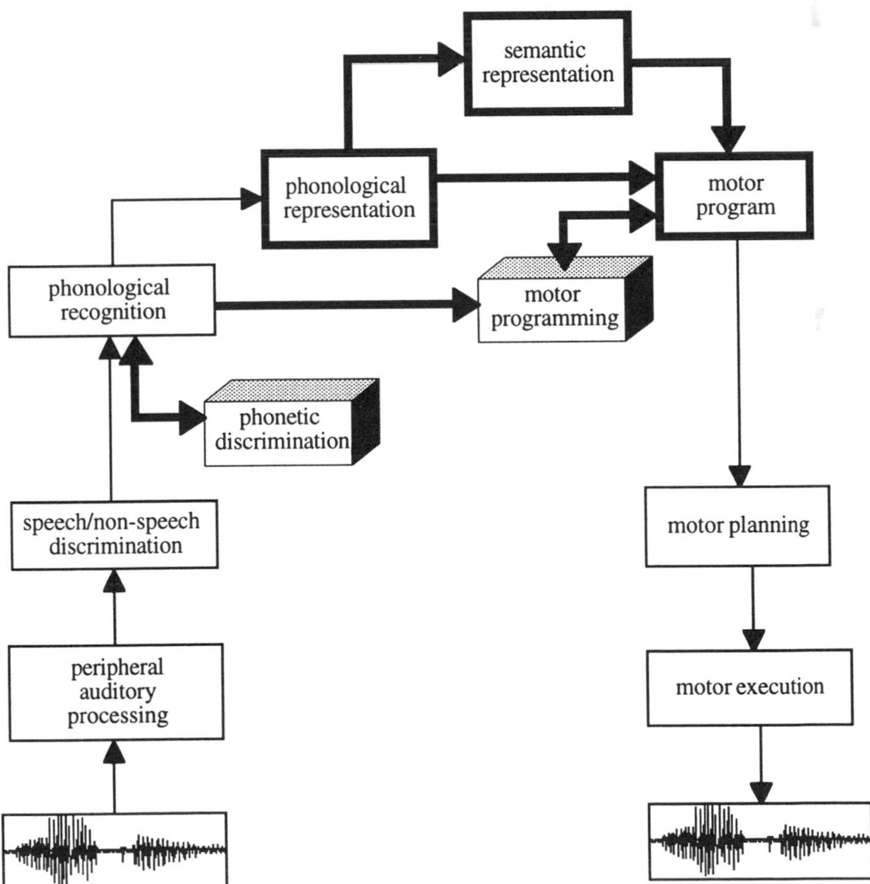

Figure 9.5: Speech processing model for Activity 9.5

as Figure 9.5, attempt to locate the deficits that you think might be responsible for Zoe's speech processing difficulties at 5;11, using the speech processing profile of Zoe from Activity 9.4 (Key to Activity 9.4). Compare your answer with the model presented in Key to Activity 9.5 at the end of this chapter, then read the following.

The level of deficit responsible for the inaccuracy of the postalveolar and affricate targets, can be hypothesized to be motor execution. This level may also be involved in the inconsistent voicing errors, though it was noted that there was also a deficit in the phonological representations, such that the voice ~ voiceless opposition was not encoded in the lexicon. Presumably this has arisen as a result of a deficit in phonological recognition, the process by which the phonological units of the language are identified from the speech stream. The cluster reduction evident in target labial + liquid clusters, but not in lingual + liquid clusters, could be attributed to a specific constraint on the motor programs that Zoe was able to produce, pointing to a deficit in motor programming. However, the possibility of a further deficit at the motor execution level cannot be ruled out, as Zoe showed no sign of being able to achieve a more accurate pronunciation when the cluster was modelled for her (see earlier: BROTHER, BRIDGE, FRUIT, BRUSHING). In other cases, Zoe could pronounce some words more accurately following modelling, e.g. the cluster in THROW and the final consonant of GOAT. This suggests a deficit in the motor program for these words which could, however, be revised in the direction of the target.

Zoe seemed to have difficulty with new multisyllabic words (e.g. PUMPKIN). This can be interpreted as a deficit in motor programming, with problems in establishing a stable new motor program. Zoe's failure on the rhyme detection task suggested that she was not yet able to segment phonological representations into their grossest constituent parts. This was reinforced by her performance on rhyme production, where she was unable to combine onsets and rhymes into new motor programs – again indicating a motor programming deficit. However, there was some evidence of awareness of the concept of segmentation: Zoe did produce a few attempts at novel syllables in the rhyme production task, even though they did not rhyme with the target; and on the rhyme detection task, she went for alliterative distractors, indicating some awareness of sound structure.

Zoe's unusual, jerky connected speech patterns can be attributed to a deficit at the level of motor planning, i.e. in the assembly of words and morphemes into fluent utterances. However, connected speech may also be affected by imprecise motor programs for individual words, e.g. lack of precise specification about the assimilatory possibilities of word-final alveolar consonants, or about the linking possibilities for final vowels.

In summary, the 'profile to model' exercise suggests that Zoe had deficits at all levels of output processing, and also, in a circumscribed way, in phonological representations. This activity has also highlighted a limitation of the data: input processing was not tested as fully as output processing. One important point that arises from the 'profile to model' activity is that it shows how different levels of deficit on the model may be responsible for different facets of Zoe's speech output problems: it has been hypothesized that phonological recognition and thence, phonological representations, are responsible for some of the voicing errors, motor programs for the cluster errors, motor planning for the connected speech problems and possibly motor execution for the affricate errors. While these suggestions are necessarily somewhat speculative given the limitations of the data available, the analysis nevertheless opens up the clinically and theoretically interesting possibility that a child's speech errors do not all have to be accounted for in terms of a single locus of deficit.

The developmental perspective on Zoe at CA 5;11

We have drawn up a psycholinguistic profile of Zoe's speech processing at 5;11 and we have interpreted the profile in terms of the speech processing model. As we did for Zoe at 3;9, we can now consider how this pattern of deficits can be related to the five phases of speech development proposed in Chapters 7 and 8: Prelexical; Whole Word; Systematic Simplification; Assembly; Metaphonological.

ACTIVITY 9.6

Aim: To interpret data about a child's speech development in terms of the five developmental phases of speech processing.

On the basis of the data presented earlier, which phase, or phases, of development, do you consider Zoe (a) to have passed through (b) not yet to have entered? From your answer, what can you conclude about her speech processing development at the age of 5;11?

Check your answer with Key to Activity 9.6 at the end of this chapter, then read the following.

The investigation of Zoe's speech processing development at 3;11 indicated that she was at a transitional point between the Whole Word Phase and the Systematic Simplification Phase. By 5;11, she had progressed to the transition between the Systematic Simplification Phase and the Assembly Phase – a point that children with normally-developing speech processing skills could be expected to reach soon after their third birthday. She had not yet entered the Metaphonological Phase, which suggested that she was at risk with regard to the development of reading and spelling. This possibility is explored further in the next chapter.

Practical Implications

Designing a therapy programme for Zoe involved addressing not only the surface patterns of simplification and error but also the source of the individual types of speech error, in speech processing terms. Zoe's therapy programme at the age of 5;11 included the following.

Auditory tasks

Auditory work was targeted specifically at the voicing opposition, working on the deficit at the levels of phonological recognition and phonological representation.

Self-monitoring work

This was targeted at Zoe's phonological retrieval errors, working on her accessing of accurate motor programs for words.

Articulatory activities

These were targeted at the postalveolar fricatives and affricates, working at the level of motor execution.

Syllable segmentation games

Games involved segmentation of the syllable into phonological constituents, including rhyme, to strengthen metaphonological awareness and thereby provide the basis for reading and spelling development. These were directed primarily at the levels of phonological recognition and motor programming.

Word segmentation games

Games involved segmentation of words into syllables, to help Zoe with the acquisition of new vocabulary, particularly polysyllabic words. Again, these were directed primarily at the levels of phonological recognition and motor programming.

These auditory, articulatory, programming and phonological awareness strands were present throughout her therapy programme (Stackhouse and Wells, 1993). As Zoe got older, the therapy focus was shifted from single words to connected speech. Junction between words was targeted and traditional voice production exercises were suggested to improve Zoe's rhythm and airflow control in her phrasing of connected speech. Specific recommendations regarding work on connected speech included the following.

Polysyllabic words

Zoe would often break up the rhythmic pattern of words of more than one syllable, particularly when the word came at the end of the utterance. This was done by combinations of features such as: insertion of a glottal stop at the end of the first syllable, lengthening of unstressed vowels and/or giving them an unreduced vowel quality, and giving equal pitch and loudness prominence to the stressed and the unstressed syllable. Some of these features are illustrated in the following examples: PUPPET → [pʊ.pɛʔ]; READY → [ʋɛʔ'tiː]; FISHES → [fɪʔʃiːs]; SUGAR → [sʊʔːkə]; BIGGER → [bɪhgɛː]. It was suggested that Zoe's awareness of the rhythmic pattern of such words in isolation, might be heightened by questions such as "Which is the big/loud/important part of the word?" in the hope that this would help Zoe to appreciate that the first syllable in such words is more prominent. It was also suggested that verse could be used to practise establishing more rhythmic patterns at the motor planning level, integrating polysyllabic words into a connected speech context.

Linking with grammar

Work on aspects of connected speech, such as rhythm, could be linked in with work on grammar. For example, if Zoe needed to practise prepositional phrases, where she frequently omitted the determiner, e.g. "with saw" – –, this could be done within an appropriate rhythmic frame, e.g. WITH A SAW ∪ ∪ –, rather than drawing atttention prosodically to the omitted determiner, which might encourage Zoe to use a more marked rhythmic pattern WITH A̲ SAW ∪ – –, thus reinforcing her habitual jerky pattern (Wells, 1994).

Resyllabification

Part of the jerkiness of Zoe's speech was attributable to her tendency not to link up a word ending with a consonant with a following word beginning with a vowel, but instead to start the second word with a glottal stop, e.g. WASH IN → [wɒʃ.ʔɪn], SET ON → [sɛʔt . ʔɒn.]. It was suggested that Zoe might initially be encouraged to transfer the final consonant of the first word to the onset of the first syllable of the second, e.g. pronounce such sequences as WASH IN → [wɒ.ʃɪn], SET ON → [sɛʔ. tɒn.]. This reinforces the point that phonological segmentation does not always reflect lexical segmentation. For a child like Zoe, who was already beginning to read, this can be reinforced visually by using plastic letters, moving the ‹t› to the start of ‹on› in SET ON, for example. Although this also leads to an artificial pronunciation, such resyllabification is found as part of normal phonological development (Stemberger, 1989), which gives the therapy programme a developmental rationale.

These therapy proposals reflect the belief that in cases such as Zoe's, it is not appropriate to treat a speech problem as a single entity. The case illustrates that a number of possible sources of difficulty may need to be tackled simultaneously in the child's therapy programme.

Summary

In this chapter we have presented detailed speech processing profiles of Zoe at two points in time, separated by over two years. The key points to emerge from the chapter are:

- The framework and profile can be used to assess the same child at different points in time and thus provide a systematic basis for examining change over time.
- The focus of speech processing assessment shifts according to the age of the child.
- The psycholinguistic framework can be used to structure findings from routine clinical assessments, as well as from specifically designed tests of speech processing.
- Detailed phonological analysis of the child's speech output can give rise to specific hypotheses about the child's speech difficulties, that can be tested out within a psycholinguistic framework.
- The results of the speech processing profile can be mapped on to an information processing model in order to identify the levels of processing deficit more precisely.
- Different aspects of a single child's speech difficulty may have their origin at different levels of speech processing.
- Assessment findings can be interpreted with reference to the five phases of development of speech processing described in Chapters 7 and 8.
- The profile, when interpreted in terms of the speech processing model and developmental phases, suggests specific objectives for therapy and teaching.

KEY TO ACTIVITY 9.1
Zoe's speech processing profile at CA 3;9

SPEECH PROCESSING PROFILE

Name: Zoe

Age: 3;9 d.o.b:

Date: October 1996

Profiler: JS/BW

Comments:

n.d., no data. Control data not available for any tasks, so number of crosses is based on impressionistic judgement.

INPUT

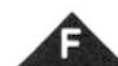

Is the child aware of the internal structure of phonological representations?

n.d

Are the child's phonological representations accurate?

✓ (except voice/voiceless)

Can the child discriminate between real words?

n.d

Does the child have language-specific representations of word structures?

n.d

Can the child discriminate speech sounds without reference to lexical representations?

n.d

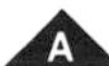

Does the child have adequate auditory perception?

✓

OUTPUT

Can the child access accurate motor programs?

✗✗✗

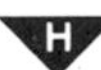

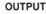

Can the child manipulate phonological units?

n.d

Can the child articulate real words accurately?

✗✗

Can the child articulate speech without reference to lexical representations?

n.d

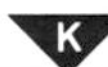

Does the child have adequate sound production skills?

✗✗

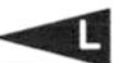

Does the child reject his/her own erroneous forms?

n.d

KEY TO ACTIVITY 9.2

Speech processing model for Zoe at CA 3;9

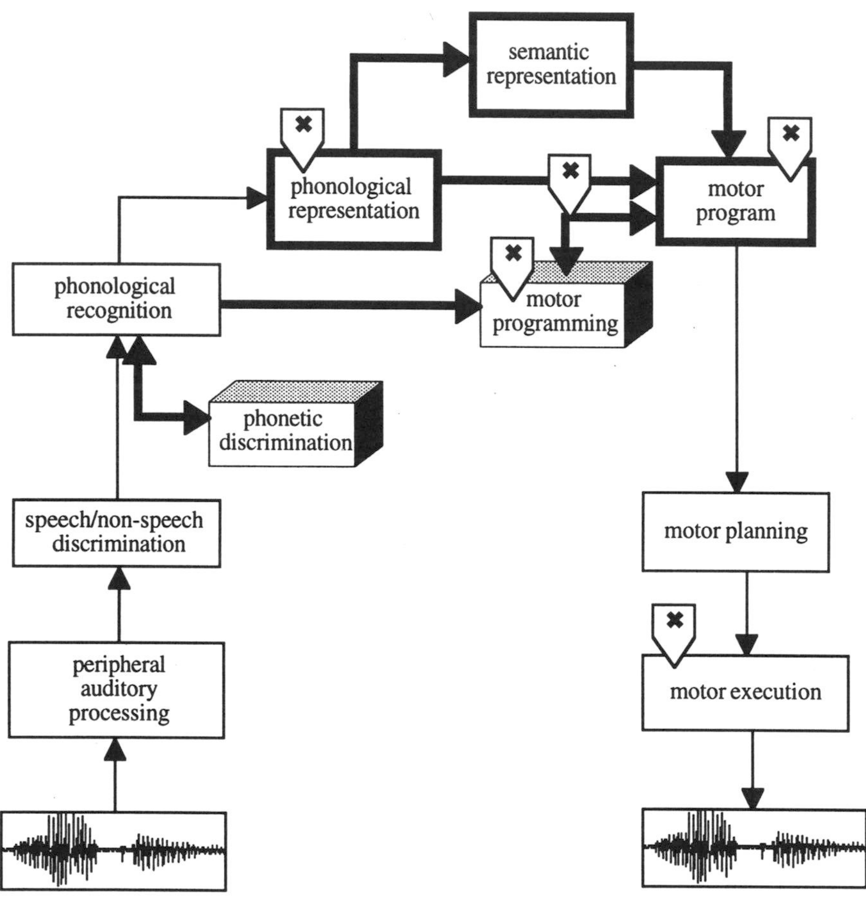

KEY TO ACTIVITY 9.3
Phases of development – Zoe at CA 3;9

(a) Zoe was producing a range of single word utterances, and had done for some time, so she could no longer be considered to be in the Prelexical Phase.

(b) There is no evidence that Zoe had entered the Metaphonological Phase and indeed this would not necessarily be expected of normally-developing children of her age.

There is no evidence that Zoe had entered the Assembly Phase either, although this would be predicted in normal development. This was because Zoe was not producing utterances of more than one word, so the features involved in linking up words in connected speech, which characterize the Assembly Phase, were not relevant. Any speech activities that involved stringing together more than one word, or even more than one place of articulation, caused Zoe great difficulty (see Nuffield assessment: Contrasting of Consonant – Vowel Structures).

KEY TO ACTIVITY 9.4
Zoe's speech processing profile at CA 5;11

SPEECH PROCESSING PROFILE

Name: Zoe

Age: 5;11 d.o.b:

Date: October 1996

Profiler: JS/BW

Comments:

n.d., no data. Control data not available for some tasks, so number of crosses is based on impressionistic judgement.

INPUT

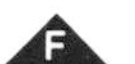

Is the child aware of the internal structure of phonological representations?
✗✗

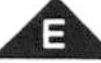

Are the child's phonological representations accurate?
✗ (particularly voice/voiceless)

Can the child discriminate between real words?
n.d

Does the child have language-specific representations of word structures?
n.d

Can the child discriminate speech sounds without reference to lexical representations?
n.d

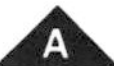

Does the child have adequate auditory perception?
✓

OUTPUT

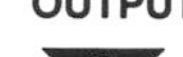

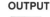

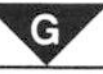

Can the child access accurate motor programs?
✗

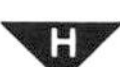

Can the child manipulate phonological units?
✗✗✗

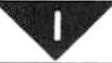

Can the child articulate real words accurately?
✗

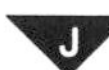

Can the child articulate speech without reference to lexical representations?
✗✗

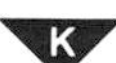

Does the child have adequate sound production skills?
✗

Does the child reject his/her own erroneous forms?
✗

KEY TO ACTIVITY 9.5
Speech processing model for Zoe at CA 5;11

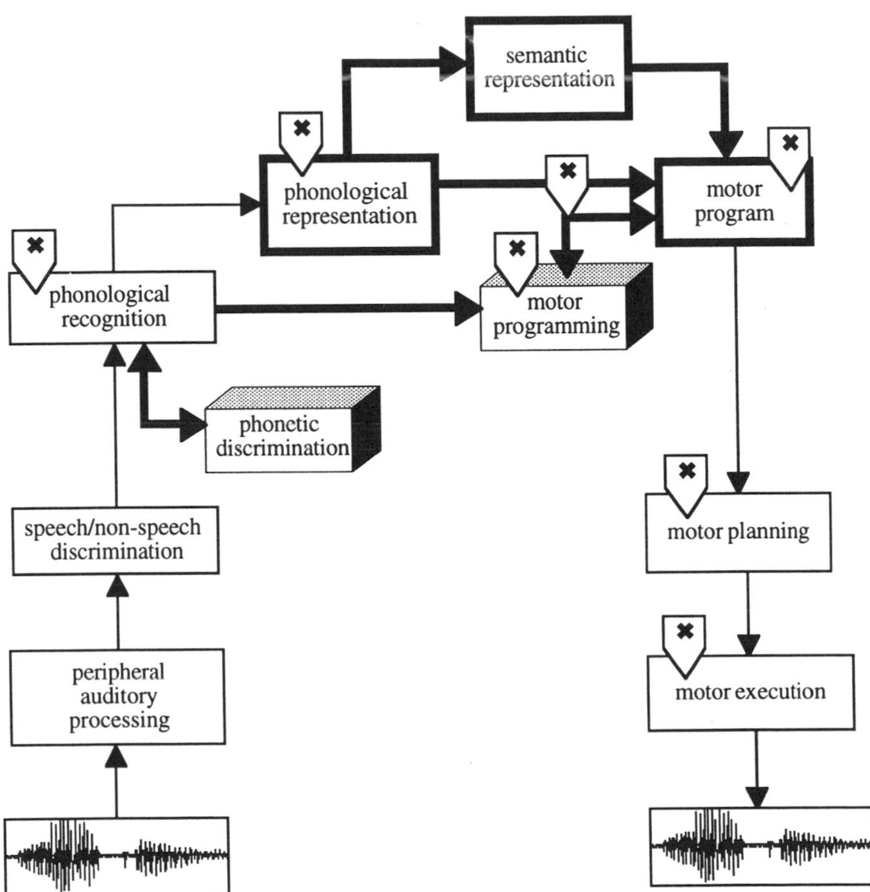

KEY TO ACTIVITY 9.6
Phases of development: Zoe at CA 5;11

(a) Zoe's single word production, though not age appropriate, was adequate in signalling many of the necessary phonological contrasts. She could no longer be described as functioning at the Whole Word Phase when producing real words, as the parametric features noted at 3;9 were no longer evident.

Her error patterns in speech output were in some aspects quite systematic, e.g. the treatment of labial consonant clusters – a pattern that in some respects is typical of the cluster reduction found in younger children with normally-developing speech. This is suggestive of the Systematic Simplification Phase, although she was no longer using earlier patterns associated with that phase, such as reduplication, consonant harmony, fronting of velars, stopping of fricatives.

(b) Deficits were evident that impacted on the production of connected speech: Zoe had only just begun to get to grips with the phonological features that characterize connected speech in English. Thus, she was not yet able to meet all the demands of the Assembly Phase.

At this point, she was showing no evidence of metaphonological skills, e.g. in her responses to rhyme tasks. This suggests that she had not progressed to the Metaphonological Phase, as would be expected by her age.

At 5;11, Zoe appeared to be around the transition between the Systematic Simplification and the Assembly Phases – a point that most children would have reached soon after their third birthday.

Chapter 10
The Unfolding Deficit II – Barriers to Literacy

In Chapter 9 we presented assessments of Zoe's speech processing skills at CA 3;9 and 5;11. At the age of 5;11, Zoe was approaching the end of her first year of formal schooling. Since we know that children such as Zoe with severe speech processing difficulties are at risk for problems with reading and spelling (cf. Chapter 1), it was relevant at this point to investigate her early reading and spelling skills. This assessment would also provide a baseline for measuring performance in later years. The purpose of this chapter is to explore the consequences of Zoe's speech processing deficits for her literacy development.

Zoe's Literacy Skills at CA 5;11

Reading

The *Schonell Graded Word Reading Test* was administered (Newton and Thomson, 1982). This involves the child reading a list of single words. Zoe recognized the word ‹little› but no others. She made a number of visual errors e.g. ‹milk› → "mum", ‹sit› → "sun". Her performance on this test put her below the 6-year level. This in itself does not constitute a problem given her age of 5;11. However, it was noted that she did not know all of the letter names and sounds and that this restricted her ability to read novel material. Zoe presented as a typical beginner reader functioning mainly in the Logographic Phase of literacy development.

Spelling

On the *Schonell Graded Word Spelling Test* (Newton and Thomson, 1982) Zoe achieved a spelling age of 5;1. She was able to spell one word correctly: IN. For the other words she tended to transcribe the initial consonant, though not always correctly.

She was asked to spell 10 further simple words. The voice/voiceless problem detected on the tests of speech and auditory discrimination (see Chapter 9) seemed to show up in her spellings, with /p/ consistently spelt ‹b›, though this could also be described as a visual or transcription error.

Spoken target	*Zoe's spelling*
PET	bt
LIP	hb
CAP	cb
FISH	fl
TENT	tt
TRAP	tb
BUMP	bb
SACK	~
NEST	ƨƨ
BANK	bt

Given the wide variation in performance in beginner readers/spellers, these results alone would not be cause for concern. However, Zoe's slow passage through the normal phases of speech development, coupled with persisting auditory discrimination difficulties and poor rhyme performance, suggested that she might find transition to the Alphabetic Phase of literacy development problematic.

Zoe continued to receive regular speech and language therapy and teaching within the language unit until the age of 7 years when she was integrated into mainstream school. When she was 9 years old there was concern about her poor literacy development and we were asked to see her again. This provided an opportunity to test out the prediction that Zoe's speech processing difficulties would interfere with the normal course of reading and spelling development.

Zoe at CA 9;8

Zoe was now attending a local junior school where she received some additional help each morning from a support worker. She was no longer receiving speech and language therapy on a regular basis but had a contact speech and language therapist, who supplied a range of test results obtained in the interim (Table 10.1).

These results confirmed that Zoe had specific expressive language and literacy difficulties in the context of normal cognitive ability. The main concern of parents and teachers at this point was Zoe's literacy difficulties, rather than her spoken language: Zoe was now intelligible and able to hold a conversation. An assessment of her speech processing and literacy skills was therefore undertaken at CA 9;8.

Table 10.1: Assesment results for Zoe at CA 7;11 and 8;9

CA 7;11		
British Picture Vocabulary Scales	Confidence band	6;8–7;9
Renfrew Word Finding Vocabulary Scales	Confidence band	7;7–7;9
Renfrew Action Picture Test	Information	8;5
	Grammar	6;5
CA 8;9		
WISC-R	Verbal IQ	95–98
	Performance IQ	105
	Full Scale	100
Burt Reading Test	Age Equivalent	7;4
BAS Word Reading Test	Age Equivalent	7;5
Schonell Test B	Age Equivalent	6;2
Bender-Gestalt	Age Equivalent	8;0–8;6

Assessment of speech processing at CA 9;8

Zoe's speech processing skills were assessed via a range of input, phonological awareness and output tasks.

Nonword auditory discrimination

This task comprised pairs of complex nonwords e.g. BESKET / BEKSET, SPODER / SPODER. Zoe was asked to say if the members of the pair were the same or different. She scored 35/40, = 87.5 per cent correct on this test. The oldest group for which control data are available is children of CA 7;0–8;0, who had a mean score of 90.7 per cent correct (s.d.7.5) (Stackhouse, 1989). She was therefore within the performance range of these normally-developing children. Two of Zoe's errors were ones often made by the normal controls (final /n/ vs /m/ and syllabic /gl̩/ vs /dl̩/) and two were made on 'same' items, which may have been due to loss of concentration. One error was on a voicing contrast item (BASKOITS / PASKOITS), echoing Zoe's auditory discrimination difficulty at 5;11. No errors were made on cluster sequence items (e.g. WESP / WEPS) or on metathetic items (e.g. IBIKUS / IKIBUS).

Auditory lexical decision

Zoe was also given an auditory lexical decision task. She had to identify if a word spoken by the tester, e.g. FIS, was the correct name for the picture presented, i.e. FISH (after Locke, 1980 a, b). Ten three- and four-syllable words were presented. Zoe made three errors on this test. Two of the errors were on the voicing contrast: [ˈkæɹəˌfæn] accepted for CARAVAN, [ˈhɛlɪˌgɒptə] accepted for HELICOPTER, out of a possible 13 voicing targets. The other error (one out of a possible four) was on the /w/ vs /r/ distinction: [ˈpæwəʃut] accepted for PARACHUTE.

Rhyme detection – auditory presentation (real words)

Zoe was assessed on four rhyme tasks, for which control data had been collected from 100 normally-developing children aged 3–7 years (Vance, Stackhouse and Wells, 1994). The tasks make use of the same or matched linguistic stimuli so that comparisons can be made across tasks. Twelve pairs of rhyming words are used for the detection tests. All words are within the vocabulary of 3-year-old children, and are monosyllabic, with no final consonant clusters, e.g. CV: CAR STAR; CVC: CAT HAT.

For the auditory test of rhyme detection (real words), a toy dog is introduced along with two bears. The dog says the stimulus item, e.g. BOAT, while each bear produces a response item, e.g. BATH, COAT . The children are asked to select the bear that produced the rhyme for the dog's word. Zoe scored 11/12 on this task, which was a similar performance to the 7-year-old controls, who were also at ceiling.

Rhyme detection – auditory presentation (nonwords)

A set of nonwords was derived from the stimuli used in the previous task, by changing the onset of each word and maintaining the rhyme, e.g. [pəut] – [həut]. The same procedure was followed as in the previous task. Again, Zoe scored like the 7-year-old controls on this task – 11/12 correct.

Rhyme detection – visual presentation

The rhyme detection task was also presented in a 'silent' condition, using pictures. For this task, 54 specially prepared photographs are used, and a vocabulary check is conducted by asking the child to name the photographs. The child is asked to select from two pictures (e.g. BOAT or GLOVE) the one that rhymes with the stimulus picture (e.g. COAT). The child posts their chosen picture in a post box. Zoe scored 12/12 correct; again like the 7-year-old controls who were also at ceiling on this task.

Zoe thus had little difficulty with the input rhyme tests in terms of accuracy of response. However, on the picture-pointing rhyme test where she had to choose one out of two pictures that rhymed with a target, she routinely made use of verbal rehearsal in order to perform this visual task. In the control study, an interesting developmental trend was observed on the visual detection task. Although this task is meant to be 'silent' in that the child is not required to produce rhyming words, the children often named the rhyme pictures as a means of rehearsal when carrying out the task. The importance of this verbal rehearsal strategy for at least some of the children was evident in the following response from one of the 4-year-olds: when asked if two pictures rhymed she replied "I don't think so yet, cos I haven't talked!" The number of children in each year band using speech output as part of their rehearsal strategies was therefore calculated. Verbal rehearsal was particularly apparent in 4-, 5- and 6-year-olds but had declined in the 7-year-olds, who were at ceiling on the task. The smallest percentage occurred in the 3-year-old group, who were only at chance level on the visual detection task.

It would appear then that from 4 to 6 years of age, as the child is grasping the task and beginning to have success, there is an increase in the use of verbal rehearsal as a strategy to assist rhyme detection. By the time the child reaches ceiling on the task at around 7 years of age, the verbal behaviour has declined. This observation shows the importance of speech as a verbal rehearsal strategy 'naturally' adopted by normally-developing children on a task that involves rhyme segmentation, even when no verbal output is required. Indeed, it was not possible for the tester to inhibit this behaviour in the children.

Zoe, at the age of 9;8, routinely made use of verbal rehearsal on the visual detection task, even though she was at ceiling on the task. In this respect she resembled the minority of the 7-year-old group, who still used verbal rehearsal. Interestingly, in the (similar) task of visual rhyme detection that Zoe had done at the age of 5;11, she had not performed above chance level, whereas on the equivalent test in the control study, the 5-year-olds were already performing above chance level. This suggests that at CA 5;11, Zoe had been performing more like children of 4 years or younger, and thus had had a distinct deficit in rhyme detection that was no longer evident at CA 9;8. Furthermore, at this earlier testing, Zoe had not made use of verbal rehearsal – again paralleling the behaviour of the youngest children in the control group. Her use of verbal rehearsal at 9;8 indicates that although Zoe could respond accurately, she was not yet able to respond automatically, and in this respect demonstrated that her rhyming skills were not yet comparable to those of most normally-developing 7-year-olds.

Rhyme production

In this task, the child is told that the dog likes words that rhyme with his name, SPOT. The child is encouraged to think of rhyming words and given corrective feedback on their productions. On subsequent items, they have to tell the dog rhyming words to the given stimuli. After some practice items, the child is given 12 test items e.g. COAT, BED, PEG, and 20 seconds per item in which to produce a rhyme string. Two measures were taken for this analysis: (1) the accuracy of the first response; and (2) the number of correct rhyme responses produced in the string. At age 9;8, Zoe had 8/12 accurate first responses. Although able to produce at least one rhyme response to nine targets, her responses were very limited. Overall, she produced a total of 20 responses which rhymed with the 12 test stimuli, less than a quarter of the total responses she gave, the remaining three-quarters being non-rhyming responses. In the control group, the ability to give an accurate first response increased progressively through the year bands. The 7-year-olds had a mean accurate first response of 11.4 (s.d. 0.86) on the rhyme production task, and were therefore at ceiling. Their mean total number of rhyming responses of 40.1 indicates that they were able to produce on average three to four rhymes per item. Zoe was thus, at 9;8, not performing as well as these 7-year-olds; her performance was in fact around the 5-year level (mean accurate responses: 6.75, s.d. 4.55; total responses: 16.95, s.d. 14.42).

One of her best responses was to the item RING. She started off well but was not able to maintain the rhyme strategy for the full 20 seconds:

RING: "ring ping ting ling
ring ping [fə'lɛ] boo
ring ping ['tɪli] boo"

This example also shows how she needed to repeat the target at regular intervals. Although this is a strategy typical of younger children, only 15 per cent of the 7-year-old children were still using it in the normative study from which these control data is taken (Vance, Stackhouse and Wells, 1994).

On a number of occasions Zoe tried a 'frame' strategy (particularly "silly old ——") to help her rhyme. Although to some extent this strategy was successful, it limited the number of correct rhyming words:

PURSE: "purse the worse the silly old turse
purse the ['lɜs ə 'lɜsi 'gæ]"

LIGHT: "light pight kite light
light pight silly old tight
light pight ['til^{j}wɛt]"

COAT: "coat a loat a potty tot
coat the pot the wotty totty"

SOCK: "sock pock silly old tock
sock tock peck too
sock ['lju 'guli gu]"

This is not typical of normally-developing children, though one 6-year-old did adopt a similar strategy in the normative study:

SOCK: "sock the wock the pit pat pock"
TWO: "two the woo the pit pat poo"

Real word repetition

Zoe's performance on repetition of complex but familiar words was tested (e.g. HELICOPTER, FEATHER, CROCODILE, SUPERMARKET – stimuli from Ryder, 1991). Zoe scored 17/24 perfectly correctly on the real word condition. A group of 20 6-year-old children tested by Ryder had a mean score of 22.3 correct. Zoe's errors were quite minor ones, e.g. CROCODILE → ['kwɒkədail], AQUARIUM → [ə'kwɛəʋiən].

Nonword repetition

Zoe was also asked to repeat nonwords matched phonetically to the real words used in the previous test (Ryder, 1991). She scored 8/24 correctly on the nonword condition. The 6-year-olds in Ryder's study had a mean score of 10.88. Examples of Zoe's errors include: /'lɛwɪˌgɒbdə/ → ['lɛʋɪˌglɒbdə]; /'vɛθə/ → ['fɛðə]; /'glɒgətail/ → ['glɒdətail]. When asked to produce a new word (i.e. a nonword) three times in succession, her responses were inconsistent, e.g. /'zubəˌbɑgɪd/ → ['zubəˌgɑdɪd], ['zubəˌgɑvɪd], ['zubəˌgʋɑbɪd].

Spontaneous speech

Zoe had made considerable progress with her speech but residual speech errors were still apparent and her speech sounded 'immature' and disjointed. There were specific lexical items that were consistently produced wrongly, e.g. the character name KIPPER in her book was consistently pronounced as [kjupə]. Otherwise, in one-and-two syllable words segmental errors were minimal. However, some immaturities remained, e.g. /r/ as in READING → [ʋidɪn], TRAP → [tʋæp]. Zoe maintained the voicing contrast more consistently than she had at CA 5;11, though very occasionally she used inappropriate aspiration, e.g. POLISH → [p̄ɒlɪʃ]. Multisyllabic words tended to have distorted articulations because of incoordination of the airflow as in REFRESHMENT → [ʋɪ'fʰʋɛʃmʰənt]. Articulatorily complex sequences were still problematic for her, for example when having to change the place of articulation, from back rounded [w] to front spread [i] in QUEEN → [kjʷɔin] or from labial to velar in PUMPKIN → ['pʌŋkɪn], or because of the syllable structure itself as in INSTRUCTED → [ɪndɪs'dʌkˌtɪd]. She would sometimes insert a glottal stop before a word final voiceless consonant at syllable boundaries within the word, e.g. HOCKEY → ['hɒʔki], BISHOP → ['bɪʔʃəp], and CASTLE → ['kæʔsʊ]; and also at the end of the word, e.g. FISH → ['fɪʔəʃ], UP → [ʌʔp], and PUPPET → ['pʌpɪʔt]. She sometimes used a glottal stop in place of voiceless consonants at the end of words, e.g. BUS → [bʌʔ]. On occasion she omitted word final consonants in connected speech, e.g. BUT SOMETIMES → [bʌ'sːʌmˌtaɪms]. This resulted in 'mumbley' speech which was difficult to understand at times.

ACTIVITY 10.1

Aim: To draw up Zoe's speech processing profile at CA 9;8.

Drawing on the assessment results just presented, fill in a speech processing profile for Zoe at 9;8, using the profile sheet in Figure10.1.

Compare your profile with the one given in Key to Activity 10.1 at the end of this chapter, then read the following.

Auditory discrimination

On the input side, there were no reported problems with hearing, so question A can be ticked. Zoe was able to complete successfully auditory discrimination of nonwords, indicating affirmative answers for question B: ***Can the child discriminate speech sounds without reference to lexical representations?***

Auditory lexical decision

On an auditory lexical decision task, addressing the accuracy of her phonological representations, Zoe made only three errors, but all three reflected her residual speech errors in voicing and /r/. Thus, compared to her performance at 5;11, the same error types were still occurring albeit more disguised. Zoe still apparently had fuzzy representations for these distinctions in some lexical items. Some doubts thus remained concerning question E: ***Are the child's phonological representations accurate?***

SPEECH PROCESSING PROFILE

Name: Zoe

Age: 9;8 d.o.b:

Date:

Profiler:

Comments:

INPUT

F — Is the child aware of the internal structure of phonological representations?

E — Are the child's phonological representations accurate?

D — Can the child discriminate between real words?

C — Does the child have language-specific representations of word structures?

B — Can the child discriminate speech sounds without reference to lexical representations?

A — Does the child have adequate auditory perception?

OUTPUT

G — Can the child access accurate motor programs?

H — Can the child manipulate phonological units?

I — Can the child articulate real words accurately?

J — Can the child articulate speech without reference to lexical representations?

K — Does the child have adequate sound production skills?

L — Does the child reject his/her own erroneous forms?

Figure 10.1: Blank profile for Activity 10.1: Zoe at CA 9;8.

Rhyme detection

Her performance on the rhyme detection task using pictures indicated that Zoe was now aware of the internal structure of phonological representations, at least as far as the onset and rhyme constituents are concerned, allowing a generally positive answer for question F: *Is the child aware of the internal structure of phonological representations?* although her dependency on vocalization suggests that this is not yet automatic. Her performance on the auditory rhyme detection tasks (real words and nonwords) allows us to tick questions B and D.

Rhyme production

Rhyme production tasks tap the ability not only to segment into onset and rhyme (as in rhyme detection) but also to manipulate these phonological constituents in order to assemble new motor programs. They thus address question H: *Can the child manipulate phonological units?* Zoe was performing at around a 5-year level on this task, showing a serious deficit which was marked by three crosses on her profile.

Spontaneous speech

Zoe's spontaneous speech production, though much improved, still showed some consistently unusual pronunciations, suggesting that her motor programs for such words are still inaccurate. A single cross was therefore put under question G: *Can the child access accurate motor programs?*

Real word repetition

Zoe made more errors on real word repetition than younger controls, suggesting that a cross should be put under question I: *Can the child articulate real words accurately?*. However, these errors are relatively minor in nature, suggesting that with familiar language material Zoe does not have great problems any more, except with some specific words (see question G).

Nonword repetition

Zoe made a large number of errors on a test of nonword repetition, some of which revealed quite serious difficulties with planning and executing unfamiliar and relatively complex articulatory sequences. Three crosses have therefore been placed under question J: *Can the child articulate speech without reference to lexical representations?* However, there was no evidence of particular difficulties with individual sounds in isolation, giving a tick under question K: *Does the child have adequate sound production skills?*

Self-monitoring

There was little evidence of Zoe correcting her own erroneous forms and so a cross has been placed under question L.

From profile to model: Zoe at 9;8

When Zoe's profile at 9;8 is compared with her profile at 5;11, the earlier deficits on the input side are less evident. On the output side, there are less marked difficulties with processing real words (G, I) but still major deficits in assembling new words, both for rhyme production (H) and for nonword repetition (J). By mapping her speech processing profile on to the speech processing model, we can see if the loci of deficits are the same as those identified at CA 5;11.

ACTIVITY 10.2

Aim: To map the results from Zoe's speech processing profile at 9;8 on to the speech processing model described in Chapter 6.

Repeat the 'profile to model' exercise that you did for Zoe at CA 3;9 and 5;11. On the speech processing model presented in Chapter 6, reproduced here as Figure 10.2, attempt to locate the deficits that you think might be responsible for Zoe's speech processing difficulties at 9;8, using the speech processing profile of Zoe from Activity 10.1 (Key to Activity 10.1).

Compare your answer with the model presented in Key to Activity 10.2, then read the following.

At 9;8, the major persisting locus of deficit was in motor programming. This is one of the capacities that is necessary to create new forms in the rhyme production task. The results suggested that Zoe's difficulty with rhyme production originated on the output side rather than with input or representations, since she performed at ceiling on all three rhyme detection tasks, indicating that she understood the concept of rhyme. More specifically, her output deficit appeared to be at the level or levels in output processing where she had to select an onset from her store of potential syllable onsets, and attach it to the rhyme that had already been segmented from the stimulus word. Furthermore, motor programming is one of the essential components involved in repeating forms heard for the first time, as in a nonword repetition task. To repeat novel stimuli, it is also necessary to be able to discriminate nonwords accurately; Zoe showed the ability to do so on the nonword discrimination task, suggesting that her problems with nonword repetition were due to deficits on the output side at the level of motor programming.

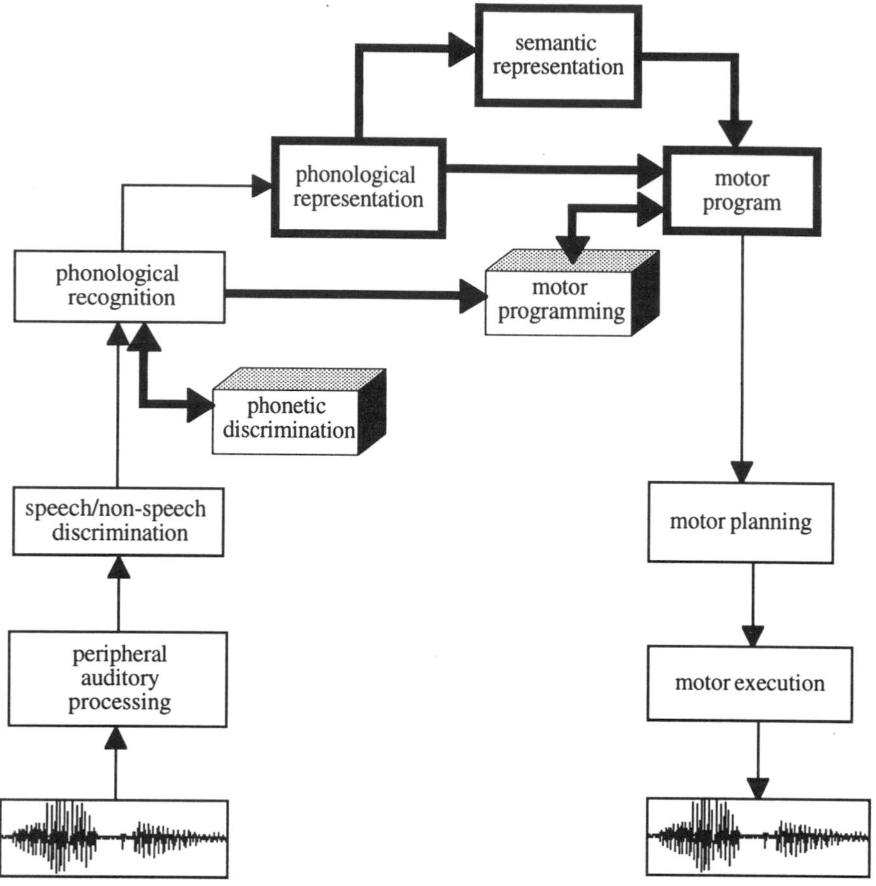

Figure 10.2: Speech processing model for Activity 10.2.

There are still some deficits in other components. In phonological recognition, phonological representations and motor programs, the deficits are not pervasive, but are restricted to particular words or phonological oppositions. The imprecise between-word junctions in connected speech suggest some remaining difficulties in motor planning.

The developmental perspective on Zoe's speech processing at CA 9;8

A profile of Zoe's speech processing at 9;8 has been drawn up (Activity 10.1), and interpreted in terms of the speech processing model (Activity 10.2). As we did for Zoe at 3;9 and at 5;11, we can now consider how this pattern of deficits can be related to the five phases of speech development proposed in Chapters 7 and 8: Prelexical; Whole Word; Systematic Simplification; Assembly ; Metaphonological.

ACTIVITY 10.3

Aim: To interpret data from Zoe at 9;8 in terms of the five developmental phases of speech processing.

On the basis of the data presented earlier, which phase, or phases, of development, do you consider Zoe (a) to have passed through (b) not yet to have entered? From your answer, what can you conclude about her speech processing development at the age of 9;8?

Check your answer with Key to Activity 10.3, then read the following.

At 5;11, Zoe was thought to be at a transitional point between the Systematic Simplification Phase and the Assembly Phase. By 9;8 she had clearly moved on: in terms of speech processing, she had reached the Metaphonological Phase, where phonological awareness skills are of paramount importance. She had not yet moved successfully through this phase, however. This was not surprising given the dependency of phonological awareness skills on the ability to create new motor programs, particularly when tasks require the child not only to manipulate phonological units silently but also to produce them in speech. Most children have moved through the Metaphonological Phase by the time they start school around their fifth birthday. Zoe was clearly behind in the development of the metaphonological skills that are prerequisite for successful learning to read and spell. In the next section we shall see what impact this had on her literacy development, about which her parents and teachers were concerned.

Zoe's Literacy Skills at CA 9;8

As the assessment of Zoe's speech processing and literacy skills at 9;8 all had to be carried out within a single day, it was only possible to administer a small number of reading and spelling tasks.

Reading

Two reading tests were administered: a test of single (real) word reading and a nonword reading test.

Single real word reading (real words)

On the *Wechsler Objective Reading Dimensions (WORD)* Basic Reading subtest (Wechsler, 1993), Zoe attained an age equivalent score of 7;6 and a standard score of 81 which is at the ninth percentile for children of her age. She was able to recognize a substantial number of the easier, more common words effortlessly but had considerable difficulty when words were unfamiliar. A few of her errors indicated that she was attempting to identify words globally, sometimes confusing them with visually similar words. For example, she read `<ruin>` as "rain" and `<pier>` as "pair". This is a common strategy amongst beginner readers who do not yet take all the letters into account when identifying words. Zoe's word attack skills were as yet poorly developed, especially on longer words, and she was unable to decode most unfamiliar words.

Single word reading (nonwords)

In order to examine decoding ability further, Zoe was asked to read a list of one- and two-syllable nonwords using the *Graded Nonword Reading Test* (Snowling, Stothard and McLean, 1996). Zoe had a great deal of difficulty with these, reading 2/10 one-syllable and 0/10 of the two-syllable nonwords correctly. On the one-syllable words she made several vowel errors e.g. <hast> read as [hɛst], <mon> read as [mɪn], <twesk> as [twɪsk]. She also occasionally omitted the final sound in consonant clusters but errors such as <drant> read as [dwant] are more likely to result from pronunciation difficulties with the /dr/ cluster. On two occasions she also read <p> as [b], a voicing error which later appeared in her spelling attempts and is likely to be connected to her speech difficulties. Although she made mistakes on these easier items, it was clear that she had learned many basic sound–letter correspondences and was often able to blend the sounds and so pronounce the item correctly.

Zoe found two-syllable nonwords much more difficult. She read the majority of the items as if they consisted of only one syllable, omitting large portions of the nonword e.g. ‹tegwop› → [twɒpf], <stansert> → [stɛnt], <chamgalp> → [ʧæmb], <balras> → ['bæwə], <molsmit> → ['məʊləz], <nolcrid> → ['nəʊtwɪd].

Spelling

Zoe was asked to spell sets of one-, two- and three-syllable words to dictation (after Snowling, 1985, reproduced in Goulandris, 1996, p.98).

Spelling of monosyllabic words

Zoe spelled 4/10 one-syllable words correctly: FAST, NEST, TENT, HAND. Errors included vowel errors in which the short vowel was represented by an incorrect letter e.g. TRIP spelled as ‹trep›, NEST spelled as ‹nast›. Here Zoe may be following what many young children do, in using the letter ‹a› to represent the short sound /ɛ/ because they hear the sound /ɛ/ at the beginning of the letter name for A (pronounced [eɪ]). An alternative explanation is that Zoe uses ‹a› when she is not sure which vowel to select. In addition, Zoe added ‹e› to the ends of some words: DRESS → ‹darse›; CARD → ‹code›; SACK → ‹sake›; BANK → ‹bake›. This may be because she is confused about the use of silent ‹e›, applying it incorrectly to words which contain short vowels, or because she is transcribing her own pronunciation as she segments the word, when the final consonant is emphasized with a schwa vowel, e.g. SACK → [s ʔaʔ kə]. Similarly, voicing errors were also apparent in one-syllable words e.g. SINK → ‹sing›, DESK → ‹Disg›.

One further spelling error was fairly consistent: inserting a vowel letter to separate the consonant letters in an initial cluster (blend). The inserted vowel is underlined in the following examples:

Spoken target		*Zoe's spelling*
CLOWN	→	‹ca̲lren›
DRESS	→	‹da̲rse›
FLOOR	→	‹fo̲le›
STAR	→	‹so̲te›
SNAIL	→	‹sa̲ne›
SMALL	→	‹se̲mll›

This splitting of the initial cluster may be due to speech difficulties encountered during the segmentation process: clusters of consonants without vowels are difficult to articulate, and had been a particular problem for Zoe at 5;11 (see Chapter 9). According to this theory, Zoe's spelling of, for example, STAR as ‹so̲te› reflects her 'sounding out' of the ST cluster, either silently or aloud, as [sə tə], leading to a spelling of ‹sote› where ‹o› represents the neutral schwa vowel. The inserted vowels in CLOWN, DRESS and SMALL can be analysed in the same way, as can SNAIL and FLOOR. This 'segmentation' analysis suggests that in three of these six examples, Zoe's spellings were attempts at the initial cluster only (FLOOR, STAR, SNAIL), while the remaining three (CLOWN, DRESS, SMALL) were attempts at the cluster plus the final consonant. An alternative explanation is that the errors are caused by visual sequencing problems, leading to confusion of letter order. This might plausibly account for FLOO̲R → ‹fo̲le› and SNA̲IL → ‹sa̲ne›, where the intrusive vowel is represented by a letter that occurs later in the target word. However, this is the less general explanation, as it does not account for the other four examples, where the inserted letter does not appear in the target spelling. Further, there was no other evidence that Zoe had any visual deficits; in fact her performance on tests of visuo-motor skill was above age appropriate.

Spelling of polysyllabic words

Zoe had difficulties when asked to spell words of more than one syllable. In a few spellings she managed to represent the correct syllabic and phonemic structure well, i.e. APPLE → ‹alpple›, PACKET → ‹pucket›. Other spellings indicated severe problems with both syllable and phoneme segmentation. Zoe's spelling of such words will be investigated in the next activity.

ACTIVITY 10.4

Aim: To analyse Zoe's spelling of two- and three-syllable words at CA 9;8.

Analyse and comment on the spelling errors presented below. Refer to the observations in the previous section about Zoe's spellings of one-syllable words, and to the profile of Zoe's speech processing skills at 9;8.

Two-syllable words		*Three-syllable words*	
Target	*Zoe's spelling*	*Target*	*Zoe's spelling*
GIRAFFE	‹gafe›	TELEPHONE	‹tlefon›
BROTHER	‹borth›	UNDERSTAND	‹undsand›
SLEEPING	‹selding›	ELEPHANT	‹enfet›
COLLAR	‹core›	UMBRELLA	‹unbe›
PUPPET	‹pue›	PYJAMAS	‹beg›

Check your answer with Key to Activity 10.4 at the end of this chapter, then read the following.

On the basis of the spelling analyses in Key to Activity 10.4, we can conclude that Zoe could usually segment the correct number of syllables in two-syllable words, but within the syllable could not always correctly match phonological constituents to appropriate graphemes or sequences of graphemes. This failure to match was compounded by residual speech errors which interfered with her rehearsal of segments within the syllable. Furthermore, she still had to learn some of the conventional rules for English spelling. When spelling three-syllable words, she had more difficulties marking the correct number of syllables. Intervention would need to target this basic structure of the word as a prerequisite for more accurate transcription of segments within the syllable.

A Developmental Perspective on Literacy and Speech Processing Skills

The speech processing assessment of Zoe at 9;8 revealed that there were still important deficits, particularly in the motor programming component, that were giving rise to difficulties with phonological awareness and processing tasks that involved the generation of novel speech ouput, such as rhyme production and nonword repetition. Developmentally, these deficits suggested that she had not yet progressed through the Metaphonological Phase. This led to the prediction that her literacy development would be seriously affected, as metaphonological skills are believed to be necessary to progress from the Logographic Phase of literacy development to the Alphabetic Phase.

Analysis of Zoe's reading and spelling performance confirmed this prediction, indicating that she was just beginning to show evidence of progressing from the Logographic Phase to the Alphabetic Phase. Zoe's performance on the reading tests, and in particular her difficulties with using phonetic strategies to decode unfamiliar words, suggested that as far as reading is concerned, she had not yet progressed from the Logographic to the Alphabetic Phase. In spelling she was slightly further on: there was evidence from her errors that she was using phonetic strategies to guide her spelling attempts, e.g. using ‹f› for PH in TELEPHONE.; splitting target consonant clusters with vowels in a way that reflected her own 'sounding out' strategy, e.g. CLOWN → ‹calren›; and her frequent success in marking the correct number of syllables by using phonetically appropriate graphemes at a sequentially appropriate places, as in UNDERSTAND → ‹un + d + sand›. The advance of spelling over reading in the transition from the Logographic Phase to the Alphabetic Phase is predicted by Frith's model (1985, p.311).

Practical Implications

Zoe had made great progress with her speech since the assessement at 5;11. At 9;8 she was intelligible, though not confident in conversation. Her intermittent unintelligibility in continuous speech was due to suprasegmental features rather than to difficulties with specific sounds. Although able to produce familiar words well, she still had an underlying specific speech disorder which affected her learning of new words. Her main level of difficulty appeared to be with creating motor programs for new and complex words. In addition, imprecise phonological representations for certain features (e.g. voicing and w/r) and for specific complex lexical items could not be ruled out. There may also have been residual lower level articulatory execution difficulties such as co-ordinating air flow for speech. In continuous speech in particular the co-occurrence of these milder but persisting speech errors could affect her intelligibility.

A more serious problem for Zoe, since it was affecting her educational progress, was her specific literacy difficulties. There is no doubt that these were related in many ways to her particular type of speech disorder. The auditory discrimination problems that were more evident in her earlier development had affected the clarity of her phonological representations. Without an accurate phonological representation, it is impossible to generate a phonetically accurate spelling for the word; if an accurate spelling is to be acquired, it will have to be by a visual, logographic strategy.

Zoe's motor programming difficulties compounded this problem since she was unable to set up stable programs quickly for new or complex material. As a consequence, she was unable to use verbal rehearsal to full effect as a strategy for practising the segmentation of words when reading, or prior to spelling them. This was demonstrated by the fact that her performance in speech and spelling deteriorated as words increased in syllable length.

In conclusion, it would be easy to underestimate the extent of Zoe's educational difficulties now that she was much more intelligible: in fact she would benefit from further specialist help. Zoe clearly knew many letter–sound relationships and could apply them quite effectively when dealing with short regular words. Considering the severity of her earlier speech difficulties, as described in Chapter 9, her grasp of letter–sound rules was impressive. However, Zoe's reading was approximately 2 years below the level expected of a child of her chronological age and her spelling was weak. It would be necessary to help Zoe develop phonological skills whilst simultaneously encouraging her to use other linguistic skills to supplement her difficulties with phonological aspects of reading and spelling.

Phonological awareness

A concentrated effort on phonological awareness training would help Zoe to refine her phonological representations, and would provide a link between speech and literacy work. A multi-sensory approach bringing in visual and kinaesthetic feedback alongside auditory/verbal work would probably be beneficial in this respect. This could involve both Zoe's teachers and a speech and language therapist working in collaboration. Rhyme activities, perhaps using plastic letters, could help Zoe to spot orthographic patterns and link them with her auditory and speech skills. Careful selection of words for rhyme production work could help to strengthen the phonological connections but needs to be accompanied by visual cueing. For further ideas see Hatcher (1994).

Zoe's severe difficulties with decoding, especially when reading longer items, indicated that she still required intensive help with phonological skills. Her weak decoding skills were preventing her from becoming an independent reader and would severely hamper her acquisition of literacy. Zoe could be taught how to discriminate short vowels by listening to words such as PEN, PAN and PIN and pointing to the correct letter from a selection of vowel cards. Clue words associated with each vowel which she could refer to when uncertain might be of assistance. Zoe could also be shown how the different vowels are actually formed in the mouth so that she could use kinaesthetic feedback to help her discriminate between them. Speech and language therapy activities and programmes such as *Cued Vowels* (Passy, 1990b) and *Auditory Discrimination in Depth* (Lindamood and Lindamood, 1975; Lindamood, Bell and Lindamood, 1997) might prove useful. It was expected that it could take Zoe a long time before short vowel discrimination became fluent.

In addition, Zoe needed to learn how to segment longer words into syllables so that she could cope with reading and spelling such words more easily. This too could be taught in the form of games, i.e. clapping the number of syllables, using games in which initial and final syllables have been divided (KIT-TEN, PUP-PY), where the child tries to locate the beginning and end portions to form a real word. Once Zoe understood about syllables it would be a relatively easy matter to help her decode longer words one syllable at a time, since she was already quite good at decoding one-syllable words.

Motor programs

The deficit in motor programming could be addressed through the learning of new vocabulary. By beginning a project or linking with an ongoing one at school, Zoe could be introduced to new vocabulary that is to be learned, spoken, read and written. She could be encouraged to reflect on word structure (how many syllables? what sounds can you hear? where are they, at the beginning or end?); then encouraged to produce it syllable by syllable (rather than sound by sound) with a normal rhythmic pattern. The written word and *Cued Articulation* (Passy, 1990a) could be used to help programme the sequence and precise phonetic content of segments. This would be coupled with writing the word and learning its spelling.

Connected speech

Traditional speech and voice production exercises focusing on rhythm and airflow would be of benefit, including work on phrasing, reducing the glottal stop within and at the end of words and on the clarity of the continuous speech. While these activities could be introduced by a speech and language therapist initially to cover some of the difficulties outlined earlier, Zoe might enjoy group drama activities where voice and presentation skills are incorporated.

The assessment described in this chapter focused on speech processing and literacy skills in particular. It would clearly be important that any programme of teaching and therapy should also be based on a language assessment that investigates verbal comprehension and expression.This would give a more balanced profile of the extent of her spoken and written language difficulties.

Summary

This chapter has illustrated the following key points.

- The framework and profile can be used to chart a child's progress from the preschool years onwards.
- The focus of the assessment shifted as Zoe got older, from speech output towards phonological awareness and literacy skills.
- The assessment of speech processing can complement and illuminate a parallel assessment of literacy skills.
- Underlying speech processing problems can create barriers to literacy development.
- Analysis of a child's spelling errors should draw on knowledge of the child's speech processing skills.
- Links can be made between the developmental phases of speech development and the developmental phases of literacy development.
- An appreciation of these links can point the way to appropriately targeted teaching and therapy.

KEY TO ACTIVITY 10.1
Zoe's speech processing at CA 9;8

SPEECH PROCESSING PROFILE

Name: Zoe

Age: 9;8 d.o.b:

Date: October 1996

Profiler: JS/BW

Comments:

n.d., no data. Control data not available for some tasks, so number of crosses is based on impressionistic judgement

INPUT

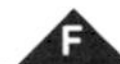

Is the child aware of the internal structure of phonological representations?
✗ (dependent on vocalization)

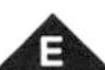

Are the child's phonological representations accurate?
✗ (for voicing and /r/)

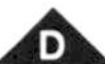

Can the child discriminate between real words?
✓

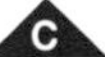

Does the child have language-specific representations of word structures?
n.d

Can the child discriminate speech sounds without reference to lexical representations?
✓

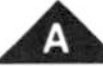

Does the child have adequate auditory perception?
✓

OUTPUT

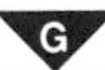

Can the child access accurate motor programs?
✗

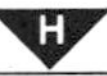

Can the child manipulate phonological units?
✗✗✗

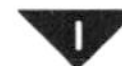

Can the child articulate real words accurately?
✗

Can the child articulate speech without reference to lexical representations?
✗✗✗

Does the child have adequate sound production skills?
✓

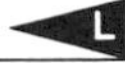

Does the child reject his/her own erroneous forms?
✗

KEY TO ACTIVITY 10.2
Speech processing model for Zoe at CA 9;8

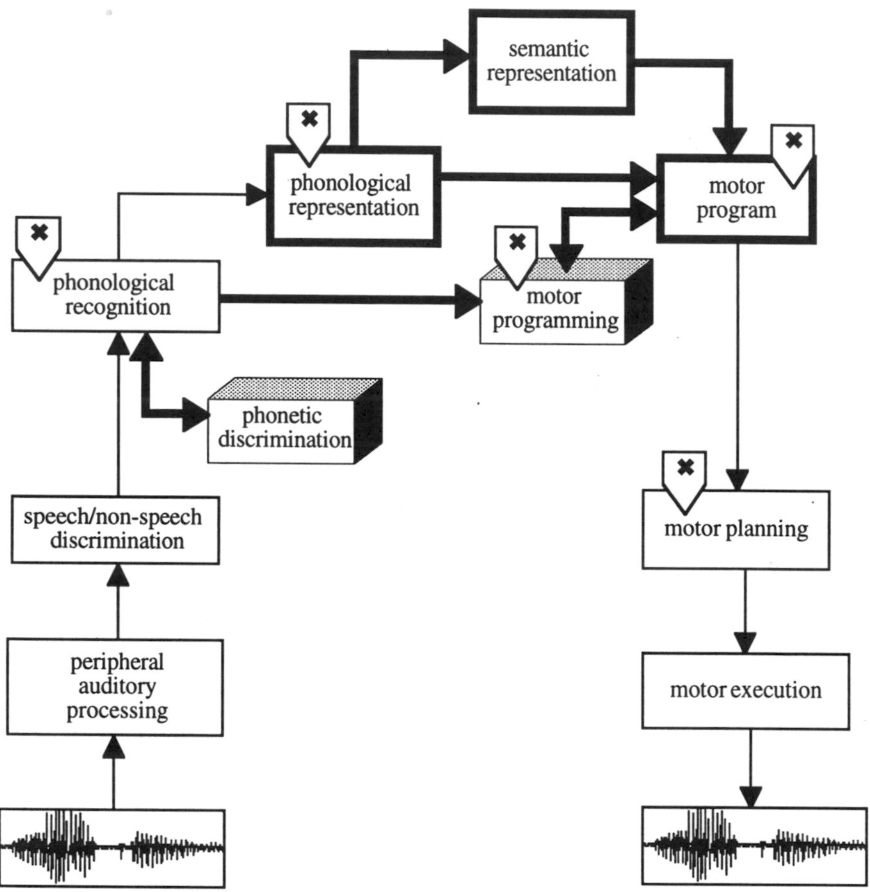

KEY TO ACTIVITY 10.3
Phases of development – Zoe at CA 9;8

With the considerable progress Zoe had made in the production of words in spontaneous speech and on the real word repetition task, it is clear that she was no longer in the Systematic Simplification Phase. The minor errors she made are not reminiscent of the classic simplifying processes.

With regard to connected speech, some residual difficulties were noted, which added up to Zoe creating the impression of 'mumbley' speech (cf. Richard in Chapter 5). This suggests that she was not completely through the Assembly Phase, though she was clearly much further on in this respect than had been the case at 5;11.

Zoe's performance on rhyme detection tasks in particular indicated that she had entered the Metaphonological Phase, though her weak performance on rhyme production, her dependence on a verbalization strategy for silent rhyme detection, and particularly her difficulties with nonword repetiton, all indicated that her ability to segment and manipulate phonological units was not fully developed. We can therefore conclude that at 9;8 Zoe was not yet through the Metaphonological Phase.

KEY TO ACTIVITY 10.4
Zoe's spellings of two- and three-syllable words

Two-syllable words

GIRAFFE → ‹gafe›. Both syllables are marked, even though the nucleus of the first, ‹i›, and the onset of the second, ‹r›, are omitted. At onset of first syllable, the ‹g› grapheme is used appropriately for /ʤ/. Nucleus ‹a› of second syllable is marked correctly, as is coda ‹fe›, apart from failure to observe spelling convention of consonant doubling.

BROTHER → ‹borth›. Both syllables are marked: ‹bor› and ‹th›, indicating successful segmentation into syllables. ‹bor› exemplifies the splitting of the onset cluster by a vowel, using a letter from later in the syllable (cf FLOOR → ‹fole› and SNAIL → ‹sane›). In the second syllable, only the onset is marked, but correctly, though the grapheme ‹th› may represent the unstressed syllable /ðə/.

SLEEPING → ‹selding›. Again, both syllables are marked, and onset cluster split by later vowel grapheme: SL → ‹sel›. The ING morpheme is transcribed accurately. A tentative explanation for /p/ → ‹d› is that Zoe's voice ~ voiceless confusion led to /p/ → [b], then the ‹b› was reversed to ‹d› in transcription.

COLLAR → ‹core›. Appears bizarre if ‹core› is read back as the real word CORE, i.e. as [kɔ]. However, [l] and [r] are commonly confused sounds in children's speech. Zoe may therefore be representing both syllables, with ‹r› representing /l/ and ‹e› representing schwa [ə] in the second syllable. Alternatively, Zoe's ‹r› may be derived from the word-final ‹r› grapheme in the target spelling; however, there is then no obvious explanation for her final ‹e›.

PUPPET → ‹pue›. First syllable marked accurately: ‹pu›. Zoe has omitted the medial ‹pp› in her spelling, but may be marking the second syllable with ‹e›. As with COLLAR, it is not certain that she is representing both syllables. In such cases, the child can be asked to beat out the number of syllables in the word, to provide an indication as to whether s/he has the correct number of syllables in her lexical representation and spelling.

Three-syllable words

TELEPHONE → ‹tlefon›. Correctly segmented, with all three syllables represented: ‹t› + ‹le› + ‹fon›. Nucleus of first syllable not marked. Final syllable shows lack of knowledge of two spelling conventions: /f/ → ‹ph› rule for words of Greek origin, and 'magic' ‹e› rule.

UNDERSTAND → ‹undsand›. Correctly segmented, with all three syllables represented: ‹un› + ‹d› + ‹sand›. Zoe's omission of nucleus of second syllable may reflect its phonetically weak position: it can be elided in casual speech (though this is also true of the second syllable of TELEPHONE). Reduction of cluster at onset of final syllable, /st/ → ‹s›, may reflect imprecise articulation and/or representation of the cluster in Zoe's speech.

ELEPHANT → ‹ehfet›. First and third syllables represented: ‹e› + ‹fet›. Omission of nasal ‹n› in coda cluster is typical of normally-developing younger spellers. Unclear whether ‹h› represents the second syllable /lə/, or is marking aspiration anticipating voiceless /f/. The vowel of second syllable of ELEPHANT is phonologically weak and subject to elision, as in TELEPHONE and UNDERSTAND.

UMBRELLA → ‹unbe›. Only the first two syllables are marked: UM → ‹un› and BRE → ‹be›. The second syllable shows cluster reduction: /br/ → [b]. Words containing both /l/ and /r/ can be particularly difficult to segment (e.g. JEWELLERY, GORILLA). It looks as though Zoe's segmentation abilities diminish when she is confronted with words that are articulatorily complex, containing clusters or other difficult sound combinations.

PYJAMAS → ‹beg›. This was the most reduced spelling of any three-syllable target word, and looks quite bizarre if read back as the real word BEG, [beg]. However, our knowledge of Zoe's speech processing and spelling can help us take a more positive view. For example, we know that she has a voice ~ voiceless confusion, so it is possible that she has analysed the initial /p/ of PYJAMAS as /b/ and transcribed it accordingly as ‹b›. The ‹g› is likely to represent the onset of the second syllable JA, i.e. pronounced [ʤ] rather than [g] (cf. GIRAFFE). She has not attempted the third syllable, however (cf. UMBRELLA above).

Chapter 11
Selecting and Designing Tests

The psycholinguistic framework for assessment that has been described in this book does not constitute a fixed and immutable set of procedures, and thus differs from a test battery. It suggests a way of thinking about, and organizing, tests and assessments that practitioners use – tests that are available in the public domain, either as packages or in research papers, and also assessments devised by the practitioner to meet the specific needs of a child or group of children. In this chapter, we explore some issues that arise when constructing and administering such assessments. The aim is twofold: firstly, to provide tools for evaluating critically tests that might be included in a psycholinguistic assessment; and secondly, to provide some food for thought for those intending to devise their own tests. It is not our aim to provide a comprehensive guide to test construction or experimental design, but rather to focus on issues that are especially relevant, and sometimes overlooked, when assessing speech processing skills in children. The following topics will be addressed: design of stimuli; matching sets of stimuli across tests; instructions and procedures; scoring; qualitative analysis of results. Issues relating to the interpretation of quantitative results in relation to control data have already been considered in Chapter 5.

Design of Stimuli

When selecting or devising stimulus words for investigating speech processing, both lexical and phonological factors need to be taken into account.

Lexical factors

The purpose of the first activity is to identify lexical factors that should be considered when devising phonological processing tasks, such as real word repetition. We might administer such a test, in conjunction with a test of nonword repetition, to see if the child has a specific problem with phonological processing when there is no access to the lexicon (nonword repetition) as opposed to possible access to the lexicon (real word repetition). Alternatively, we might administer such a test in conjunction with a confrontation naming test, to see if a child has greater difficulty when entirely dependent upon his / her own lexical representations (naming) than when s/he also has access to the acoustic signal (real word repetition) (cf. Chapter 2).

ACTIVITY 11.1

Aim: To identify lexical factors that need to be taken into account when devising lists of stimuli for speech processing tasks such as real word repetition.

Compare the following alternative lists of 10 items, to be used as a test of real word repetition with children aged 3 to 7 years.

(a) What are the main similarities and differences between the two lists?

(b) Given the possible reasons for administering a test of real word repetition, are there any grounds for preferring one list to the other?

	(i)	(ii)
(1)	DOG	KEY
(2)	ELEPHANT	TELEPHONE
(3)	FOX	LOCKS
(4)	GIRAFFE	BEHIND
(5)	HIPPOPOTAMUS	EXCAVATOR
(6)	MONKEY	PURPLE
(7)	PENGUIN	PLAYING
(8)	RABBIT	QUICKLY
(9)	RHINOCEROS	POCAHONTAS
(10)	SQUIRREL	STRONGER

Check your answer with Key to Activity 11.1 at the end of this chapter, then read the following.

If the test is of real word repetition as distinct from nonword repetition, it is crucial that the items in the test should indeed be real words for the children to be tested, i.e. that they should be comprehended by the youngest children. If a word is unknown, it is effectively a 'nonword', and thus will interfere with the comparison of results across real and nonword conditions. In set (ii), it is quite possible that EXCAVATOR is a nonword, that might for example be lexicalized by a child to ESCALATOR if s/he knows that word. It is also possible that some of the animals in set (i) would be unknown to 3-year-olds. It would therefore be important to test the child's comprehension of the items before administering the test.

If results of the repetition test are to be compared to results from a test of confrontation naming, to determine whether there is a dissociation in performance across the two tasks, it is desirable to use the same set of items for the two tests. Otherwise, it is not possible to tell whether the dissociation is genuinely the result of a differential ability in processing via the two different routes, or whether it is merely caused by one set of words being inherently more difficult than the other. If the set of words is thus to be used for picture-naming as well, each item will need to be depicted in an unambiguous way, so that the picture will only elicit the word required. On these grounds, list (i) is clearly preferable: it contains items which are all nouns, depicting different animals. List (ii) contains a number of words which are much harder to depict in an unambiguous way: STRONGER; PLAYING; BEHIND; QUICKLY for instance. Even apparently unambiguous objects can be problematic, if there are alternative ways of referring to them. Thus, a picture depicting TELEPHONE in list (ii), would very likely elicit PHONE in confrontation naming.

One reason why some of the words in (ii) are harder to depict is that they do not represent objects. Grammatically, some are not nouns, but belong to a range of other grammatical categories: comparative adjective; verb; preposition; adverb. The grammatical status and morphological make-up of stimulus items are variables that are normally best controlled for, not only because of the picturability issue, but also because different word classes may have different phonological characteristics. For example a child may persistently use 'fronting', pronouncing /g/ as [d], at the beginning of the target word GOING when it functions as an auxiliary, as in I'M GOING TO SEE HIM TOMORROW, but not when it functions as a lexical verb, as in I'M GOING TO THE SEASIDE TOMORROW. Similarly, in list (ii) some words consist of more than one morpheme: STRONG + ER, PLAY + ING, LOCK+S. Again, there are children who pronounce phonological items differently according to whether or not they represent separate morphemes; thus a child may omit the /s/ at the end of LOCKS (which could represent a plural marker, for example), but not the /s/ at the end of FOX, even though in the adult language FOX rhymes with LOCKS. (In another context, there may be very good reasons for wanting to investigate such differences, in which case items such as FOX and LOCKS could be matched across lists.) In these respects (i) is clearly preferable to (ii). However, (i) is not unproblematic either: drawing all words from the same, quite narrow, semantic field, might result in priming, whereby the child is led to access items more rapidly and easily, having just heard a related item. This might lead to better responses than would otherwise be the case.

Phonological factors

So far we have considered factors relating to vocabulary, grammar and morphology, and have found that list (i) is superior in most respects. Turning to phonological variables, the situation is less clear cut. In the next activity, there is no need to compare the two lists, as both illustrate the same points.

ACTIVITY 11.2

Aim: To identify phonological factors that need to be taken into account when devising lists of stimuli for speech processing tasks.

What are the main phonological differences between items in list (i)?

Check your answer with Key to Activity 11.2 at the end of this chapter, then read the following.

There may be good reasons for using a short list of words of varying length, as in list (i), for example as a screening test. However, research has shown that the number of syllables in the word is an important variable affecting accuracy of response on repetition tests, and is developmentally sensitive (Gathercole et al., 1994; Vance, Stackhouse and Wells, 1995). For this reason, repetition and naming tests (of both real and nonwords) often control for number of syllables, having within the test separate lists of one-, two-, three-, four- and even five-syllable words. However, there are other phonological variables that need to be considered. These are explored in the next activity, which focuses on a set of three-syllable words.

ACTIVITY 11.3

Aim: To identify factors that determine number of syllables in multisyllabic words.

List (iii) is a candidate set of three-syllable words for a word repetition test which controls for number of syllables, to be used with children aged 3 to 7 years.

(a) Count the number of syllables in your own pronunciation of each word. Are all the words properly described as having three syllables?

(b) Mark the stressed syllable in each word by putting a stress mark ˈ before it. What is the role of stress in determining the number of syllables in pronunciation?

(iii)
BANANA
BIRTHDAYCAKE
ELEPHANT
KANGAROO
LIBRARY
POLICEMAN
POTATO
PYJAMAS
TELEPHONE

Check your answer with Key to Activity 11.3 at the end of this chapter, then read the following.

The inherent 'weakness' of the elided syllables is evident in the way they are treated by young children learning English: the initial syllable of BANANA, POTATO, PYJAMAS, is often omitted completely, giving NANA [nɑnə], TATO [teitəu], JAMAS. [dʒɑməz]. The propensity for a syllable to be elided is not, however, simply a function of its position in the word: if it were, we might expect the first syllable of LIBRARY and ELEPHANT to be elided or omitted, as happens with BANANA and PYJAMAS. The crucial factor is whether or not the syllable is stressed: the syllables that get elided are unstressed. However, this is not the whole story either: position is also important. For example, we find 'NANA ['nɑnə] or B'NANA, ['bnɑnə] but not BA'NAN [bə'nɑn]. Typically, it is an unstressed syllable preceding a stressed syllable which is subject to elision; and also an unstressed syllable following a stressed syllable but preceding another syllable – like the middle syllable of LIBRARY and TELEPHONE (Gimson, 1989). The importance of stress as a variable in determining both how a word is pronounced by adults, and also how a word's pronunciation can be simplified by children, means that in a test of repetition it is sometimes desirable to stick to a single stress pattern.

Phonological variables in phonological awareness tasks

Let us now turn to some phonological variables that can arise in tests of rhyme skills.

ACTIVITY 11.4

Aim: To identify phonological factors that need to be taken into account in rhyme tests.

Here are two items from each of two tests of rhyme detection, of the kind described in Chapter 3. In each test, one of the two items is phonologically flawed. Which is it, and why?

Test 1	*Stimulus*	*Rhyme target*	*Semantic distractor*
Item (a)	COAT	BOAT	GLOVE
Item (b)	SHOE	TWO	BOOT

Test 2	*Stimulus*	*Rhyme target*	*Alliterative distractor*
Item (a)	PEG	LEG	PEAR
Item (b)	DOOR	SAW	DUCK

Check your answer with Key to Activity 11.4 at the end of this chapter, and read the following.

This activity has pointed up accent differences as a possible confounding variable. Many of the potential pitfalls that involve accent differences relate to vowels and particularly their lexical distribution. Thus, CALF and LAUGH rhyme for speakers from the south of England, but not in the north, where the /a/ vowel is found in some words for which southern accents have /ɑ/, including LAUGH, BATH, GRASS. In some accents of English, POOR, POUR and PAW all rhyme, in others only the first two rhyme, and in others still, none of them rhyme.

Accent differences of this kind are relevant not only to rhyme tasks. The number of phonetic segments in a word can vary according to accent, which can be relevant to segmentation and blending tasks. For example, words such as RING have a single consonant [ŋ] in coda (final) position in many accents of English, but in others there is a cluster [ŋg]. Similar examples of accent differences can be found in relation to the number of syllables in the word, and the position of the stress. Thus, SECRETARY regularly has four syllables in General American, but three in British English. ARISTOCRAT has the main stress on the second syllable in some accents, but on the first in others. In fact, accent differences are so pervasive that it is not practical to avoid all potential confusions. What is important is for the practitioner who is selecting a test or devising one to be aware of the possible differences, and to take account of them, for example when using the test with a different population from the one for which it has been originally designed, or on which it has been standardized.

Other potential phonological pitfalls arise if we are not sufficiently aware of the ways in which pronunciation can diverge from spelling. Some of these are relevant to tests of segmentation, as the next activity shows.

ACTIVITY 11.5

Aim: To explore ways in which the orthographic form of a word can be phonologically misleading.

This activity derives from a study investigating segmentation skills in a group of normally-developing children with a mean CA of 3;10 and in older language-disordered children. The task required the child to divide bisyllabic words into monosyllabic words. Every bisyllabic word was said to contain at least one real monosyllabic word (e.g. PENCIL includes the word PEN). There were eight monosyllabic words to correspond to the eight bisyllabic words, as listed below.

For which words in the following list is it inaccurate to state that the bisyllabic word 'contains' the corresponding monosyllabic word? Why?

AIRPLANE	PLANE
FOOTBALL	FOOT
HOTDOG	HOT
PANCAKE	CAKE
DOCTOR	DOCK
MONKEY	KEY
PENCIL	PEN
WINDOW	DOUGH

Check your answer with Key to Activity 11.5 at the end of this chapter, then read the following.

The question, and indeed the segmentation task itself, begs the further question 'What is a word?' We can use 'word' in at least three senses: in relation to its meaning and grammatical form (morphological word); in relation to its spelling (orthographic word) and in relation to its sound (phonological word). The word in its most general semantic sense, that is able to take different forms, is often referred to as a lexeme. Thus, the lexeme RED refers to a particular colour and is, most commonly, an adjective (morphological word); it has a phonological form /rɛd/, which it shares with the past form of the verb READ; and an orthographic form of three letters: ‹r› ‹e› ‹d›.

First let us consider the orthographic word. We can rephrase the question posed for this activity as: does each of the bisyllabic words in the list contain the corresponding monosyllabic word in its correct orthographic form (irrespective of pronunciation and meaning)? The answer is 'Yes' for six of the words : PLANE, FOOT, HOT, CAKE, KEY, PEN, but 'No' for DOUGH and DOCK, as the correct spellings for the corresponding bisyllabic words are not DOCKTOR and WINDOUGH. If we adopt an orthographic criterion, there is then some inconsistency. Furthermore, it would seem a surprising criterion to use for this study, where the control children to be tested were under 4 years, and thus would not be expected to have orthographic knowledge.

Next, consider the phonological form. The sound sequence of PLANE is virtually identical to the second syllable of AIRPLANE. Similarly, the sound sequence of PEN can be virtually identical to the first syllable of PENCIL. For most of the other items, however, the situation is less clear. For example, the first syllable of FOOTBALL ends not with [t] (as at the end of FOOT), but, for many speakers, with something more like [p] – a place of articulation that anticipates the initial [b] of the second syllable. There is thus a phonetic difference between the monosyllabic word and the first syllable of the bisyllabic word. In terms of the adult language, the [p] pronunciation for a word with final /t/ before an initial /b/ is phonologically predictable, and so for adults it could be argued that the monosyllable is 'the same word' as is found in the first syllable of football. However, it is arguable whether 3-year-old children have access to this knowledge yet. Similar problems arise with DOCTOR and HOTDOG, where the final consonant of the first syllable is often pronounced as a glottal stop, and as such is not unambiguously identifiable as /t/ or /k/. Finally, in the case of MONKEY, there are virtually no phonetic or phonological grounds for identifying the second syllable, which is unstressed, and normally has an unaspirated [k] and a short vowel, with the monosyllabic word KEY, which has an aspirated [k], and a longer, closer vowel in many accents.

Finally, consider the morphological word: does the morpheme represented in the monosyllabic word also appear within the bisyllabic word? It clearly does, in some cases. PLANE has the same meaning on its own as it does in AIRPLANE. The FOOT in FOOTBALL preserves the meaning of the monosyllabic item, and this is also evident in HOTDOG, PANCAKE, and, possibly, PENCIL. However, DOCK, KEY and DOUGH clearly have no relationship of meaning or grammatical form with the corresponding syllable in the paired bisyllabic word.

In conclusion, this activity has demonstrated that there are considerable complexities lurking behind apparently straightforward concepts such as 'word'. Some awareness of these complexities is needed when investigating the development of children's metaphonological skills. We have also seen how misleading the orthographic form of a word can be when it comes to pronunciation. This underlines the importance of using a phonetic notation, not merely the conventional spelling, when presenting both real and nonword stimuli in published form (Wells, 1995).

Phonological legality

Earlier in this chapter we considered some of the issues surrounding the use of nonwords, for example in tests of repetition, or auditory lexical decision. In the assessment framework in Chapter 4, a further distinction was made between nonwords that are phonologically legal, i.e. possible, but not actual, words of English; and nonwords that are phonologically illegal – not actual words of English, and not possible words either. Why might it be useful to contrast a child's ability to process legal nonwords and illegal nonwords? One reason was discussed in Chapter 6: if the child performs no better on legal nonwords than on illegal nonwords, it suggests that s/he is not yet tuned in to language-specific phonological features.

In order to compile contrasting lists of legal and illegal nonwords, we need to be clear about what makes a nonword illegal. This is the purpose of the next activity.

ACTIVITY 11.6

Aim: To determine what makes a nonword legal or illegal.

Decide whether the following are legal or illegal nonwords for English. On what grounds have you made your decision?

(1) [wax]
(2) [pstrux]
(3) [bɛʔ]
(4) [ʒain]
(5) [maiʃ]
(6) [bɛ]
(7) [bnɛk]
(8) [sfil]
(9) [aba]
(10) [pətəkə]
(11) [ˌsupəkalɪˌfradʒɪlɪstɪkˌɛkspɪjalɪ'dəuʃəs]

Check your answer with Key to Activity 11.6 at the end of this chapter, then read the following.

The most obvious reason for categorizing a word as illegal is that it contains items which do not occur in the phonological inventory of English. An example is the voiceless velar fricative at the end of [pstrux] and [wax]. Words containing such exotic sound types are therefore illegal. However, even this criterion is problematic, since regional accents of English can contain sound types that are exotic to the standard variety. For example, the voiceless velar fricative in coda position is commonplace in Scouse, the Liverpool accent, in words where in other accents a voiceless velar plosive is found, e.g. WACK is pronounced [wax]. While the word can be considered illegal for most accents of English, it is legal in Liverpool. The same point arises with [bɛʔ], which is common as a realization of BET in a number of accents, including that of London. So the claim that the words in the list are illegal, has to be qualified by 'in the Southern British Standard Accent'.

Another criterion for categorizing a word as illegal is that it contains an English phonological item, but in an illegal position. An example is the initial [ʒ] in [ʒain]. [ʒ] is found in English between vowels, as in MEASURE ['mɛʒə], but not in initial or final position. This criterion is not always easy to apply, however. Take the case of [maiʃ]. Many people would consider this word to be legal, since [mai] is obviously legal (= MY), and [ʃ] occurs at coda position, as in MESH. However, there are no words in English where [ʃ] follows [ai]. More generally, [ʃ] is very rare after any dipthong or long vowel, and most of the words in which it does occur are recently borrowed from French, e.g. GAUCHE, NICHE, QUICHE, which have a low frequency. This observation points to the fact that legality, in phonology as in life, is not a clearcut affair. The 'phonological system' of English is made up of several subsystems, some containing a very large number of words, others very few, like the 'recent French borrowing' subsystem just illustrated. The exotic nature of this combination for English speakers is attested by the way in which some borrowings of this type are treated when they become well established and more frequent in the language: many speakers pronounce NICHE as [nɪʧ], to rhyme with PITCH [pɪʧ] and HITCH [hɪʧ], conforming to a more widespread English phonotactic pattern.

A slightly different instance is provided by the onsets of [pstrux] and [bnɛk]. Here, the individual consonants are all legal in English, but not in that sequence at the onset position. This type of restriction is sometimes referred to as a phonotactic constraint. Again, legality is not a clearcut issue. Take the case of [sfil]. [sf] is not normally included in the inventory of English onset two-item clusters with /s/: /sp-, st-, sk-, sl-, sn-, sm- /. Nevertheless, it is found in a small subset of words, such as SPHERE [sfɪə] and SPHINX [sfɪŋks], derived from Greek. Another example of a legal item in an illegal position is provided by [bɛ]. In English there is a general constraint that word-final stressed syllables cannot end with a short vowel such as [ɛ]: either there is a coda consonant (as in BET), or the vowel is long or diphthongal (as in BEE, BEAR).

The role of stress is important for appreciating why two other items in the list are illegal. [aba] is illegal since it is a bisyllabic word for which the stress pattern is not indicated. If the stress were on the initial syllable, the vowel in the second syllable would be the central vowel known as schwa, i.e. ['abə] (cf. the English pronunciation of the Swedish rock band Abba). If the stress were final, it would violate the rule discussed in relation to [bɛ], and would need a final consonant. In the case of [pətəkə], again stress is not marked. For it to be a legal English word, one syllable would have to be stressed and thus contain a vowel other than schwa, since schwa can only occur in unstressed syllables. [pətəkə] is a sequence often given to children to repeat as part of assessment of verbal praxis (cf. Question K on the assessment framework). From a psycholinguistic perspective, such a task can be viewed as an illegal nonword repetition test.

The remaining word in the list, [ˌsupəkalɪˌfradʒɪlɪstɪkˌɛkspɪjalɪˈdəuʃəs], does not violate any of the phonological constraints that have been mentioned so far. Nevertheless, its length makes it unusual as a candidate word of English. Possible word length does vary from language to language, in much the same way as the other phonological constraints that have been discussed are language-specific, and as we have seen, phonological legality is more a continuum than a clearcut issue. On these grounds it could be argued that this word too is in breach of the laws of English word phonology. After all, as Mary Poppins comments, 'the sound of this is something quite atrocious'!

To summarize the chapter to this point: we have considered lexical and phonological factors that need to be taken into account when devising individual stimuli and sets of stimuli for speech processing tasks, including real and nonword repetition, rhyme and segmentation. Factors that have been highlighted include the variability between different accents of English; the relationship between spelling and pronunciation; the importance of stress; and the fact that the vocabulary of English consists of a number of subsystems that have slightly different phonological 'rules'. In the next section, we will consider issues that arise when drawing up matched sets of stimuli for use on related speech processing tasks.

Matching Sets of Stimuli

One of the key tenets of a psycholinguistic approach to the assessment of speech disorders is that an isolated test of one aspect of speech processing tells us relatively little. What is revealing is the pattern of association and dissociation of a child's performance across more than one test. As well as requiring careful control of variables within an individual test, this approach to assessment requires careful matching *across* subtests, since this increases the strength of the conclusions that can be drawn from dissociations of performance. To take a simple example first: we may hypothesize that a child has more speech processing difficulties the greater the length of the word involved. In order to test the hypothesis, we may define word length in terms of number of syllables, and measure the accuracy of the child's production when repeating nonwords of one vs two vs three vs four vs five syllables. To do this we can construct five lists, each with the same number of words (cf. Gathercole and Baddeley, 1996). However, we would probably wish to take further precautions to ensure that the word lists are comparable in all respects other than the variable of number of syllables. For example, the results could be affected if the words in one list contained a much greater number of consonant clusters than those in the other lists, since clusters are likely to reduce accuracy of production independent of number of syllables. Similarly, major differences in the stress patterns found in multisyllabic words, of the type discussed in the previous section, could have an effect on production accuracy. On such a test it is therefore important to match across word lists as far as is possible, to minimize the possible effects of unwanted variables. If a statistically significant difference between performance on the different lists is then found, we can be all the more confident that this really is an effect of word length (as defined by number of syllables), rather than any other factor. If closely matched or identical stimuli are to be used in different tests, it is, however, important to ensure the tests are administered on separate occasions, in order to minimize the risk of practice effects.

The same kind of reasoning can be applied when constructing tests involving nonwords, performance on which is to be compared to a real word test. When constructing a test of nonword repetition or nonword auditory discrimination, the nonwords can be derived systematically from the set of words to be used in the parallel real word test, in order to guarantee close matching betweeen the two sets.

ACTIVITY 11.7

Aim: To consider ways in which nonword-stimuli can be systematically derived from real word stimuli to create phonologically matched lists.

How have the following sets of nonwords been derived from the real words?

(i)

TELEPHONE	/ˈtɒləˌfain/
FEATHER	/ˈfæðɪ/
CROCODILE	/ ˈkrɪkəˌdəʊl/
HELICOPTER	/ ˈhɪləˌkæptɪ/
BUTTERFLY	/ ˈbatəˌfləʊ/
PARACHUTE	/ ˈpɛrəˌʃit/

(ii)

TELEPHONE	/ˈdɛwəˌvəʊd/
FEATHER	/ˈvɛθə/
CROCODILE	/ˈglɒgətˌail/
HELICOPTER	/ˈlɛwɪˌgɒbdə/
LABRADOR	/ ˈwapləṭɔ/
SUPERMARKET	/ ˈzubəˌbɑgɪd/

Compare your answer with Key to Activity 11.7 at the end of this chapter, then read the following.

In both lists, the alterations are arbitrary (except insofar as they are designed to avoid the creation of illegal nonwords), but at the same time they are systematic: all members of a sound class are treated in the same way. This ensures as far as possible that unpredictable interfering factors are excluded. As a consequence, when the results of the real and nonword tests are compared, we can be reasonably confident that any differences are due to the variable of word type (real vs nonword), rather than to any extraneous phonological variables.

In some cases, matching can be total: identical stimuli can be used for different tests. For example, exactly the same list can be used for real word repetition as for confrontation naming; or for repetition as single words vs repetition in a connected speech context (Vance, Stackhouse and Wells, 1995). Similarly, words used for speech tasks can also be used for tasks of auditory lexical decision, or for blending tasks. In tests of rhyme and segmentation, the same items can be used for spoken tasks as for silent tasks (e.g. rhyme judgement from pictures only). There can be partial overlap: for example, the stimulus item for a rhyme production task can be used as the target item in a rhyme judgement task (Vance, Stackhouse and Wells, 1994). Finally, stimuli used for speech or auditory tasks can also be used for tests of reading or spelling.

In constructing sets of items for a particular subtest, in addition to the specific linguistic factors already discussed, basic considerations of experimental design need to be borne in mind. Firstly, each subtest has to contain enough items for statistical analysis to be feasible. How many items this is obviously depends on the type of test, and on what is being measured. The general principle is: the more items the better, from a statistical standpoint; however, this has to be set against effects of fatigue on young children. As a rule of thumb, at least 12 items per experimental condition is a bare minimum. Secondly, it is important to avoid excessive memory load in tests which are not designed to include memory as a variable. For instance, children may fail a test of auditory discrimination of the ABCX type, not because they are unable to discriminate between the targeted phonetic difference, but because they are unable to hold all four items in store long enough to perform the comparison needed (cf. Richard's performance on the *Sound Categorisation Test* (Bradley, 1984), described in Chapter 5).

Test Instructions and Procedures

The psycholinguistic assessment framework presented in this book involves the administration of tests that differ from one another in quite subtle ways and which can make use of the same or very similar stimuli, e.g. rhyme judgement from auditory stimuli vs rhyme judgement from visual stimuli (pictures); repetition of real words vs repetition of matched nonwords. It is therefore particularly important that the instructions given to the child should be clear and unambiguous.

ACTIVITY 11.8

Aim: To consider the psycholinguistic implications of the wording of test instructions.

Imagine that you are administering a test of nonword repetition to a 5-year-old child. The test consists of 20 legal nonwords. How do you introduce the test to the child, and what instructions do you give?

Check your answer with Key to Activity 11.8 at the end of this chapter, then read the following.

There are at least two strategies that the child can adopt when presented with a legal nonword to repeat.

(a) Attempt to mimic the presenter's pronunciation as accurately as possible. This would be a *phonetic* strategy.

(b) Treat the stimulus as a new or potential word of English, and reproduce it in terms of his/her own system (including regional accent, and also stage of phonological development in the case of young children). This would be a *phonological* strategy.

In terms of the model presented in Chapter 6, the phonetic strategy (a) does not involve the lexicon: a motor program is created for a one-off production, but is not stored for future reference. This is comparable to the situation where a student of phonetics is asked to reproduce as accurately as possible an 'exotic' word spoken by the tutor. The phonological strategy (b), on the other hand, involves the creation of a new lexical entry with a new phonological representation (even though it has no semantic representation). This is comparable to the situation where the child hears a new word in conversation, is unable yet to assign a meaning to it, but nevertheless creates a new lexical entry with phonological representation, in the expectation that the semantics can be added later.

It is not yet clear what factors induce a child to follow one strategy as opposed to the other. However, it has been noted that some children will mimic the tester's pronunciation if the tester has an accent different to that of the subject, suggesting that the phonetic familiarity of the input is one factor. A study of normally-developing (London) children's repetition of real words presented in an unfamiliar (Glaswegian) accent indicated that this may change with age (Nathan, Wells and Donlan, 1996). Four-year-old children attempted to imitate the word in the original Glaswegian accent, if they did not recognize what lexeme it was; whereas 7-year-olds were more likely to repeat such words using their own accent, whether or not they identified the lexeme correctly. In psycholinguistic assessment, we therefore need to minimize uncertainty as to which strategy the subject has used. Publications reporting the administration of nonword repetition tests do not always indicate the precise wording of the instructions. The element of uncertainty can be reduced if instructions are worded along the following lines, in recognition of the fact that there are two distinct tasks that the child could be asked to perform.

(a) *Phonetic imitation task:* 'I am going to say some strange words that you won't have heard before. Try and copy exactly what I say.'
(b) *Phonological repetition task:* 'I am going to say some new English words that you won't have heard before. Say them after me.'

Within the psycholinguistic framework we are usually more interested in (b), since we are interested in nonword repetition performance as an indicator of how the child is able to handle the learning of new words. The psycholinguistic importance of children's performance on type (a) tasks is an important area for future research, since it may provide insights into how the child can handle 'exotic' phonetic material, as required when making sense of unfamiliar accents of his or her own language, and when learning a second language.

The stimuli themselves can be presented from prerecorded tape, or spoken live by the tester. Live presentation is more 'friendly' and familiar for young children, and also preserves important visual information about pronunciation. On the other hand, audiotape presentation allows for standardized presentation across children and avoids the situation of the tester making mistakes or slips of tongue – easily done in nonword tests. It also allows use of a voice different to that of the tester. Stimuli can be presented on videotape, thereby preserving visual information. If either video or audiotape is used, it is critical that the quality of the tape and the machine is such as to ensure excellent sound quality.

Recording of Data

In the case of tests that require analysis of the child's spoken response, it is essential to record the responses for subsequent listening and transcription, ideally using a video recorder together with a good quality audio recorder with carefully positioned external microphone, in a quiet room. It is advisable to make a simultaneous phonetic transcription at the time of testing, noting any visual features of the pronunciation that will not be accessible subsequently if only an audio recording has been made. As well as providing a basis for phonetic transcription, a high quality audio recording can be analysed acoustically, in order to measure selected phonetic parameters. Other, more invasive types of recording such as electropalatography, where tongue contact is recorded on an artificial palate, can be very useful in particular situations to shed light on the child's underlying phonological system, as in the study by Gibbon (1990) which was described in Chapter 7.

Scoring of Results

The kind of scoring used depends firstly on the nature of the test, and secondly on the type of analysis that is to be carried out. Responses on input tests, such as auditory discrimination, auditory lexical decision or rhyme judgement, will be marked initially as right or wrong, giving a quantitative measure that can be used for statistical analysis. Further, more qualitative analysis is usually possible too: for example, in the case of a rhyme detection task, a child may consistently choose semantic distractors rather than alliterative distractors, indicating that s/he has not yet developed awareness of sound similarity between words.

Sometimes a test throws up interesting data that have not been predicted. For example, in a test of purportedly 'silent' rhyme detection, where for each item the children had to identify two of three pictures that rhymed, it was observed that many children were unable to perform the task without saying the words aloud, even when requested not to (Wells, Stackhouse and Vance, 1996). As described in Chapter 10, subsequent analysis revealed that there was a developmental pattern to this behaviour: the words were spoken aloud by the 4-, 5- and 6-year-olds, but not by the youngest children (aged 3), who could not do the task at all, nor by the oldest (aged 7), who made virtually no mistakes. This suggested that the process of learning to do rhyme detection includes a stage of speaking the words aloud. This finding was not predicted in the design of the study, and emerged as the result of *post hoc* qualitative analysis.

In the case of output tasks, there are generally two levels of scoring. Initially, it is useful to score the child's production of a word as either right or wrong, (on tests of naming, repetition or blending for example) since this provides straightforward data for subsequent statistical analysis. Even at this level, however, scoring is not always straightforward.

ACTIVITY 11.9

Aim: To determine what counts as a 'correct' pronunciation for testing purposes.

In their responses to a nonword repetition test, MB and JM, who were in their early teens, both gave different pronunciations of GLISTERING, in a nonword repetition test (Wells, 1995):

MB: ['glɪstɹɪŋ]
JM: ['glɪstəʋɪn 'glɪstəɹɪn]

Would you score these pronunciations as right or wrong? Why?

Now read the following.

All three transcriptions represent widespread pronunciations of such phonological sequences in English. In order to score a phonological repetition, whether real word or legal nonword, as incorrect, it is necessary to know about the phonological system that the child is learning, and (in the case of younger children) about the normal path of phonological development for a child acquiring that system. For example, JM's realisation of /ɪŋ/ as [ɪn] is common in many accents, as is the realization of /r/ as labiodental [ʋ] rather than postalveolar [ɹ]. In a still wider range of accents, the labiodental realization of /r/ is found in normal phonological development (Lodge, 1984). MB's realization conforms more closely to the pronunciation of educated speakers of Southern British English, yet it has only two syllables, even though the target word appears under the three-syllable set in the word list. In fact, a two-syllable realization of similar words (e.g. BLISTERING) is a very common variant in most accents of English (cf. the discussion in the first section of this chapter).

If the test is designed to elicit phonetic imitations, rather than phonological repetitions, thorough phonetic training for the tester is an obvious requirement. A phonetically trained analyst (such as a speech and language therapist) should be able to make an auditory judgement as to whether or not the target pronunciation has been achieved, and to score it as right or wrong accordingly. For many purposes this method of scoring will suffice, although the absolute accuracy of the phonetician's auditory judgement is open to question. If greater accuracy is needed, instrumental methods such as electropalatography may be required. The reliability of procedures for assessing speech output is thus dependent on the phonetic skills of the tester.

Rather than scoring an entire pronunciation as right or wrong, it is often helpful to carry out a more fine-grained quantitative analysis of errors, particularly when the child is making so many errors that virtually all the responses would be scored as wrong on a simple right/wrong basis. Alternative methods include: scoring the number of target segments that are correctly realized; or scoring the number of phonetic features that are correctly realized in each target segment (Bryan and Howard, 1992; Stackhouse and Snowling, 1992b).

In addition to quantitative scoring, more detailed qualitative analysis of the speech patterns found in the child's responses can give insights into the speech processing difficulties underlying the child's speech production difficulties. The data can be examined to see whether the child's errors are systematic. Do they affect a particular set of consonants or vowels; or particular phonetic features (e.g. voicing, place of articulation)? Do they mainly occur at particular positions in the word or syllable e.g. in unstressed syllables, or word finally, or in coda position? Do they involve simplification of the phonological structure e.g. by cluster reduction, weak syllable deletion? Such fine-grained analysis can suggest hypotheses about the nature of a child's speech processing difficulties, as was illustrated with reference to Zoe in Chapter 9. Detailed phonological analysis calls for phonetic skill on the part of the analyst, in preparing impressionistic phonetic records using auditory and, where appropriate, instrumental techniques; and then phonological skills, to interpret the phonetic data in terms of its implications for the child's ability to realize the phonological structures and systems of his or her language.

Summary

This chapter has highlighted a number of variables that need to be taken into account when designing, administering and scoring speech processing tests for the purposes of psycholinguistic investigation. On most occasions practitioners will inevitably be using tests that are imperfect from some points of view. Awareness of these imperfections can inform the interpretation of the test results, so that we are not led to make stronger claims about the child's profile of speech processing abilities than are warranted by the data available.

A number of points have been raised.

- For tests of real word processing the test items need to be within the child's vocabulary.
- When compiling lists of real word items for speech processing tasks, grammatical and semantic factors need to be considered as well as phonological factors.

- The accents of the tester and of the children being tested need to be taken into account when selecting items.
- The written form of a word may be an inaccurate guide to the spoken form of the word, e.g. with regard to number of syllables, pronunciation of consonant sequences and of unstressed vowels.
- The position of word stress is an important factor when devising lists of matched words.
- The distinction between 'legal' and 'illegal' nonwords is not clearcut.
- The vocabulary of English consists of a number of subsystems that differ from one another in some phonological respects, e.g. range of consonant clusters permitted.
- Nonwords can be derived systematically from real words to provide closely matched word lists.
- The precise wording of test instructions may determine the processing route used by the child.
- It is important to note visual as well as auditory phonetic features of the child's responses and to make a permanent record using audio and / or video tape.
- The scoring of speech production tests such as real word and nonword repetition tasks is not straightforward and calls for awareness of developmental and accent factors.
- Administration of speech production tests is not a substitute for phonological analysis of a child's speech.

KEY TO ACTIVITY 11.1

Lexical factors

Similarities

Both lists contain words of varying length, and stress patterns. In fact, most pairs of items are matched across lists on these two variables.

Differences

The words in (i) belong to the same semantic field (animals), while the words in (ii) are not semantically linked. The words in (i) are likely to be in the vocabulary of most 3-year-olds, while some words in (ii) may not be. All the words in (i) are singular animate nouns, while the words in (ii) represent different grammatical classes:

common (inanimate) noun	singular	KEY TELEPHONE, EXCAVATOR
common (inanimate) noun	plural	LOCKS

proper noun		POCAHONTAS
adjective		PURPLE
adjective	comparative	STRONGER
adverb		QUICKLY
preposition		BEHIND
verb		PLAYING

KEY TO ACTIVITY 11.2
Phonological factors

The most striking phonological differences between items in list (i) are as follows

(a) Word length. There are words of one syllable (DOG, FOX), two (GIRAFFE, MONKEY, PENGUIN, RABBIT, SQUIRREL), three (ELEPHANT), four (RHINOCEROS) and five (HIPPOPOTAMUS).

(b) Stress. Stress can appear on the first syllable (e.g. PENGUIN), the second (e.g. GIRAFFE), or the third, e.g. HIPPOPOTAMUS.

(c) Phonotactic structure. For example, some onsets consist of consonant clusters, as in the first syllable of SQUIRREL or the second syllable of PENGUIN, while others have a singleton consonant, as in the first syllable of PENGUIN or the second syllable of SQUIRREL.

KEY TO ACTIVITY 11.3
Elision and stress

(a) For many speakers, several words in the list are not pronounced with three syllables. Many speakers of British English regularly elide the middle syllable of LIBRARY, even in quite slow and formal speech. The same can happen to TELEPHONE, with the middle vowel being elided, though only in more casual speech. The initial vowel in words such as BANANA, POLICEMAN, POTATO, PYJAMAS, is also regularly elided by many speakers, giving what is phonetically more of a bisyllabic pronunciation, even though, when asked, such speakers will probably agree that the word has three syllables in more careful speech.

(b) The most common stress patterns for the words in the list are as follows:

BA'NANA
'BIRTHDAYCAKE
'ELEPHANT
KANGA'ROO

'LIBRARY
PO'LICEMAN
PO'TATO
PYJ'AMAS
'TELEPHONE

Stressed syllables do not get elided. Unstressed syllables are most likely to be elided when following a stressed syllable and preceding another syllable (e.g. LIBRARY); the vowel of an unstressed syllable is also susceptible to elision when it is word initial, preceding a stressed syllable: BA'NANA, PO'LICEMAN, PO'TATO, PYJ'AMAS.

KEY TO ACTIVITY 11.4
Phonological factors in rhyme tests

In both cases, (a) is preferable to (b).

In Test 1(b), the semantic distractor BOOT, as well as being related to the stimulus SHOE semantically, also has the same vowel [u], and is thus a 'half-rhyme'. This might interfere with the child's identification of TWO as the correct rhyme for SHOE.

In Test 2(b), SAW rhymes with DOOR only in 'non-rhotic' accents of English, such as Southern British Standard or Australian, i.e. accents in which /r/ is not pronounced after a vowel unless it is followed by another vowel. There are, however, many rhotic accents of English, such as Scottish, Northern Irish, General American, in which /r/ is always pronounced in words with 'r' in the spelling. Items with dialectal variables of this kind should therefore be avoided if there is the possibility that the child to be tested is from such an accent group.

KEY TO ACTIVITY 11.5
Orthographic factors

It could be argued that only PLANE and PEN are 'contained' in the corresponding bisyllabic word. See text for discussion.

KEY TO ACTIVITY 11.6
Legal vs illegal nonwords

In the standard variety of Southern British English, there is a case for arguing that all are illegal, except [ˌsupəkaliˌfradʒilistikˌɛkspijali'dəuʃəs]. See text for discussion.

KEY TO ACTIVITY 11.7
Matching nonwords to real words

In (i), the consonants and syllable structure of the real word have been retained, but the vowels have been changed to create nonwords. Certain restrictions on vowel substitution have been observed: long vowels and diphthongs have been replaced by long vowels and diphthongs, short vowels by short vowels .

In (ii), the vowels and syllable structure of the real word have been retained, but this time the consonants have been changed. This has been done by a systematic alteration of phonetic features, e.g. voiceless plosives and fricatives become voiced (/k/ → /g/, /s/ → /z/), and vice versa (/b/ → /p/); nasals are converted to the corresponding voiced oral stop: /m/ → /b/; approximants are interchanged: /l/ → /w/ and so on.

KEY TO ACTIVITY 11.8
Test instructions

The following instruction is suggested (see text for discussion):

> 'I am going to say some new English words that you won't have heard before. Say them after me.'

Chapter 12
A Framework for Practice and Research

This book has presented a psycholinguistic assessment framework, a theoretical model of speech processing, and a developmental phase model for speech and metaphonological awareness. A systematic hypothesis testing approach to the investigation of speech processing skills in children has been elaborated through a series of activities and illustrated through case studies. This approach is not tied to any specific clinical entity but can be used with any child who presents with speech and/or literacy problems. Further, the approach is equally well suited to the investigation of speech and literacy skills in normally-developing children. This allows for a developmental perspective on children with difficulties and for direct comparisons between normal and atypical development to be made.

A speech processing model has been used throughout this book to show what skills are necessary for normal speech development and how these skills are also the foundation for children's literacy development. In particular, phonological awareness is interpreted within the speech processing model in order to emphasize that it is not an entirely distinct area, but rather an extension of children's speech processing development. The case of Zoe presented in Chapters 9 and 10 demonstrates the connection between speech processing, phonological awareness and literacy development.

A phase model of speech development was presented in Chapters 7 and 8. It comprises five phases: Prelexical; Whole Word; Systematic Simplification; Assembly; and Metaphonological. It is proposed that normally-developing children move through these phases smoothly and, as a consequence, develop the skills necessary to perform phonological awareness and literacy tasks. In contrast, children with speech difficulties have trouble with one or more of these phases. Further, the precise nature of their speech difficulties will depend on which particular developmental phase (or phases) is troublesome for them, as is shown in Figure 12.1.

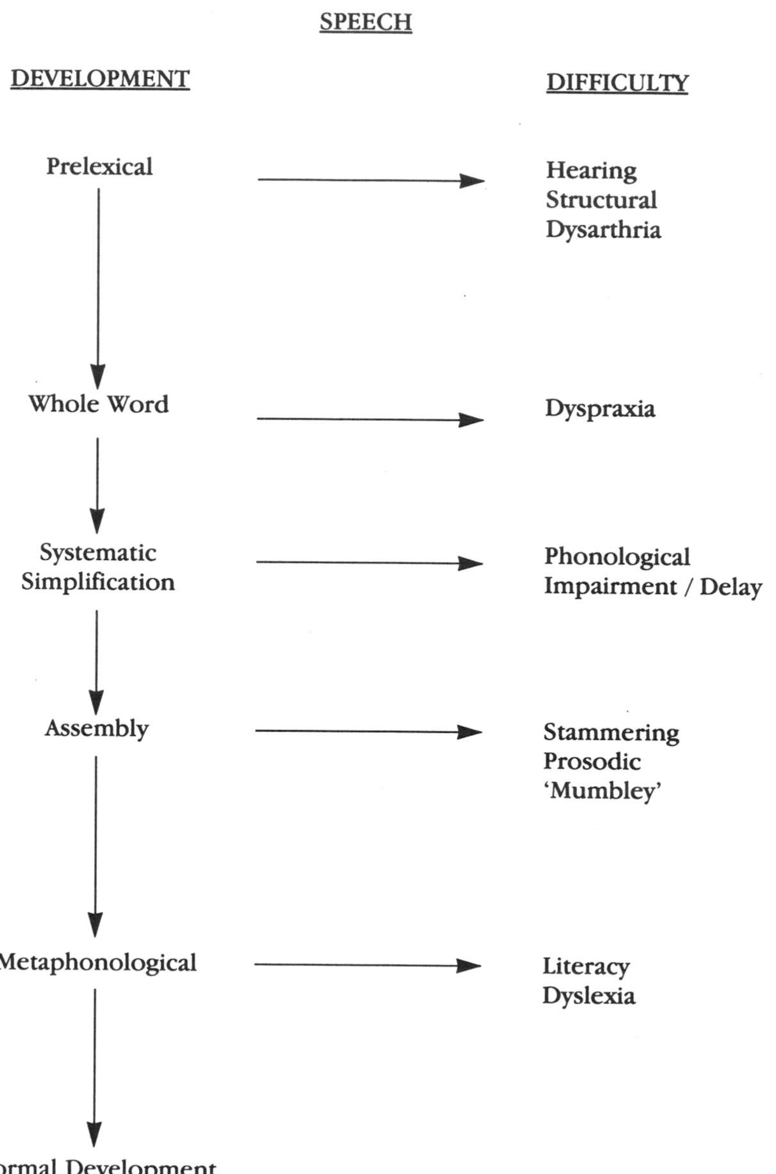

Figure 12.1: A developmental phase perspective on speech difficulties

In Chapter 8, this phase model of speech development was compared with Frith's phase model of literacy development. In both models, words are first dealt with as wholes, whether it be for speech (Whole Word Phase) or for literacy (Logographic Phase). This is followed by phases in which children become increasingly sensitive to the constituents of words. This begins to happen in speech development ~~nally around the age of 2;0, when children move into the Systematic

Simplification Phase – a necessary step if children are to develop the phonological awareness skills characteristic of the Alphabetic Phase of literacy development. The phases of speech development culminate in the Metaphonological Phase (around the age of 4;0 to 5;0) after which the child is ready to break through to the Alphabetic Phase of literacy development and make sense of literacy instruction. The relationship between phases of speech development and phases of literacy development is set out in Figure 12.2.

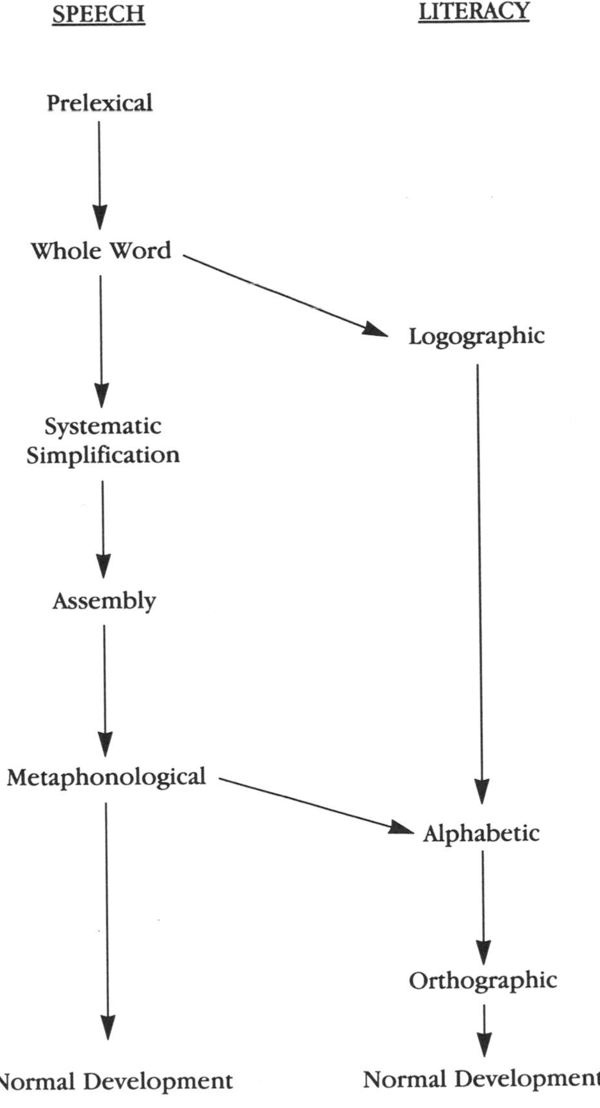

Figure 12.2: The relationship between the phases of speech and literacy development

Children who have difficulties moving through the normal phases of speech development, either because they get stuck at the Whole Word Phase (as in developmental verbal dyspraxia) or who are delayed reaching and/or moving on from the Systematic Simplification Phase (as in phonological impairment or delay), have poorly developed phonological awareness skills. These phonological awareness skills are dependent on a smooth transition through the Systematic Simplification Phase to the Metaphonological Phase of speech development. Without this transition children will also have trouble with the Alphabetic Phase of literacy development. Thus, taking a developmental perspective explains why the most serious forms of phonological dyslexia (defined by Frith, 1985 as arrested development within the Logographic Phase of literacy development) have been found in children with developmental verbal dyspraxia, whose speech difficulties arise in the stage prior to the Systematic Simplification Phase (Stackhouse and Snowling, 1992b; Snowling, Goulandris and Stackhouse, 1994). It also explains why children who have speech problems persisting beyond the age of 5;6 are at risk for literacy problems (Bishop and Adams, 1990; Bird, Bishop and Freeman, 1995): they have not moved into the Metaphonological Phase in time to take full advantage of the literacy instruction offered at school. For some, this means a slow start to their literacy development, following which satisfactory progress is made; for others the slow start is followed by slow or atypical progress and associated educational problems.

Use of the Framework in Practice

Investigating children's speech difficulties within the psycholinguistic framework has highlighted a number of factors which not only affect children's individual therapy / teaching programmes but also raise questions about service delivery and the role of the professionals involved.

The same speech error, e.g. voicing confusion, can arise at either the input side, for example with auditory discrimination affecting lexical representations, as with Zoe (Stackhouse and Wells, 1993; Chapters 9 and 10, this volume); or at the output side, for example with articulatory incoordination, as with JM (Snowling, Hulme, Wells, et al., 1992) and John (Chapter 1, this volume). This finding calls into question the traditional practice of organizing therapy groups on the basis of the surface speech error, e.g. voicing groups, stopping groups, fronting groups, in which all of the children in the group follow the same programme. By taking into account the precise locus of each child's difficulty the therapy can be targeted at individual children's needs more specifically within the group setting.

The discovery that different speech errors co-occurring within the same child can have different loci of origin (Chiat, 1983; Brett, Chiat and Pilcher, 1987; Stackhouse and Wells, 1993; Chapters 9 and 10, this volume) suggests that it is necessary to go beyond general statements about a child's auditory discrimination skills or articulatory skills. In order to understand why a child's speech problem is persisting and what aspects of their problem will create barriers to literacy development, a more precise testing of input and output skills targeting the different error types needs to be carried out.

Applying the psycholinguistic framework approach to assessment in practice is likely to uncover more cases of children with hidden speech and language problems such as Richard, the 11-year-old boy with dyslexia presented in Chapter 5. This raises important issues about service delivery models and how children with persisting speech and language problems can be supported in mainstream school. Undoubtedly, collaborative work between professionals and carers is the key, not only to managing such ongoing cases (Wright, 1992, 1996; Hatcher, 1994), but also to setting up preventive programmes in the preschool years (Layton and Deeney, 1996).

The psycholinguistic framework makes explicit why and how speech and language therapists might be involved with children with literacy problems. Because the framework emphasizes the centrality of speech processing skills in literacy development, it shows why speech and language therapists are well suited to work on the prerequisite as well as the ongoing 'back-up' skills necessary for literacy development. In collaboration with the teacher and psychologist, the speech and language therapist can make an important contribution in assessing how a child's speech processing profile performance may impact on literacy development. The role of the speech and language therapist with children who have literacy problems can be summed up as follows:

> 'The role of the speech and language therapist does not include teaching reading and spelling which is traditionally and rightly the teacher's domain. Rather, the role is one of identification and promoting the underlying skills that contribute to literacy development.'
>
> Snowling and Stackhouse (1996, p.240)

However, in order to identify and monitor older children with speech and literacy problems we need to change the long-held view that a speech problem is only at the segmental level (i.e. with 'sounds'). This view may be the reason why many older children are not referred for a speech and language therapy assessment. Children with dyslexia, for example, can often pronounce all 'sounds' perfectly well but have persisting speech problems in connected speech, at the junctions between words and on specific lexical items (Stackhouse, 1996). Traditional therapy approaches to intelligibility have tended to focus on targeting speech sounds or processes but we also need to develop children's speech skills beyond the segment (Wells, 1994).

In terms of how the psycholinguistic framework will affect a child's therapy and teaching programmes, there seems little doubt that a greater understanding of an individual's difficulties will result in a more suitable therapy and teaching programme. However, a psycholinguistic investigation in itself may not be sufficient to plan the detailed programme necessary for children with persisting speech problems. In Chapter 1 we introduced the psycholinguistic perspective by comparing it with two other perspectives commonly taken on children with speech difficulties: the medical and the linguistic. Each has a role to play in managing children's speech and literacy problems but there will be a mixture in the balance of contributions from these perspectives depending on the nature of the child's difficulties. For example, if the child has a structural abnormality which is causing speech difficulties, then intervention may be primarily via surgery. If successful, the child may not need any further investigation from a linguistic or psycholinguistic perspective.

The linguistic and psycholinguistic perspectives are much more dependent on each other, however. For example, the case of Jenny in Chapter 5 illustrated that although we could identify areas for therapy we could not complete our therapy plan without including the phonological analysis of her speech errors, derived from the linguistic perspective. Without this detail we could not devise the appropriate stimuli to include in the tasks we wanted to administer. Compare this case with Zoe at 5;11, in Chapter 9, where detailed linguistic and psycholinguistic investigations were reported. Because Zoe's speech errors had been related to her psycholinguistic profile, it was possible to make precise suggestions about what stimuli should be used in therapy activities, e.g. stimuli incorporating the voice/voiceless contrast were used specifically in auditory lexical tasks. In summary, the psycholinguistic perspective on a case contributes to the understanding of the nature of a child's spoken difficulties and how these may affect literacy development. It shows a child's processing strengths and weaknesses and therefore influences when a top-down or bottom-up approach needs to be taken in therapy/teaching tasks. In a similar way, it suggests how tasks should be presented in terms of appropriate modalities. What it does not do is reveal precisely what stimuli would be appropriate in terms of e.g. segments, lexical items or sentence structure for an individual child. For this level of detail, a linguistic analysis of a child's spoken and/or written language output is necessary.

Use of the Framework in Research

The framework and models presented in this book are suitable for both small- and large-scale research projects. Clinical application issues as well as theoretical questions can be addressed. Broadly, the research to date can be divided into (a) case studies, some longitudinal, of children with speech and literacy problems and (b) group studies of normally-developing children for the purposes of studying normal development in its own right, as well as for identifying atypical development.

Although the framework was originally devised to assess children with verbal dyspraxia and dyslexia, the range of case studies has now expanded. For example, investigations have been carried out into the nature of speech problems in children with Down's syndrome (Coffield, 1994) and the phonological awareness skills of children who stammer (Forth, Stackhouse, Vance *et al.*, 1996). The framework has been extended to investigate the nature of developmental word-finding difficulties in children (Constable, Stackhouse and Wells, in press) and also word-finding difficulties in children with acquired language problems following road traffic accidents (Onslow, 1995). Current projects include children with dysarthria, hearing loss, epilepsy and various syndromes.

Comparing speech processing profiles over time through longitudinal case studies helps us to understand the unfolding nature of children's difficulties, and in particular how a speech problem may interfere with phonological awareness and literacy development (cf. Chapter 10). The prognostic implications of different types of profiles are not yet clear. Some young children with severe speech difficulties have made remarkable progress while others with apparently less serious difficulties continue to have wide-ranging problems. Clearly, prognostic indicators are much broader than psycholinguistic factors alone, and include educational and teaching opportunities, availability of speech and language therapy and medical factors. However, in general the more pervasive the speech processing deficit (i.e. affecting input, representation and output processing) and the longer it persists (e.g. beyond the age of 5;6) the more likely it is that educational problems will ensue.

Research looking at the early identification of at-risk children is essential if intervention and prevention are to be effective. Psycholinguistic profiling has something to offer here. As more longitudinal studies of children with speech disorders are completed, the more retrospective information we will have about the significance of a child's preschool speech processing profile for later speech, language and literacy development.

Clinical issues such as the relationship between oral–motor skills and intelligibility have been explored through the psycholinguistic framework (Evans, 1994; Williams, 1996) and questions about theoretical models are also being addressed. One investigation, for example, is examining the relationship between speech processing skills and memory by analysing performance on experimental memory tasks in terms of the speech processing model (Vance, Donlan and Stackhouse, 1996). Instrumentation techniques have also been combined with psycholinguistic assessment procedures. For example, electropalatography data collected on a 9-year-old boy with speech and language problems have been interpreted within a psycholinguistic framework in order to evaluate theoretical speech processing models (Dent and Clarke, 1996).

A developmental perspective is necessary when working with children (Frith, 1985; Stackhouse and Wells, 1996; Vance, 1996b; Bishop, 1997) and has been stressed throughout this book. It is still an important aspect even when working with adults with developmental speech and literacy problems and children with acquired problems. The developmental perspective is achieved by administering tests that are developmentally appropriate for the child and for which normal control data are available. Group studies of speech processing skills in normally-developing children are essential for understanding the nature of speech and literacy problems in children (see Bishop, 1997 for further discussion).

The Way Forward

This book has set out a means of collating children's assessment results in a systematic way. Collected together, profile sheets of individual cases provide a useful database on the nature of children's speech processing difficulties and how they change over time. Such a database can be used to address theoretical and management issues such as the relationship between speech and literacy difficulties in children, early identification, prognosis and treatment efficacy. Further, working within a common framework such as this can facilitate research, practice and communication between professionals, to the benefit of children with speech and literacy difficulties.

Appendices

APPENDIX 1

Phonetic Symbols and Diacritics

The phonetic symbols and diacritics that occur in the book are listed in this Appendix. For a full description of phonetic symbols and terminology, see Laver (1994). The reference accent used here is that of the standard variety of Southern British English, as described for example by Cruttenden (1994) to whose description the reader is referred for further details. Each consonant and vowel symbol has a phonetic value broadly equivalent to that found in the corresponding word pronounced in the reference accent, unless otherwise indicated. If no such key word is provided, the sound type represented by the symbol is not found in that accent.

Prosodic notation

Nuclear tones in the reference accent, as follows:
ˋ fall; ˆ rise-fall; ˊ rise; ˇ fall-rise

Relative pitch height and on-syllable pitch movement are represented impressionistically between staves, above the transcription.

Pauses between or within utterances are represented in tenths of a second, e.g. (0.5). (.) indicates a pause of a tenth of a second or less; or alternatively, – indicates a silent beat.

: indicates a sustention of the preceding sound.

[represents the point at which simultaneous speech begins.

{*f* } represents notable loudness.

◡ = rhythmically short.

– = rhythmically long.

ˈ indicates that in a real English word, e.g. BAˈNANA, the following syllable bears the main lexical stress; in a nonword target, e.g. /bəˈkɑtə/, it indicates where the main stress is intended to be. In transcriptions of spoken utterances, it represents perceived prominence, mainly of loudness and pitch, e.g. [bəˈnɑnə].

ˌ indicates that the following syllable bears secondary lexical stress e.g. ˌHIPPOˈPOTAMUS.

̩ indicates that a consonant forms the nucleus of the syllable: e.g. BUTTON ⟶ [bʌtn̩].

$ = syllable boundary.

Vowel symbols

Diphthongs have the quality of the two constituent vowel symbols pronounced in sequence, the first longer than the second.

ə	mid-central unrounded	SOFA, ABOUT, BUTTERCUP
ɪ	centralized close–mid front spread	BIT
ɛ	open-mid front spread	BET
æ	raised open front unrounded	BAT
a	open front unrounded	BAT (Northern English)
ʌ	raised open central unrounded	BUG
ɒ	open back rounded	POT
ʊ	centralized close–mid back rounded	PUT
ɵ	mid central rounded	
u	close back rounded	BOOT, SHOE
aʊ	diphthong	BOUT, COW
əʊ	diphthong	BOAT, LOW
ʉ	close central rounded	
i	close front spread	BEAT, BEE
eɪ	diphthong	BAIT, BAY
aɪ	diphthong	BITE, BUY
ɒɪ	diphthong	NOISE, BOY
ɑ	open back unrounded	PARK, BAR
ɔ	open–mid back rounded	SORT, SAW
ɜ	midcentral unrounded	BIRD, FUR
ɪə	diphthong	BEARD, BEER
ɛə	diphthong	BEAR

Consonant symbols: plosives, affricates, nasals

p	voiceless bilabial plosive	PIN
b	voiced bilabial plosive	BIN
t	voiceless alveolar plosive	TIN
d	voiced alveolar plosive	DIN

c	voiceless palatal plosive	THANKYOU
ɟ	voiced palatal plosive	EGGYOLK
k	voiceless velar plosive	COAT
g	voiced velar plosive	GOAT
ʔ	glottal stop	WATER (Cockney pronunciation)

tɕ	voiceless alveolo-palatal affricate	
dʑ	voiced alveolo-palatal affricate	
ʧ	voiceless postalveolar affricate	CHEESE, NATURE
ʤ	voiced postalveolar affricate	GEM, MAJOR

m	voiced bilabial nasal	MAJOR
n	voiced alveolar nasal	NATURE
ɲ	voiced palatal nasal	AGNEAU (French)
ŋ	voiced velar nasal	SINGING

Consonant symbols: fricatives

ɸ	voiceless bilabial	
β	voiced bilabial	
θ	voiceless dental	THIN, MOTH
ð	voiced dental	THIS, MOTHER
s	voiceless alveolar	SEA, RICE
z	voiced alveolar	ZOO, LOSE
ɬ	voiceless alveolar lateral	LLANDUDNO (Welsh)
ɮ	voiced alveolar lateral	
ʃ	voiceless postalveolar	SHOE, NATION
ʒ	voiced postalveolar	MEASURE
ɕ	voiceless alveolo-palatal	
ʑ	voiced alveolo-palatal	
ç	voiceless palatal	MICH (German)
x	voiceless velar	BUCH (German)
h	voiceless glottal	HAT

Symbols and diacritics: approximants, secondary articulations etc.

l	voiced alveolar lateral approximant	LOCK
w	voiced labial-velar approximant	WATER
ʋ	voiced labiodental approximant	
ɹ	voiced postalveolar approximant	RIGHT, CARRY
ɾ	voiced alveolar tap	BETTER (American pronunciation)
r	cover symbol for different pronunciations of this phonological item in different varieties of English	

j	voiced palatal approximant	Y̲ELLOW
ʲ	palatal resonance / secondary articulation	
̟	advanced tongue position / front resonance	
̠	retracted tongue position / back resonance	
̝	close articulation	
̥	voiceless	POTATO → [pə̥tʰeɪtəʊ]
ʰ	aspirated	PET → [pʰɛt]
˭	unaspirated	STAR → [st˭ɑ]
̃	nasalized	VIN (French) → [vɛ̃]

APPENDIX 2

Examples of Tests for Each Question in the Psycholinguistic Assessment Framework

(Presented in top to bottom order for both input and output sides of the model. Space has been left at the end of each question to enable you to add your own test examples.)

INPUT

F. Is the child aware of the internal structure of phonological representations?

Picture onset detection: identification of pictures that begin with the same 'sound', e.g. KEY, KITE, SHOE. The tester does not name the pictures (e.g. *PhAB* subtest: Alliteration Part 2, Frederickson, 1995).

Picture rhyme detection: identification of pictures that rhyme, e.g. RING, SWING, DUCK. The tester does not name the pictures (Vance, Stackhouse and Wells, 1994).

Picture rhyme judgement: two pictures presented, tester asks "Do these pictures rhyme?", e.g. KEY~TREE, SHOE~BIKE. The tester does not name the pictures (Vance, Stackhouse and Wells, 1994).

E. Are the child's phonological representations accurate?

Silent blending: identification of a picture that corresponds with the tester's spoken presentation of segments, e.g. onset + nucleus + coda : /pr/ + /æ/ + /m/; onset + r̩ime: /pr/ + /æm/, (Counsel, 1993). Sound Recognition subtest (Goldman, Fristoe and Woodcock, 1978).

Auditory detection of speech 'errors', e.g. child looks at picture of a FISH. Tester asks "Is this a PISH?"; "Is this a FISH?"; "Is this a FIS?" (Locke, 1980a, b).

Minimal pair picture discrimination: identification of the picture that corresponds with the tester's spoken presentation of stimuli, e.g. in connected speech: I LIKE THE COAT WITH THE LONG FUR ~ I LIKE THE GOAT WITH THE LONG FUR (Cassidy, 1994); and in single words: CLOWN VS CROWN (MorganBarry, 1988).

D. Can the child discriminate between real words?

Minimal pair auditory discrimination: clusters. Same / Different discrimination, e.g. LOST VS LOTS (Bridgeman and Snowling, 1988).

Auditory rhyme detection, e.g. Three finger puppets presented; the tester speaks a word for each one (JAM, FISH, PRAM). Child points to the two puppets which said the rhyming words (Vance, Stackhouse and Wells, 1994).

Auditory rhyme judgement, e.g. Tester asks, "Do BOAT and COAT rhyme?" (Vance, Stackhouse and Wells, 1994).

Minimal pair auditory discrimination: CVC. Same/different discrimination e.g. PIN~BIN (e.g. Wepman and Reynolds, 1987).

C. Does the child have language-specific representations of word structures?

Auditory discrimination of legal from illegal nonwords, e.g. BLICK VS BNICK (Waterson, 1981; Stackhouse, 1989).

Auditory discrimination of legal from exotic nonwords, e.g. [sɒf] vs [ɬɒf].

B. Can the child discriminate speech sounds without reference to lexical representations?

Auditory discrimination of complex nonwords, e.g. IBIKUS vs IKIBUS (Stackhouse, 1989).
Auditory discrimination of clusters in nonwords, e.g. VOST vs VOTS (Bridgeman and Snowling, 1988).

ABX auditory nonword discrimination, e.g Two puppets presented; tester says "This puppet says BRISH. This puppet says BRIS. Which puppet said BRIS?" (Locke, 1980a, b; Vance, 1996a).

Rhyme judgement of nonwords, e.g. "Do POAT and HOAT rhyme?" (Vance, Stackhouse and Wells, 1994).

A. Does the child have adequate auditory perception?

Auditory fusion: judge when two nonspeech sounds (e.g. 'beeps') are heard as one (McCroskey, 1984).

Pitch change detection – judge if two nonspeech sounds are the same or different in terms of their pitch (Tallal and Piercy, 1980).

Hearing tests, e.g. audiometry.

OUTPUT

G. Can the child access accurate motor programs?

Production of segments from a picture: e.g. Coda supply: child looks at picture (FISH), tester produces "fi-" [fɪ], child supplies "sh" [ʃ] (Muter, Snowling and Taylor, 1994).

Spontaneous speech data.

Picture Description data (e.g. Goldman and Fristoe, 1969; Stackhouse and Snowling, 1992b).

Naming tests:
- (a) lexical (e.g. Renfrew 1972; German, 1989);
- (b) accuracy (e.g. Anthony, Bogle, Ingram, et al., 1971; Goldman and Fristoe, 1969; Grunwell and Harding, 1995).

H. Can the child manipulate phonological units?

Spoonerism test, e.g. BOB DYLAN → "Dob Bylan" (Perin, 1983; *PhAB*, Frederikson, 1995).

Onset string production, e.g."Tell me as many words as you can that begin with /k/" (e.g. Alliteration Fluency subtest on the *PhAB*, Frederikson, 1995).

Rhyme String Production, e.g. "Tell me as many words as you can that rhyme with CAT" (e.g. Vance, Stackhouse and Wells, 1994; Rhyme Fluency subtest on the *PhAB*, Frederikson, 1995).

I. Can the child articulate real words accurately?

Sound blending of real words from verbally presented segments, e.g. /pr/ + /a/ + /m/ → "pram" (Hatcher, 1994; real word items on the blending subtest from the *Aston Index*, Newton and Thomson, 1982).

Repetition tasks:

(a) Connected speech, e.g. repetition of sentence: HIS UMBRELLA IS YELLOW (Vance, Stackhouse and Wells, 1995).

(b) Real words on more than one occasion e.g. 'Say CATERPILLAR three times' (e.g. *Nuffield Centre Dyspraxia Programme*, Connery, 1992).

(c) Real words of increasing syllable length, with and without clusters, e.g. with clusters: GLOVE; TRACTOR; UMBRELLA (Vance, Stackhouse and Wells, 1995).

J. Can the child articulate speech without reference to lexical representations?

Nonword blending from verbally presented segments, e.g D-U-P; T-I-S-E-K. (nonword items in blending subtest on the *Aston Index*, Newton and Thomson, 1982).

Repetition of nonwords on more than one occasion, e.g. "Say KUDIGAN /ˈkudɪgən/ three times" (Williams, 1996).

Repetition of nonwords with increasing syllable length, with and without clusters, e.g. with clusters GLEV /glɛv/; TRECTEE /ˈtrɛkti/; AMBRAHLI /æmˈbrɑli/ (Snowling, Stackhouse and Rack, 1986; Ryder, 1991; Vance, Stackhouse and Wells, 1995; Gathercole and Baddeley, 1996).

K. Does the child have adequate sound production skills?

Diadochokinetic rates: Repeated imitation of sounds in isolation, e.g. [p] and in sequences e.g. [pə pə pə]; [pə tə kə] (Fletcher, 1978; Henry, 1990; Williams, 1996).

Oral examination of structure and function (Huskie, 1989; *POSP*, Brindley *et al*., 1996.).

L. Does the child reject his /her own erroneous forms?

Tester observes if child attempts to correct his/her own speech output spontaneously.

Appendix 3
For Photocopying

SPEECH PROCESSING PROFILE

SPEECH PROCESSING PROFILE

Name: Comments:

Age: d.o.b:

Date:

Profiler:

INPUT

F

Is the child aware of the internal structure of phonological representations?

E

Are the child's phonological representations accurate?

D

Can the child discriminate between real words?

C

Does the child have language-specific representations of word structures?

B

Can the child discriminate speech sounds without reference to lexical representations?

A

Does the child have adequate auditory perception?

OUTPUT

G

Can the child access accurate motor programs?

H

Can the child manipulate phonological units

I

Can the child articulate real words accurately?

J

Can the child articulate speech without reference to lexical representations?

K

Does the child have adequate sound production skills?

L

Does the child reject his/her own erroneous forms?

Appendix 4
For Photocopying

SPEECH PROCESSING MODEL

SPEECH PROCESSING MODEL

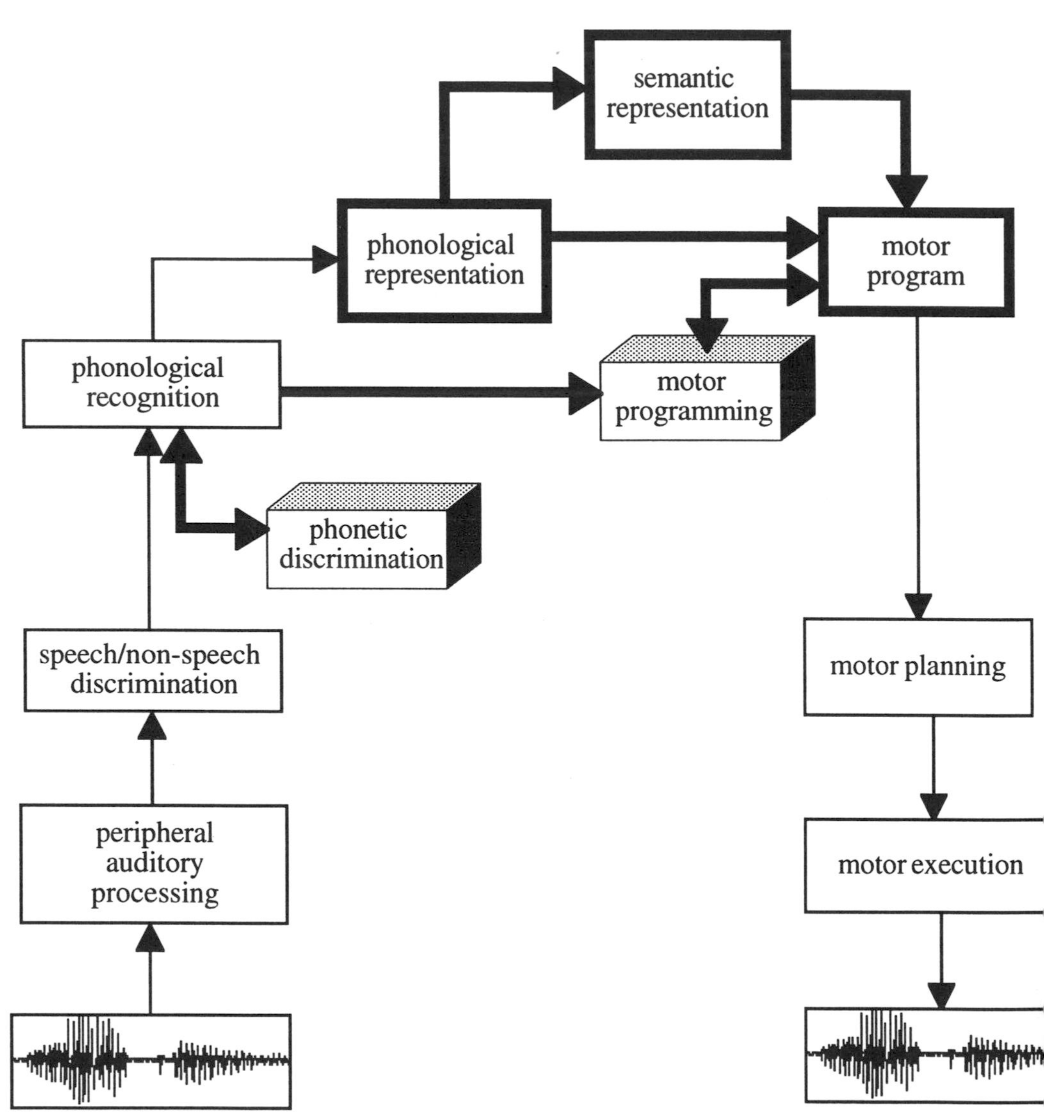

References

Adams, M.J. (1990) *Beginning To Read: Learning and Thinking about Print.* Cambridge, MA: MIT Press.

Aitchison, J. (1987) *Words in the Mind: An Introduction to the Mental Lexicon.* Oxford: Basil Blackwell.

Aitchison, J. (1989) *The Articulate Mammal: An Introduction to Psycholinguistics*, 3rd edition. London:Hutchinson; New York: Universe.

Anthony, A., Bogle, D., Ingram, D., McIsaac, M.W. (1971) *The Edinburgh Articulation Test.* Edinburgh: Churchill Livingstone.

Barton, D. (1976) *The Role of Perception in the Acquisition of Phonology.* Unpublished doctoral dissertation, University of London. (Reprinted by the Indiana University Linguistics Club, 1978.)

Benedict, H. (1979) Early lexical development: Comprehension and production. *Journal of Child Language* **6**: 183–200.

Berko, J. (1958) The child's learning of English morphology. *Word* **14**: 150–177.

Bernstein Ratner, N. (1994) Stuttering and language. In Starkweather, C.W., Peters, H. (Eds) *Stuttering: Proceedings of the First World Congress on Fluency Disorders*, pp. 87–92. The International Fluency Association. Nijmegen: University Press.

Bird, J., Bishop, D.V.M. (1992) Perception and awareness of phonemes in phonologically impaired children. *European Journal of Disorders of Communication* **27**: 289–311.

Bird, J., Bishop D.V.M., Freeman, N.H. (1995) Phonological awareness and literacy development in children with expressive phonological impairments. *Journal of Speech and Hearing Research* **38:** 446–462.

Bishop, D.V.M. (1985) Spelling ability in congenital dysarthria: Evidence against articulatory coding in translating between phonemes and graphemes. *Cognitive Neuropsychology* **2**: 229–251.

Bishop, D.V.M. (1989) *Test for Reception of Grammar*, 2nd edition. Manchester: Department of Psychology, University of Manchester.

Bishop, D.V.M. (1992) The underlying nature of specific language impairment. *Journal of Child Psychology and Psychiatry* **33**(1): 3–66.

Bishop, D.V.M. (in press) *Uncommon Understanding.* Hove, Sussex: Psychology Press.

Bishop, D.V.M., Adams, C. (1990) A prospective study of the relationship between specific language impairment, phonological disorders and reading retardation. *Journal of Child Psychology and Psychiatry* **31**: 1027–1050.

Bishop, D.V.M., Robson, J. (1989) Unimpaired short-term memory and rhyme judgement in congenitally speechless individuals. Implications for the notion of articulatory coding. *Quarterly Journal of Experimental Psychology* **41A(1)**: 123–140.

Bishop, D.V.M., Rosenbloom, L. (1987) Classification of childhood language disorders. In Yule, W., Rutter, M. (Eds) *Language Development and Disorders* pp. 16–41). Oxford: Blackwell Scientific.

Boberg, E. (Ed) (1993) *The Neuropsychology of Stuttering*. Alberta: The University of Alberta Press.

Boysson-Bardies, B. de , Halle, P., Sagart, L., Durand, C. (1989) A cross-linguistic investigation of vowel formants in babbling. *Journal of Child Language* **16** : 1–17.

Bradley, L. (1984) *Assessing Reading Difficulties: A Diagnostic and Remedial Approach*, 2nd edition. London: Macmillan Education.

Bradley, L., Bryant, P. (1983) Categorising sounds and learning to read: A causal connection. *Nature* **301**: 419–421.

Brett, L., Chiat, S., Pilcher, C. (1987) Stages and units in output processing: some evidence from voicing and fronting processes in children. *Language and Cognitive Processes* **3(4)**: 165–177.

Bridgeman, E., Snowling, M. (1988) The perception of phoneme sequence: a comparison of dyspraxic and normal children. *British Journal of Disorders of Communication* **23(3)**: 245–252.

Brindley, C., Cave, D., Crane, S., Lees, J., Moffat, V. (1996) *Paediatric Oral Skills Package (POSP)*. London: Whurr Publishers.

Bryan, A., Howard, D. (1992) Frozen phonology thawed: the analysis and remediation of a developmental disorder of lexical phonology. *European Journal of Disorders of Communication* **27(4)**: 343–365.

Bryant, P.E., Nunes, T. (1997) Spelling and grammar. Paper presented at *Integrating Research and Practice in Literacy*. An International Symposium.

Bryant, P.E., MacLean, M., Bradley, L., Crossland, J. (1989). Nursery rhymes, phonological skills and reading. *Journal of Child Language* **16**: 407–428.

Campbell, R. (1983) Writing nonwords to dictation. *Brain and Language* **19**: 153–179.

Campbell, R., Wright, H. (1988) Deafness, spelling and rhyme. *Quarterly Journal of Experimental Psychology* **40 A**: 771–780.

Cassidy, B. (1994) *An Investigation into the Auditory Discrimination Skills of Normally Developing Children Using Single Word and Sentence Stimuli*. Unpublished M.Sc thesis. National Hospital's College of Speech Sciences/Institute of Neurology, London University.

Catts, H.W. (1993) The relationship between speech–language impairments and reading disabilities. *Journal of Speech and Hearing Research* **36**: 948–958.

Catts, H.W., Vartiainen, T. (1993) *Sounds Abound*. East Moline Ill: Linguisystems.

Catts, H.W., Hu, C-F., Larrivee, L., Swank, L. (1994) Early identification of reading disabilities. In Watkins, R.V., Rice, M. (Eds) *Specific Language Impairments in Children. Communication and Language Intervention Series 4*. London: Paul H. Brookes.

Chaney, C. (1992) Language development, metalinguistic skills and print awareness in 3 year old children. *Applied Psycholinguistics* **13**: 485–514.

Chiat, S. (1983) 'Why Mikey's right and my key's wrong': the significance of stress and word boundaries in a child's output system. *Cognition* **14**: 275–300.

Chiat, S. (1989) The relation between prosodic structure, syllabification and segmental realization: evidence from a child with fricative stopping. *Clinical Linguistics and Phonetics* **3(3)**: 223–242.

Chukovsky, K. (1963) *From Two to Five*. Berkeley, CA: University of California Press.

Clarke-Klein, S., Hodson, B. (1995) A phonologically based analysis of misspellings by third graders with disordered-phonology histories. *Journal of Speech and Hearing Research* **38**: 839–849.

Coffield, C. (1994) *An Investigation into the Speech Output of Four Down's Syndrome Adolescents*. Unpublished M.Sc. thesis, London: National Hospital's College of Speech Sciences/Institute of Neurology.

Coltheart, M. (1980) *Analysing Acquired Disorders of Reading*. Clinical Tests. London: Birkbeck College.

Connery, V. (1992) *Nuffield Centre Dyspraxia Programme.* London: Nuffield Hearing and Speech Centre, Royal National Throat, Nose and Ear Hospital.

Constable, A., Stackhouse, J., Wells, B. (in press) Developmental word finding difficulties and phonological processing: the case of the missing handcuffs. *Applied Psycholinguistics*.

Conture, E., Yaruss, J., Edwards, M. (1995) Childhood stuttering and disordered phonology. In Starkweather, C.W., Peters, H. (Eds) *Stuttering: Proceedings of the First World Congress On Fluency Disorders.* The International Fluency Association. Nijmegen: University Press.

Counsel, J. (1993) *Oral Language Deficits in Reading Impaired Children.* M.Sc. thesis, Department of Human Communication Science. University College London.

Crary, M. (1984) Neurolinguistic perspective on developmental verbal dyspraxia. *Communicative Disorders* **9**: 33–49.

Cruttenden, A. (1994) *Gimson's Pronunciation of English,* (5th Edition). London: Edward Arnold.

Crystal, D., Varley, R. (1993) *Introduction to Language Pathology*. 3rd Edition. London: Whurr Publishers.

Crystal, D., Garman, M., Fletcher, P. (1989) *The Grammatical Analysis of Language Disability,* 2nd edition. London: Whurr Publishers.

Darili, E. (1994) *An Investigation into the Lexical-phonological Representations of Normal Nursery Children.* M.Sc. thesis. Department of Human Communication Science, University College London.

Dent, H., Clarke, R. (1996) A two-pronged approach to assessment: combining psycholinguistic and instrumental procedures in the investigation of a developmental speech and language disorder. Department of Human Communication, University College, London. *Work In Progress* **6**: 44–54.

Dodd, B. (1975) Children's understanding of their own phonological forms. *Quarterly Journal of Experimental Psychology* **27**: 165–172

Dodd, B. (1995) *Differential Diagnosis and Treatment of Children with Speech Disorder*. London: Whurr Publishers.

Dodd, B., Gillon, G., Oerlemans, M., Russell, T., Syrmis, M., Wilson, H. (1995) Phonological disorder and the acquisition of literacy. In Dodd, B (Ed) *Differential Diagnosis and Treatment of Children with Speech Disorder*. London: Whurr Publishers.

Dollaghan, C.A., Biber, M.E., Campbell, T.F. (1995) Lexical influences on nonword repetition. *Applied Psycholinguistics* **16**: 211–222.

Duncan, D.M. (Ed) (1990) *Working with Bilingual Language Disability*. New York and London: Chapman & Hall.

Dunn, L.M., Dunn, L., Whetton, C., Pintillie, D. (1982) *British Picture Vocabulary Scales*. Windsor: NFER-Nelson.

Ehri, L.C., Wilce, L.S. (1980) The influence of orthography on readers' conceptualisation of the phonemic structure of words. *Applied Psycholinguistics* **1(4)**: 371–386.

Eilers, R. E., Oller, D.K. (1976) The role of speech discrimination in developmental sound substitutions. *Journal of Child Language* **3**: 319–329.

Elliott, C.D., Murray, D.J., Pearson, L.S. (1983) *British Ability Scales*. Windsor: NFER-Nelson

Ellis, A.W., Young, A.W. (1988) *Human Cognitive Neuropsychology*. London: Lawrence Erlbaum.

Evans, A. (1994) *The Relationship Between Oral-motor Skills and Intelligibility in Speech Disordered Children.* M.Sc. thesis. Department of Human Communication Science, University College London.

Ferguson, C.A., Farwell, C. B. (1975) Words and sounds in early language acquisition. *Language* **51**: 419–439.

Ferguson, C., Menn , L., and Stoel-Gammon, C. (1992) *Phonological Development: Models, Research, Implications.* Timonium, MD: York Press.

Fletcher, P. (1985) *A Child's Learning of English.* Oxford: Basil Blackwell.

Fletcher, S.G. (1978) *The Fletcher Time-by-Count Test of Diadochokinetic Syllable Rate.* Tigard Oregon: C.C. Publications.

Forth, T., Stackhouse, J., Vance, M., Nicholson, A., Cook, F. (1996) Can Stammerers Rhyme? Department of Human Communication Science, University College London. *Work in Progress*, **6**: 59–77.

Fowler, A.E. (1991) How early phonological development may set the stage for phoneme awareness. In Brady, S.A., Shankweiler, D.P. (Eds) *Phonological Processes in Literacy: A Tribute to Isabelle Y. Liberman.* Hillsdale, NJ: Lawrence Erlbaum.

Fox, B., & Routh, D.K. (1984) Phonemic analysis and synthesis as word attack skills: Revisited. *Journal of Educational Psychology* **76**, (6): 1059–1064.

Frederikson, N. (Ed.) (1995) *Phonological Assessment Battery (PhAB)*. Windsor: NFER-Nelson.

Frith, U. (1985) Beneath the surface of developmental dyslexia. In Patterson, K.E., Marshall, J.C., Coltheart, M. (Eds) *Surface Dyslexia,* pp. 301–330. London: Routledge and Kegan Paul.

Garman, M. (1990) *Psycholinguistics*. Cambridge: Cambridge University Press.

Gathercole, S.E. (1993) Word learning in language-impaired children. *Child Language Teaching and Therapy* **9** (3), 187–199.

Gathercole, S., Baddeley, A. (1996) *The Children's Test of Nonword Repetition (CN Rep)*. London: The Psychological Corporation.

Gathercole, S., Willis, C.S., Baddeley, A.D., Emslie, H. (1994) The Children's Test of nonword repetition: A test of phonological working memory. *Memory* **2**(2): 103–127.

German, D. (1989) *Test of Word Finding.* Leicester: Taskmaster.

German, D. (1990) *Test of Adolescent Word Finding.* Leicester: Taskmaster.

German, D. (1991) *Test of Word Finding in Discourse*. Leicester: Taskmaster.

Gibbon, F. (1990) Lingual activity in two speech-disordered children's attempts to produce stop consonants: evidence from electropalatographic (EPG) data. *British Journal of Disorders of Communication* **25**: 329–340.

Gibbon, F., Dent, H., Hardcastle, W. (1993) Diagnosis and therapy of abnormal alveolar stops in a speech-disordered child using electropalatography. *Clinical Linguistics and Phonetics* **7**(4): 247–268.

Gimson, A.C. (1989) *An Introduction to the Pronunciation of English,* 4th edition. London: Edward Arnold.

Goldman, R., Fristoe, M. (1969) *Goldman–Fristoe Test of Articulation.* Windsor: NFER-Nelson.

Goldman, R., Fristoe, M., Woodcock, R. (1978) *Goldman–Fristoe–Woodcock Auditory Skills Test Battery, revised edition.* Windsor: NFER-Nelson

Goodglass, H., Kaplan, E., Weintraub, S. (1983) *The Boston Naming Test.* Philadelphia, PA: Lea and Febiger.

Gordon, P. (1995) Childhood stuttering and language: research and clinical application. In Starkweather, C.W., Peters, H. (Eds) *Stuttering: Proceedings of the First World Congress On Fluency Disorders*, pp. 81–86. The International Fluency Association. Nijmegen: University Press.

Gordon, P., Luper, H. (1989) The effects of syntactic complexity on the occurrence of disfluencies in five-year-old nonstutterers. *Journal of Fluency Disorders* **14**: 429–445.

Goswami, U. (1990) A special link between rhyming skills and the use of orthographic analogies by beginning readers. *Journal of Child Psychology and Psychiatry* **31**: 301–311.

Goswami, U. (1994) The role of analogies in reading development. *Support for Learning* **9**: 22–25.

Goswami, U., Bryant, P. E. (1990) *Phonological Skills and Learning to Read.* Hove: Lawrence Erlbaum.

Goulandris, N. (1996) Assessing reading and spelling skills. In Snowling, M., Stackhouse, J. (Eds) *Dyslexia, Speech and Language: A Practitioner's Handbook.* London: Whurr Publishers.

Grunwell, P. (1985) *PACS: Phonological Assessment of Child Speech.* Windsor: NFER-Nelson.

Grunwell, P. (1987) *Clinical Phonology,* 2nd edition. London: Croom Helm.

Grunwell, P. (1992) Principled decision making in the remediation of children with phonological disability. In Fletcher, P., Hall, D. (Eds) *Specific Speech and Language Disorders in Children.* London: Whurr Publishers.

Grunwell, P., Yavas, M. (1988) Phonotactic restrictions in disordered child phonology: a case study. *Clinical Linguistics and Phonetics* **2**(1): 1–16.

Grunwell, P., Harding, A. (1995) *PACS TOYS.* Windsor, UK: NFER-Nelson.

Haege, A. (1995) Cognitive abilities and interactional variables in young stutterers. In Starkweather, C.W., Peters, H. (Eds) *Stuttering: Proceedings of the First World Congress On Fluency Disorders*, pp. 162–167. The International Fluency Association. Nijmegen: University Press.

Harris, J., Cottam, P. (1985) Phonetic features and phonological features in speech assessment. *British Journal of Disorders of Communication* **20**(1): 61–74.

Hatcher, P.J. (1994) *Sound Linkage: An Integrated Programme for Overcoming Reading Difficulties.* London : Whurr Publishers.

Hatcher, P. J. (1996) Practising sound links in reading intervention with the school-age child. In Snowling, M., Stackhouse, J. (Eds) *Dyslexia, Speech and Language: A Practitioner's Handbook.* London: Whurr Publishers.

Hatcher, P.J., Hulme, C., Ellis, A.W. (1994) Ameliorating early reading failure by integrating the teaching of reading and phonological skills: The phonological linkage hypothesis. *Child Development* **65**: 41–57.

Henry, C. (1990) The development of oral diadochokinesis and non-linguistic rhythmic skills in normal and speech-disordered young children. *Clinical Linguistics and Phonetics* **4**(2): 121–138.

Hewlett, N. (1990) Processes of development and production. In Grunwell, P. (Ed.) *Developmental Speech Disorders*, pp.15–38. London: Whurr Publishers.

Hodson, B., Paden, E. (1991) *Targeting Intelligible Speech: A Phonological Approach to Remediation.* 2nd edition, Austin,TX: Pro-Ed.

Hogg, R., McCully, C. (1987) *Metrical Phonology: A Coursebook.* Cambridge: Cambridge University Press.

Howell, J., Dean, E. (1994) *Treating Phonological Disorders in Children: Metaphon - Theory to Practice,* 2nd edition. London: Whurr Publishers.

Howlin, P., Cross, P. (1994) The variability of language test scores in 3- and 4-year-old children of normal non-verbal intelligence: a brief research report. *European Journal of Disorders of Communication* **29**(3): 279–288.

Hughes, R. (1983) The internal representation of word-final phonemes in phonologically disordered children. *British Journal of Disorders of Communication* **18**: 78–88.

Hulme, C., Snowling, M. (1992) Deficits in output phonology: a cause of reading failure? *Cognitive Neuropsychology* **9**: 47–72.

Huskie C.F. (1989) Assessment of speech and language status: subjective and objective approaches to appraisal of vocal tract structure and function. In Stengelhofen, J. (Ed) *Cleft Palate – The Nature and Remediation of Communication Problems*. London: Whurr Publishers.

Huttenlocher, J. (1974) The origins of language comprehension. In R. Solso (Ed) *Theories in Cognitive Psychology,* pp. 331–368. New York: Lawrence Erlbaum.

Ingram, D. (1989) *First Language Acquisition: Method, Description and Explanation.* Cambridge: Cambridge University Press.

Jenkins, J.J. (1966) Reflections on the conference. In Smith F, Miller GA (Eds.) *The Genesis of Language: A psycholinguistic approach*. Cambridge MA: MIT Press.

Jusczyk, P.W. (1992) Developing phonological categories from the speech signal. In Ferguson, C.A., Menn, L., Stoel-Gammon, C. (Eds) *Phonological Development: Models, Research, Implications*. Timonium, MD: York Press.

Jusczyk, P.W., Aslin, R.N. (1995) Infants' detection of the sound pattern of words in fluent speech. *Cognitive Psychology* **29**: 1–23.

Jusczyk, P.W., Cutler, A., Redanz, N.J. (1993) Infants' preference for the predominant stress patterns of English words. *Child Development* **64**: 675–687.

Jusczyk, P.W., Luce, P.A., Charles-Luce, J. (1994) Infants' sensitivity to phonotactic patterns in the native language. *Journal of Memory and Language* **33**: 630–645.

Jusczyk, P.W., Friederici, A.D., Wessels, J., Svenkerud, V.Y., Juszcyk, A.M. (1993). Infants' sensitivity to the sound patterns of native language words. *Journal of Memory and Language* **32**: 402–420.

Kay, J., Lesser, R., Coltheart, M. (1992) *Psycholinguistic Assessments of Language Processing in Aphasia (PALPA)*. Hove: Lawrence Erlbaum.

Kelly, J., Local, J. (1989) *Doing Phonology.* Manchester: Manchester University Press.

Kent, R. (1992). The biology of phonological development. In Ferguson, C.A., Menn, L., Stoel-Gammon, C. (Eds) *Phonological Development: Models, Research, Implications*. Timonium, MD: York Press.

Kirtley, C., Bryant, P., MacLean, M., Bradley, L. (1989) Rhyme, rime, and the onset of reading. *Journal of Experimental Child Psychology* **48**: 224–245.

Klein, H., Constable, A., Goulandris, N., Stackhouse, J., Tarplee, C. (1994) *Clinical Evaluation of Language Fundamentals (CELF-R:UK).* UK Examiners Manual-Supplement. London: The Psychological Corporation.

Laver, J. (1994) *Principles of Phonetics.* Cambridge: Cambridge University Press.

Layton, L., Deeney, K. (1996) Promoting phonological awareness in preschool children. In Snowling, M., Stackhouse, J. (Eds) *Dyslexia, Speech and Language: A Practitioner's Handbook.* London: Whurr Publishers.

Lees, J. (1993) *Children with Acquired Aphasias.* London: Whurr Publishers.

Leonard, L., McGregor, K. (1991) Unusual phonological patterns and their underlying representations: a case study. *Journal of Child Language* **18**: 261–271.

Letterland: Further information from, Letterland Ltd, Barton, Cambridge CB3 7AY, UK.

Levelt, W. (1989) *Speaking – From Intention to Articulation.* Cambridge, MA: MIT Press.

Lewis B.A., Freebairn, L. (1992) Residual effects of preschool phonology disorders in grade school adolescence and adulthood. *Journal of Speech and Hearing Research* 35:819–831.

Lewkowicz, N.K. (1980) Phonemic awareness training: What to teach and how to teach it. *Journal of Educational Psychology* **72**: 686–700.

Liberman, I.Y., Shankweiler, D., Fischer, F.W., Carter, B. (1974) Reading and the awareness of linguistic segments. *Journal of Experimental Child Psychology* **18**: 201–212.

Lindamood, C., Lindamood, P. (1975) *Auditory Discrimination in Depth.* Colombus OH: Macmillan/McGraw Hill.

Lindamood, P., Bell, N. and Lindamood, P. (1997) Achieving competence in language and literacy by training in phonemic awareness, concept imagery and comparator function. In Hulme, C. Snowling, M. (Eds) *Dyslexia: Biology, Cognition and Intervention.* London: Whurr Publishers.

Local, J. K. (1992) Modelling assimilation in a non-segmental rule-free phonology. In Docherty, G.J., Ladd, D.R. (Eds): *Papers in Laboratory Phonology II*, pp. 190–223. Cambridge: Cambridge University Press.

Locke, J.L. (1980a) The inference of speech perception in the phonologically disordered child. Part I: The rationale, some criteria, the conventional tests. *Journal of Speech and Hearing Disorders* **45**: 431–444.

Locke, J.L. (1980b) The inference of speech perception in the phonologically disordered child. Part II: Some clinically novel procedures, their use, some findings. *Journal of Speech and Hearing Disorders* **45**: 445–468.

Locke, J.L. (1983) *Phonological Acquisition and Change.* New York: Academic Press.

Lodge, K. (1984) *Studies in the Phonology of Colloquial English* London: Croom Helm

Louko, J.L. (1995) Phonological characteristics of young children who stutter. *Topics in Language Disorders* **15**(3): 48–59.

Lowe, M., Costello, A. (1988) *Symbolic Play Test.* 2nd Edition. Windsor Berks: NFER-Nelson.

Macken, M.A. (1980) The child's representation: the 'puzzle-puddle-pickle' evidence. *Journal of Linguistics* **16**: 1–17.

Macken, M.A. (1992) Where's phonology? In Ferguson, C.A., Menn, L., Stoel-Gammon, C. (Eds) *Phonological Development: Models, Research, Implications.* Timonium, MD: York Press.

MacLean, M., Bryant, P.E., Bradley, L. (1987) Rhymes, nursery rhymes and reading in early childhood. *Merrill-Palmer Quarterly* **33**: 255–281.

Magnusson, E., Naucler, K. (1990) Reading and spelling in language disordered children - linguistic and metalinguistic prerequisites: report on a longitudinal study. *Clinical Linguistics and Phonetics* **4**(1): 49–61.

Mann, V.A. (1986) Phonological awareness: The role of reading experience. *Cognition* **24**: 65–92.

Marion, M.J., Sussman, H.M., Marquardt, T.P. (1993) The perception and production of rhyme in normal and developmentally apraxic children. *Journal of Communication Disorders* **26**: 129–160.

Masterson, J., Hazan, V., Wijayatilake, L. (1995) Phonemic processing problems in developmental phonological dyslexia. *Cognitive Neuropsychology* **12**(3): 233–259.

McCrosky, R.L. (1984) *Wichita Auditory Processing Test.* Oklahoma: Modern Education Corporation.

McGregor, K., Schwartz, R. (1992) Converging evidence for underlying phonological representation in a child who misarticulates. *Journal of Speech and Hearing Research* **35**: 596–603.

Menyuk, P., Chesnick, M., Liebergott, J.W., Korngold, B., D'Agnostino, R., Belanger, A. (1991) Predicting reading problems in at-risk children. *Journal of Speech and Hearing Research* **34**: 893–903.

Merzenich, M.M., Jenkins, W.M., Johnston, P., Schreiner, C., Miller, S.L., Tallal, P. (1996) Temporal processing deficits of language impaired children ameliorated by training. *Science* **271**: 77–80.

Milloy, N., MorganBarry, R. (1990) Developmental neurological disorders. In Grunwell P. (Ed) *Developmental Speech Disorders.* London: Whurr Publishers

MorganBarry, R. (1989) *The Auditory Discrimination and Attention Test.* Windsor: NFER-Nelson.

Muter, V. (1996) Predicting children's reading and spelling difficulties. In Snowling, M., Stackhouse, J. (Eds) *Dyslexia, Speech and Language: A Practitioner's Handbook*. London: Whurr Publishers.

Muter, V., Snowling, M., Taylor, S. (1994) Orthographic analogies and phonological awareness: Their role and significance in early reading development. *Journal of Child Psychology and Psychiatry* **35**: 293–310.

Nathan, L., Wells, B., Donlan, C. (1996) A developmental study of the effects of accent variation on single-word comprehension. Department of Human Communication Science, University College London: *Work in Progress* **6**: 78–93.

Newton, C. (1997) *The development of between-word processes in the connected speech of children aged between 3 and 7.* MS Department. of Human Communication Science, University College, London.

Newton, M., Thomson, M. (1982) *Aston Index.* Wisbech: LDA.

Nippold, M.A. (1990) Concomitant speech and language disorders in stuttering children: A critique of the literature. *Journal of Speech and Hearing Disorders* **55**(1): 51–60.

Oller, D.K., Eilers, R.E., Bull, D., Carney, A. (1985) Prespeech vocalisations of a deaf infant: a comparison with normal metaphonological development. *Journal of Speech and Hearing Research* **28**: 47–63.

Olson, R.K., Wise, B.W., Conners, F., Rack, J., Fulker, D. (1989) Specific deficits in reading and component language skills: Genetic and environmental influences. *Journal of Learning Disabilities* **22**: 339–348.

Onslow, D. (1995) *Investigating Word Finding Difficulties in Children with Developmental and Acquired Language Disorders.* M.Sc. thesis. Department of Human Communication Science, University College London.

Ozanne, A. (1992) Normative data for sequenced oral movements and movements in context for children aged three to five years. *Australian Journal of Human Communication Disorders* **20**: 47–63.

Ozanne, A. (1995) The search for developmental verbal dyspraxia. In Dodd, B. (Ed) *Differential Diagnosis and Treatment of Children with Speech Disorder.* London: Whurr Publishers.

Parker, A., Rose, H. (1990) Deaf children's phonological development. In Grunwell P. (Ed) *Developmental Speech Disorders.* London: Whurr Publishers.

Passy, J. (1990a) *Cued Articulation*. Ponteland, Northumberland: STASS Publications.

Passy, J. (1990b) *Cued Vowels.* Ponteland, Northumberland: STASS Publications.

Perfetti, C.A., Beck, I., Bell, L., Hughes, C. (1987) Phonemic knowledge and learning to read are reciprocal: A longitudinal study of first grade children. *Merrill-Palmer Quarterly* **33**: 283–319.

Perin, D. (1983) Phonemic segmentation and spelling. *British Journal of Psychology* **74**: 129–144.

Plunkett, K. (1995) Connectionism and language acquisition. In Fletcher, P., McWhinney, B. (Eds) *The Handbook of Child Language*, pp. 36–71. Oxford: Blackwell.

Popple, J., Wellington, W. (1996) Collaborative working within a psycholinguistic framework. *Child Language Teaching and Therapy* **12**(1): 60–70.

Pring, L., Snowling, M. (1986) Developmental changes in word recognition: an information processing account. *Quarterly Journal of Experimental Psychology* **38A**: 395–418.

Raaymakers, E., Crul, T. (1988) Perception and production of the final /s - ts/ contrast in Dutch by misarticulating children. *Journal of Speech and Hearing Disorders* **53**: 262–270.

Raine, A., Hulme, C., Chadderton, H., Bailey, P. (1991) Verbal short-term memory span in speech-disordered children: Implications for Articulatory coding in short-term memory. *Child Development* **62**: 415–423.

Read, C., Yun-Fei Zhang., Hong-Yin Nie., Bao-Qing Ding. (1986) The ability to manipulate speech sounds depends on knowing alphabetic writing. *Cognition* **24**: 31–44.

Reid, J., Grieve, R., Dean, E.C., Donaldson, M.L., Howell, J. (1993) Linguistic awareness in young children. In Clibbens, J. (Ed) *Proceedings of the Child Language Seminar*, University of Plymouth.

Renfrew, C. E. (1972) *Word-Finding Vocabulary Scale*. Available from C.E. Renfrew, North Place, Old Headington, Oxford.

Renfrew, C.E. (1989) *Renfrew Action Picture Test,* 3rd edition. Available from C.E. Renfrew, North Place, Old Headington, Oxford.

Renfrew, C. E. (1991) *The Bus Story - A Test of Continuous Speech,* 2nd edition . Available from C.E. Renfrew, North Place, Old Headington, Oxford.

Reynell, J., Huntley, M. (1985) *Reynell Developmental Language Scales*, revised edition. Windsor: NFER-Nelson.

Robinson, P., Beresford, R., Dodd, B. (1982) Spelling errors made by phonologically disordered children. *Spelling Progress Bulletin* **22**: 19–20.

Rustin, L. (Ed) (1991) *Parents, Families and the Stuttering Child*. London: Whurr Publishers.

Ryder, R. (1991) *Word and Non-Word Repetition in Normally Developing Children.* Unpublished M.Sc. thesis, Department of Human Communication Science, University College London.

Scarborough, H. (1990) Very early language deficits in dyslexic children. *Child Development* **61**: 1728–1743.

Schwartz, R., Leonard, L. (1982) Do children pick and choose? An examination of phonological selection and avoidance in early acquisition. *Journal of Child Language* **9**: 319–336.

Semel, E., Wiig, E.H., Secord, W. (1987) *Clinical Evaluation of Language Fundamentals, revised.* London: The Psychological Corporation.

Smith, N. (1973) *The Acquisition of Phonology: A Case Study*. Cambridge: Cambridge University Press.

Snowling, M. (1985) *Children's Written Language Difficulties*. Windsor, NFER-Nelson.

Snowling, M. (1987) *Dyslexia. A Cognitive Developmental Perspective*. Oxford: Basil Blackwell.

Snowling, M. (1996) Developmental dyslexia: an introduction and theoretical overview. In Snowling, M., Stackhouse, J. (Eds) *Dyslexia, Speech and Language: A Practitioner's Handbook*. London: Whurr Publishers.

Snowling, M., Frith, U. (1986) Comprehension in 'hyperlexic' readers. *Journal of Experimental Child Psychology* **42**: 392–415.

Snowling, M., Hulme, C. (1989) A longitudinal case study of developmental phonological dyslexia. *Cognitive Neuropsychology* **6**: 379–401.

Snowling, M., Hulme, C. (1994) The development of phonological skills. *Transactions of the Royal Society* **B346**: 21–28.

Snowling, M., Stackhouse, J. (1983) Spelling performance of children with developmental verbal dyspraxia. *Developmental Medicine and Child Neurology* **25**: 430–437.

Snowling, M., Stackhouse, J. (Eds) (1996) *Dyslexia, Speech and Language: A Practitioner's Handbook*. London: Whurr Publishers.

Snowling, M., Goulandris, N., Stackhouse, J. (1994) Phonological constraints on learning to read: evidence from single case studies of reading difficulty. In Hulme C., Snowling M. (Eds) *Reading Development and Dyslexia*. London: Whurr Publishers.

Snowling, M., Hulme, C., Wells, B., Goulandris, N. (1992) Continuities between speech and spelling in a case of developmental dyslexia *Reading and Writing* **4**: 19–31.

Snowling, M., Stothard, S.E., McLean, J. (1996) *The Graded Nonword Reading Test*. Bury St Edmunds: Thames Valley Test Company.

Snowling, M., Stackhouse, J., Rack, J. (1986) Phonological dyslexia and dysgraphia – a developmental analysis. *Cognitive Neuropsychology* **3**(3): 309–340

Spencer, A. (1988) A phonological theory of phonological development. In Ball, M. (Ed) *Theoretical Linguistics and Disordered Language*. London: Croom Helm.

Stackhouse, J. (1980) Speech difficulties associated with dental problems. *General Dental Practice* **5(A)** (4.3): 5–16.

Stackhouse, J. (1982) An investigation of reading and spelling performance in speech disordered children, *British Journal of Disorders of Communication* **17**(2): 53–60.

Stackhouse, J. (1989) *Phonological Dyslexia in Children with Developmental Verbal Dyspraxia*. PhD Thesis, Psychology Department, University College London.

Stackhouse, J. (1990) Phonological deficits in developmental reading and spelling disorders. In Grunwell P. (Ed), *Developmental Speech Disorders*. London: Whurr Publishers.

Stackhouse, J. (1992a) Developmental verbal dyspraxia: a longitudinal case study. In Campbell, R. (Ed), *Mental Lives: Case Studies in Cognition*. Oxford: Blackwell.

Stackhouse, J. (1992b) Developmental verbal dyspraxia I: A review and critique. *European Journal of Disorders of Communication* **27**: 19–34.

Stackhouse, J. (1992c) Promoting reading and spelling skills through speech therapy. In Fletcher, P., Hall, D., (Eds) *Specific Speech and Language Disorders in Children*, London: Whurr Publishers.

Stackhouse, J. (1993) Phonological disorder and lexical development: two case studies. *Child Language, Teaching and Therapy* **9**(3): 230–241.

Stackhouse, J. (1996) Speech, spelling and reading: who is at risk and why? In Snowling, M., Stackhouse, J. (Eds) *Dyslexia, Speech and Language: A Practitioner's Handbook*. London: Whurr Publishers.

Stackhouse, J. (1997) Phonological awareness: connecting speech and literacy problems. In Hodson, B., Edwards, M.L. (Eds) *Perspectives in Applied Phonology*. Gaithensburg, Maryland, MD: Aspen Publishers.

Stackhouse, J., Snowling, M. (1992a) Barriers to literacy development in two cases of developmental verbal dyspraxia. *Cognitive Neuropsychology* **9**(4): 272–299.

Stackhouse, J., Snowling, M. (1992b) Developmental verbal dyspraxia II: a developmental perspective. *European Journal of Disorders of Communication* **27**: 35–54.

Stackhouse, J., Wells, B. (1991) Dyslexia: the obvious and hidden speech and language disorder. In Snowling, M., Thomson, M. (Eds) *Dyslexia: Integrating Theory and Practice*. London: Whurr Publishers. (Reprinted in *Speech Therapy in Practice* 7(**1**), August 1991.)

Stackhouse, J., Wells, B. (1993) Psycholinguistic assessment of developmental speech disorders. *European Journal of Disorders of Communication* **28**: 331–348

Stackhouse, J., Wells, B. (1996) Developmental supermodels. *Bulletin of the Royal College of Speech and Language Therapists*. No 527: 9–10.

Stanovich, K.E. (1994) Does dyslexia exist? *Journal of Child Psychology and Psychiatry* **35**: 579–596.

Stemberger, J.P. (1989) Speech errors in early child language production. *Journal of Memory and Language* **28**: 164–188

Stengelhofen, J. (Ed) (1989) *Cleft Palate: The Nature and Remediation of Communication Problems*. London: Whurr Publishers

Stoel-Gammon, C., Cooper, J.A. (1984) Patterns of early lexical and phonological development. *Journal of Child Language* **11**: 247–271.

Stothard, S.E. (1996) Assessing reading comprehension. In Snowling, M., Stackhouse, J. (Eds) *Dyslexia, Speech and Language: A Practitioner's Handbook*. London: Whurr Publishers.

Stothard, S.E., Snowling, M.J., Hulme, C. (1996) Deficits in phonology but not dyslexic? *Cognitive Neuropsychology* **13 (5)**: 641–672.

Stuart, M., Coltheart, M. (1988) Does reading develop in a sequence of stages? *Cognition* **30**: 139–181.

Studdert-Kennedy, M., Whitney Goodell, E. (1995) Gestures, features and segments in early child speech. In de Gelder, B., Morais, J. (Eds) *Speech and Reading: A Comparative Approach*. London: Taylor & Francis.

Tallal, P. (1980) Auditory temporal perception, phonics and reading disability in children. *Brain and Language* **9**: 182–198.

Tallal, P., Piercy, M. (1980) Defects of auditory perception in children with developmental dysphasia. In Wyke, M.A. (Ed). *Developmental Dysphasia*. New York: Academic Press.

Tallal, P., Stark, R.E., Mellits, D. (1985) The relationship between auditory temporal analysis and receptive language development: evidence from studies of developmental language disorder. *Neuropsychologia* **23**(4): 527–534.

Taylor, J. (1996) Developing handwriting skills. In Snowling, M., Stackhouse, J. (Eds) *Dyslexia, Speech and Language: A Practitioner's Handbook*. London: Whurr Publishers.

Thorum, A.R. (1986) *The Fullerton Language Test For Adolescents*. Palo Alto, CA: Consulting Psychologists Press.

Treiman, R. (1993) *Beginning to Spell. A Study of First Grade Children*. New York: Oxford University Press.

Treiman, R., Zukowski, A. (1996) Children's sensitivity to syllables, onsets, rimes and phones. *Journal of Experimental Child Psychology* **61**: 193–225.

van der Lely, H., Howard, D. (1995) Specific language impairment in children: Response to Gathercole and Baddeley. *Journal of Speech and Hearing Research* **38**: 466–472.

Vance, M. (1991) Educational and therapeutic approaches used with a child presenting with acquired aphasia with convulsive disorder (Landau-Kleffner syndrome). *Child Language Teaching and Therapy* 7: 41–60.

Vance, M. (1994) Phonological processing, verbal comprehension and lexical representation. Proceedings of NAPLIC Conference: *Understanding Comprehension: Perspectives on Children's Difficulties with Interpretation of Spoken Language*, Birmingham.

Vance, M. (1996a) Assessing speech processing skills in children: a task analysis. In Snowling, M., Stackhouse, J. (Eds) *Dyslexia, Speech and Language: A Practitioner's Handbook*. London: Whurr Publishers.

Vance, M. (1996b) Investigating speech processing skills in young children. In *Caring to Communicate: Proceedings of the Royal College of Speech and Language Therapists' Golden Jubilee Conference, York*. London: Royal College of Speech and Language Therapists.

Vance, M., Donlan, C., Stackhouse, J. (1996) Speech processing limitations on non-word repetition in children. Department of Human Communication Science, University College London: *Work in Progress* **6**: 94–101.

Vance, M., Stackhouse, J., Wells, B. (1994) 'Sock the wock the pit-pat- pock'– Children's responses to measures of rhyming ability, 3–7 years. Department of Human Communication Sciences, University College London: *Work in Progress* **4**: 171–185.

Vance, M., Stackhouse, J., Wells, B. (1995) The relationship between naming and word repetition skills in children age 3–7 years. Department of Human Communication Science, University College London: *Work in Progress* **5**: 127–133.

Vellutino, F. (1979) *Dyslexia: Theory and Research*. Cambridge, MA: MIT Press.

Vellutino, F.R., Harding, C.J., Phillips, F., Steger, J.A. (1975) Differential transfer in poor and normal readers. *Journal of Genetic Psychology* **126**: 3–18.

Vihman, M.M. (1996) *Phonological Development: The Origins of Language in the Child*. Oxford: Blackwell.

Vint, D. (1993) *Spoonerisms: A Study of the Development of Phonological Awareness in Older Children*. B.Sc. thesis, Department of Human Communication Science, University College London.

Waterson, N. (1976) Perception and production in the acquisition of phonology. In: von Raffler-Engel, W., Lebrun, Y. (Eds) *Baby Talk and Infant Speech*. Amsterdam: Swets & Zeitleinger. Reprinted in Waterson, (1987).

Waterson, N. (1978) Growth of complexity in phonological development. In: Waterson, N., Snow, C. (Eds) *The Development of Communication*. Chichester & New York: John Wiley & Sons. Reprinted in Waterson, (1987).

Waterson, N. (1981) A tentative developmental model of phonological representation. In: Myers, T., Laver, J., Anderson, J. (Eds) *The Cognitive Representation of Speech*. Amsterdam: North Holland. (Reprinted in Waterson, 1987).

Waterson, N. (1987) *Prosodic Phonology: The Theory and its Application to Language Acquisition and Speech Processing*. Newcastle upon Tyne: Grevatt & Grevatt.

Webster, P.E., Plante, A.S. (1992) Effects of phonological impairment on word, syllable, and phoneme segmentation and reading. *Language, Speech and Hearing Services in Schools* **23**: 176–182.

Wechsler, D. (1993) *Wechsler Objective Reading Dimensions (WORD)*. New York: The Psychological Corporation.

Weiner, F. (1979) *Phonological Process Analysis.* Baltimore, MD: University Park Press.

Wells, B. (1994) Junction in developmental speech disorder: a case study. *Clinical Linguistics and Phonetics* **8(1)**: 1–25.

Wells, B. (1995) Phonological considerations in repetition tests. *Cognitive Neuropsychology* **12**(8): 847–855.

Wells, B., Local. J. (1993) The sense of an ending: a case of prosodic delay. *Clinical Linguistics and Phonetics* **6**(4): 59–73.

Wells, B., Peppé S., Vance, M. (1995) Linguistic assessment of prosody. In Grundy, K. (Ed) *Linguistics in Clinical Practice,* 2nd edition. London: Whurr Publishers.

Wells, B., Stackhouse, J., Vance, M. (1996) A specific deficit in onset-rhyme assembly in a 9-year-old child with speech and literacy difficulties. In Powell, T.W. (Ed) *Pathology of Speech and Language: Contributions of Clinical Phonetics and Linguistics.* New Orleans, LA: ICPLA.

Wepman, J.M., Reynolds, W.M. (1987) *Wepman's Auditory Discrimination Test,* 2nd edition. Los Angeles: Western Psychological Services.

Williams, P. (1996) *Diadochokinetic Rates in Children with Normal and Atypical Speech Development.* M.Sc. thesis. Department of Human Communication Science, University College London.

Wise, B., Olson, R., Treiman, R. (1990) Subsyllabic units as aids in beginning readers' word learning: onset-rime vs. post-vowel segmentation. *Journal of Experimental Child Psychology* **49**: 1–19.

Wolk, L., Conture, E.G., Edwards, M.L. (1990) Comorbidity of stuttering and disorderd phonology in young children. *South African Journal of Communication Disorders* **37**: 15–20.

Wright, J. (1992) Collaboration between speech and language therapists and teachers. In Fletcher, P., Hall, D. (Eds) *Specific Speech and Language Disorders in Children*. London: Whurr Publishers.

Wright, J. (1996) Teachers and therapists: The evolution of a partnership. *Child Language Teaching and Therapy* **12**(1): 3–16.

Zhurova, L.E. (1963) The development of analysis of words into their sounds by preschool children. *Soviet Psychology and Psychiatry* **2**: 17–27.

Index